Handb

Handbook of Pediatric Oncology

University of Texas
M. D. Anderson Cancer Center

Edited by
Roberta A. Gottlieb, M.D.
Fellow, Department of Pediatric Hematology and Oncology,
University of Texas M. D. Anderson Cancer Center, Houston

Donald Pinkel, M.D.
Professor of Pediatrics, University of Texas Medical School at Houston;
Pediatrician and Director, Pediatric Leukemia Research Program,
University of Texas M. D. Anderson Cancer Center, Houston

Little, Brown and Company
Boston/Toronto/London

Library of Congress Catalog Card No. 89-80903

ISBN 0-316-32169-9

Printed in the United States of America

FG

Contents

Contributing Authors

Joann L. Ater, M.D.
Assistant Professor of Pediatrics, University of Texas Medical School at Houston; Assistant Pediatrician, University of Texas M. D. Anderson Cancer Center, Houston

C. Thomas Black, M.D.
Assistant Professor of Surgery and Pediatrics, University of Texas Medical School at Houston; Attending Surgeon, The Hermann Hospital and University of Texas M. D. Anderson Cancer Center, Houston

A. Bruce Carter, D.D.S.
Chief, Dental Clinic, Texas Children's Hospital; Clinical Assistant Dental Oncologist, University of Texas M. D. Anderson Cancer Center, Houston

Karen R. Cleary, M.D.
Assistant Professor of Pathology, University of Texas Medical School at Houston; Assistant Pathologist, University of Texas M. D. Anderson Cancer Center, Houston

Donna R. Copeland, Ph.D.
Associate Professor of Pediatrics (Psychology), University of Texas Medical School at Houston; Associate Psychologist, University of Texas M. D. Anderson Cancer Center, Houston

Steven J. Culbert, M.D.
Associate Professor of Pediatrics, University of Texas Medical School at Houston; Associate Pediatrician, University of Texas M. D. Anderson Cancer Center, Houston

Laura E. Ferguson, M.D.
Pediatrician, The Stephenville Clinic, Stephenville, Texas

Robert W. Frenck, Jr., M.D.
Instructor, Department of Pediatrics, University of Texas Medical School at Houston

Roberta A. Gottlieb, M.D.
Fellow, Department of Pediatric Hematology and Oncology, University of Texas M. D. Anderson Cancer Center, Houston

Joshua Halpern, M.D.
Senior Clinical Fellow, Department of Radiotherapy, University of Texas M. D. Anderson Cancer Center, Houston

Melissa M. Hudson, M.D.
Assistant Professor of Pediatrics, University of Tennessee, Memphis, College of Medicine; Assistant Member, Department of Hematology and Oncology, Saint Jude Children's Research Hospital, Memphis

Sima Jeha, M.D.
Fellow, Department of Pediatric Hematology and Oncology, University of Texas M. D. Anderson Cancer Center, Houston

Keith F. Jorgenson, M.D., Ph.D.
Fellow, Department of Pediatric Hematology and Oncology,
University of Texas M. D. Anderson Cancer Center, Houston

Moshe H. Maor, M.D.
Professor of Radiotherapy, University of Texas Medical School at
Houston; Radiotherapist, University of Texas M. D. Anderson
Cancer Center, Houston

Bernard L. Maria, M.D.
Assistant Professor, University of Toronto Faculty of Medicine;
Paediatrician, Department of Paediatric Neurology and
Haematology/Oncology, Hospital for Sick Children, Toronto

Robert N. Marshall, M.D.
Associate Professor of Pediatrics (Endocrinology), University of
Texas Medical School at Houston; Associate Pediatrician, The
Hermann Hospital, Houston

J. Arly Nelson, Ph.D.
Associate Professor of Pharmacology, University of Texas Medical
School at Houston; Associate Pharmacologist, Department of
Experimental Pediatrics, University of Texas M. D. Anderson
Cancer Center, Houston

Kevin P. O'Brien, M.D.
Pediatrician, Southeast Permanente Medical Group, Atlanta

Nancy Collins O'Brien, M.D.
Assistant Professor of Pediatrics, University of Texas Medical
School at Houston; Assistant Pediatrician, University of Texas
M. D. Anderson Cancer Center, Houston

Donald Pinkel, M.D.
Professor of Pediatrics, University of Texas Medical School at
Houston; Pediatrician and Director, Pediatric Leukemia Research
Program, University of Texas M. D. Anderson Cancer Center,
Houston

Maureen S. Sanger, Ph.D.
Fellow in Behavioral Pediatrics, Vanderbilt University School of
Medicine and John F. Kennedy Center for Research on Education
and Human Development, George Peabody College, Nashville

Allison Stovall, M.S.W.
Social Work Supervisor, University of Texas M. D. Anderson
Cancer Center, Houston

Louise C. Strong, M.D.
Associate Professor of Genetics and Sue and Radcliffe Killam
Professor of Experimental Pediatrics, University of Texas Medical
School at Houston; Associate Geneticist, University of Texas
M. D. Anderson Cancer Center, Houston

Margaret P. Sullivan, M.D.
Professor of Pediatrics, University of Texas Medical School at
Houston; Pediatrician and Interim Chairman, Department of
Pediatrics, University of Texas M. D. Anderson Cancer Center,
Houston

Cynthia J. Tifft, M.D., Ph.D.
Medical Staff Fellow, Interinstitute Genetics Program, National Institutes of Health, Bethesda, Maryland

Béla B. Toth, M.S., D.D.S.
Associate Professor of Dental Oncology and Chief, Chemotherapy and Pediatric Patient Support Section, University of Texas M. D. Anderson Cancer Center, Houston

Robert A. Weisgrau, M.D.
Fellow in Cross-Sectional Imaging, Department of Radiology, Baylor College of Medicine, Houston; Clinical Assistant Professor, Section of Angiography/Interventional Radiology, University of Texas Medical School at Houston

Preface

This handbook had its inception during internship, when one first encounters many of the problems in clinical management that are unique to children with cancer. That most of the crises seem to arise at night brings to mind an old Cornish prayer:

From ghoulies and ghaisties,
   and long-leggity beasties,
   and things that go BUMP! in the night,
May the good Lord preserve us.

This handbook provides a straightforward and practical approach to the management of "things that go bump in the night" and will be useful to medical students, residents, and fellows. Private practitioners will also find it useful, especially as more children are referred back to their community pediatricians for continuation of cancer treatment.

The handbook is divided into five parts, which address (1) the approach to common tumors, (2) the role of pathology, (3) therapeutic interventions (including a section on immunotherapy and growth factors), (4) complications of therapy (organized by organ system), and (5) an up-to-date review of the genetics of cancer. It is intended to serve as a quick reference for management of specific problems, as well as to provide a brief background for issues unique to the specialty. We have attempted to avoid institutional biases and did not include treatment protocols, which vary with time and among institutions.

It is hoped that this handbook will provide a knowledge base and practical guidance for all physicians and nurses who face the challenge of caring for children with cancer. Humbly offered, this book is for the children.

R. A. G.
D. P.

Acknowledgments

This book would not have been possible without the input of the house staff, who used a trial version of this handbook over the last four years, as well as the encouragement and thoughtful suggestions of the pediatric faculty at the University of Texas M. D. Anderson Cancer Center and the University of Texas Medical School at Houston. Dr. Joseph Wiley of the Johns Hopkins Oncology Center provided many constructive recommendations. I am especially grateful to Renee Shapiro for her unflagging dedication and cheerful expertise throughout the preparation of the manuscript. Last, but not least, I thank my husband, Robert Weisgrau, for his unwavering support, patience, and culinary expertise.

R. A. G.

Handbook of Pediatric Oncology

Approach to Common Malignancies

1

Leukemia and Classification of Hematopoietic Malignancies in Children

Leukemia
Kevin P. O'Brien

PERSPECTIVE
Leukemia is the most common malignancy in children, with an incidence of 4 per 100,000 children. Peak incidence is at 2 to 6 years of age, with slightly increased occurrence in boys (male-female ratio 1.3 : 1). Acute lymphoid leukemia (ALL) accounts for 80 percent of childhood leukemias. Leukemia is more common in children with Down's or Bloom's syndrome. Preleukemic syndromes of variable pancytopenia are unusual in children.

SIGNS AND SYMPTOMS
Fever and easy bruising or bleeding are presenting symptoms in 50 to 60 percent of children with leukemia. Pallor, lethargy, recurrent infection, hepatosplenomegaly, and lymphadenopathy may also be present. Retroorbital infiltration may cause proptosis, and abdominal nodal involvement (as in Burkitt's lymphoma) or hepatosplenomegaly may cause abdominal distention. Bone pain, arthralgias, and fever may lead to the mistaken diagnosis of juvenile rheumatoid arthritis.

EVALUATION
1. History taking and physical examination are primary.
2. Obtain a complete blood cell count, platelet and reticulocyte counts, and a differential count. Leukemic blast cells may be seen on peripheral smear. Thrombocytopenia and anemia are common.
3. A chemistry panel and electrolytes should be analyzed. Lactate dehydrogenase is often elevated. Rapid turnover of leukemic cells leads to increased production of urates, phosphates, and potassium (see Tumor Lysis Syndrome in Chap. 19).
4. Obtain a coagulation profile plus fibrinogen and fibrin split products. Coagulopathy is especially common with acute promyelocytic leukemia.
5. Blood typing and cross-matching should be done in anticipation of a need for transfusion.
6. Urinalysis may reflect the excessive urate load or, rarely, leukemic infiltration.
7. Chest radiography may reveal thymic enlargement, which may be a life-threatening feature of T-cell leukemia and lymphoma.
8. If anthracyclines will be used during induction, baseline cardiac evaluation should include electrocardiogram and echocardiogram.
9. Baseline studies include a hepatitis panel and viral titers for

varicella, cytomegalovirus, Epstein-Barr virus, and herpes simplex virus type 1. A tuberculin skin test and tetanus control should be performed.

10. Bone marrow aspirate provides adequate material for full characterization of leukemic cells. Spinal fluid examination (including opening pressure) may be followed by the administration of intrathecal chemotherapy.

11. Dental evaluation and therapeutic intervention is essential to reduce caries decay and bacterial seeding during episodes of immunosuppression and mucositis caused by chemotherapy.

12. Ophthalmologic examination provides baseline information and may reveal leukemic involvement of the eye.

DISEASE CLASSIFICATION

Classification of the leukemias is based on the morphologic features of blast cells, enzyme markers, and immunologic markers.

Acute Lymphoid Leukemia

The French-American-British (FAB) classification of acute lymphoid (L) leukemia is as follows:

L_1: Small cells, regular nuclei, rare nucleoli, homogeneous chromatin, scant cytoplasm

L_2: Large heterogeneous cells, irregular nuclei, one or more nucleoli, heterogeneous chromatin, moderate cytoplasm, variable to deep basophilic staining

L_3: Large homogeneous cells with regular nuclei, prominent nucleoli, finely stippled chromatin, and abundant basophilic cytoplasm with prominent vacuoles

The immunologic classification of ALL is shown in Table 1-1.

Nonlymphoid Leukemia

The FAB classification of nonlymphoid (myeloid [M]) leukemia is as follows:

M_1: Undifferentiated myeloid, peroxidase positive, more than 90 percent blast cells

M_2: Differentiated myeloid, peroxidase positive, 30 to 90 percent blast cells

M_3: Promyeloid, peroxidase positive, heavily granulated, many Auer rods

Table 1-1. Immunologic classification of acute lymphoid leukemia (ALL)

Type of ALL	Surface Ig	Cytoplasmic Ig	CALLA	HLA-DR	E-rosette
Common ALL	−	−	+	+	
Unclassified	−	−	−	+	
Pre-B cell	−	+	+	+	
B cell	+	+	< 10%+	+	
T cell	−	−	< 10%	< 10%+	50%+

Key: Ig = immunoglobulin; CALLA = common acute lymphoid leukemia antigen; − = negative; + = positive.

M_4: Esterase positive, more than 30 percent blast cells, monocytoid features in 20 to 80 percent of cells

M_{5a}: Esterase positive, 90 percent blast cells, monocytoid features in more than 80 percent of cells

M_{5b}: Esterase positive, 30 to 90 percent blast cells, monocytoid features

M_6: Erythroid predominance, 30 percent blast cells

M_7: Megakaryocytoid leukemia, undifferentiated or differentiated

MDS: Myelodysplastic syndromes (refractory anemia with or without blast cells)

TREATMENT

Leukemia is treated with chemotherapy. Selection of drugs is based on classification of the leukemia. Initial management should also address the likelihood of an immunocompromised host, tumor lysis, and renal failure, as well as coagulopathy and hyperviscosity syndromes. Thus, early management includes hydration, alkalinization treatment with allopurinol, and prevention or treatment of specific infections.

Therapy is divided into three phases. First, remission must be induced in all cases of ALL over a period of 4 to 6 weeks. Mainstays of therapy are prednisone and vincristine as well as triple intrathecal therapy to treat or prevent central nervous system involvement. L-Asparaginase is frequently employed. Second, consolidation or intensification therapy (for approximately 2 months) is intended to eradicate residual leukemic cells after induction therapy. Third, less intensive combination chemotherapy, primarily on an outpatient basis, is continued for months to years and includes intrathecal chemotherapy.

Because intrathecal chemotherapy is part of many treatment protocols, a description of the technique is presented here. The dosages of methotrexate, cytarabine, and hydrocortisone are determined in relation to patient age. The drug diluent is preservative-free buffered saline or Elliott's B solution. Volume is determined as approximately 10 percent of the cerebrospinal fluid (CSF) volume. The chemotherapeutic agents are prepared by fresh aseptic technique, with millipore filtration and at room temperature. Intrathecal administration requires the patient to be in a lateral recumbent position. Atraumatic lumbar puncture is accomplished to allow free CSF flow of one-half of the injection volume. Drugs are instilled by gradual steady injection, avoiding aspiration. After drug administration, the patient should remain prone with his or her head lowered for 30 minutes. There must be no vincristine in the room.

Classification of Hematopoietic Malignancies in Children

Donald Pinkel

Malignant neoplasms of hematopoietic cells account for one-half of childhood cancer. Classification methods and nomenclature vary widely among institutions and among hematologists, oncologists, and pathologists. It must be kept in mind that cancer represents *disorderly* cell proliferation and differentiation. By its nature it defies orderly classification. The following is a tentative system we currently find useful in the care of patients.

LYMPHOID CELLS

Malignant neoplasms of lymphoid cells represent approximately 80 percent of hematopoietic malignancies in children. When the bone marrow contains 25 percent or greater neoplastic cells, the cancer is considered acute lymphoid leukemia (ALL). When lymph nodes, viscera, thymus, or other tissues are involved but there are less than 25 percent neoplastic cells in the marrow, the cancer is called a lymphoid lymphoma. For subclassification of lymphoid leukemia and lymphoma, we currently use immunophenotypic criteria as determined by testing of cell surface "cluster of differentiation (CD)" antigens with monoclonal antibodies. Clinical features, light and electron microscopy, cytochemical stains, combined microscopy and immunochemistry, and cytogenetic study also contribute to classification.

Chronic lymphoid leukemia is not observed in children and adolescents.

Early Pre-B (Common) Acute Lymphoid Leukemia

Early pre-B (common) ALL is the most frequent lymphoid cancer in children. It usually originates in bone marrow and causes pancytopenia, bone and joint symptoms, and enlarged lymph nodes, liver, and spleen. Occasionally it arises in subcutaneous and peripheral lymph node sites and presents as a lymphoma when detected early.

The risk of early pre-B ALL is highest in preschool children from privileged families, which accounts for the high frequency of leukemia in children between ages 2 and 6 years in developed nations. The cure rate of early pre-B ALL at present is the best of all leukemias—about 70 percent.

The immunophenotypic markers are those of early pre-B lymphoid lineage with expression of the DR antigen and common acute lymphocytic leukemia antigen (CALLA) but no evidence of immunoglobulin formation. Chemical stains generally indicate periodic acid-Schiff (PAS)–positive cytoplasmic granules and terminal deoxycytidine transferase (TdT) activity. Chromosomal analysis often reveals hyperdiploidy—a finding associated with a high cure rate—but occasionally a Philadelphia-like chromosome, t(9;22), which is associated with more aggressive disease and usually a rapid, fatal course.

Pre-B Acute Lymphoid Leukemia

Pre-B ALL presents like early pre-B ALL but is noted more frequently in black and Hispanic children than in white children. The difference may be relative, based on a lower incidence of early pre-B ALL.

The morphology, cytochemistry, and immunophenotypic markers are similar to those of early pre-B ALL but with the additional finding of intracytoplasmic immunoglobulin by immunofluorescent antibody stains. Chromosomal analysis frequently reveals pseudodiploidy, particularly a t(1;19) translocation, which is associated with a low cure rate.

Early Pre-B/Monocytoid (Null) Acute Lymphoid Leukemia

Early pre-B/monocytoid (null) ALL usually occurs in infants, adolescents, and adults. It tends to have an explosive onset, rapid course, and very low cure rate. Although lymphoid on light microscopy, it may have monocytoid features by electron microscopy and special stains. Immunophenotypically, it lacks CALLA antigen but often demonstrates the DR antigen and frequently myeloid or myelomonocytoid antigens. Chromosomal analysis usually reveals pseudodiploidy, principally translocations involving chromosome 11 band q 23.

Thymic Cell (T Cell) Acute Lymphoid Leukemia/Lymphoma

Thymic cell (T cell) ALL/lymphoma demonstrates features of thymus-derived cells, both clinically and biologically. It appears largely in thymus and lymph nodes, where it is called T cell lymphoma or lymphoblastic lymphoma. When the bone marrow contains 25 percent or greater T-lymphoma cells, it is called T cell ALL. T cell ALL/lymphoma occurs more frequently in boys and usually in children past six years old. It tends to progress rapidly from normal peripheral blood counts to high leukemia cell levels in the peripheral blood and early invasion of the arachnoid meninges. Thymic enlargement can result in superior vena cava syndrome and suffocation.

T cell ALL/lymphoma can be associated with excessive T cell helper or suppressor function or with parathormone-like osteoclastic activity and consequent hypercalcemia. Metabolic problems, such as hyperuricemia, hyperkalemia, and hyperphosphatemia, are also frequent, particularly after inauguration of therapy.

Light microscopy features resemble those of early pre-B and pre-B ALL. Acid phosphatase stain is usually positive and TdT present. Immunophenotyping reveals T cell surface antigens and heat-stable rosettes with sheep red blood cells. Chromosome analysis often reveals translocations or inversions involving chromosome 14 band q 11 or chromosome 7 band q 36, the regions encoding respectively the alpha and the beta chains of T cell receptor antigen.

B Cell Acute Lymphoid Leukemia/Lymphoma

B cell ALL/lymphoma is the most rapidly growing human cancer. It arises from submucosal lymphoid tissue, lymph nodes, abdominal viscera, and bones and progresses to bone marrow and the central nervous system. It most often appears as a local or regional lymphoma, particularly in the abdomen. It is the major cause of intussusception in the older child. Renal insufficiency can result from renal infiltration, hyperuricemia, or both. When the marrow aspirate contains 25 percent or greater neoplastic cells, it is called B cell ALL. Pathologists use the term *Burkitt's lymphoma* or *Burkitt's leukemia* because of its resemblance to Burkitt's tumor, an African lymphoma associated with Epstein-Barr virus infection.

Microscopy reveals distinctive cytologic features such as deeply basophilic cytoplasm and abundant vacuoles (French-American-British [FAB] L-3 morphology). The distinctive immunophenotypic feature is secretion of immunoglobulin on the cell surface. Chromosome analysis reveals consistent translocation of band q 24 of chromosome 8 to regions on chromosome 2, 14, or 22 that encode immunoglobulin chains. The translocated band contains a deregulated *myc* oncogene.

MYELOID CELLS

Malignant neoplasms of myeloid cells usually arise from bone marrow and are called leukemia. When clinically localized to bone, lymph node, or some other extramedullary site, they are called chloroma. Most myeloid leukemias in children and adolescents are acute, but chronic myeloid leukemia of the adult or juvenile type can also occur.

Light and electron microscopy, cytochemical stains, and cytogenetics are the most useful methods of classifying myeloid leukemias. Immunophenotype is of little help.

Acute Myeloid Leukemia

Acute myeloid leukemia (AML) has a steady incidence throughout childhood but occurs more frequently during adolescence. The undifferentiated form (FAB M-1) can be identified by positive myeloperoxidase and Sudan black stains and by ultrastructure. The differentiated form (FAB M-2) is readily diagnosed by light microscopy. Auer rods, when present, are pathognomonic of AML. Chromosome analysis often reveals a t(8;21) translocation in differentiated AML, a finding associated with an appreciable cure rate on modern chemotherapy.

Acute Promyeloid Leukemia

Acute promyeloid leukemia (APL) demonstrates a predominance of cells resembling promyelocytes but with distinctive abnormalities such as hypergranularity and numerous Auer rods (FAB M-3). Light microscopy is usually sufficient for diagnosis, although ultrastructure is helpful when granules are less distinct. Patients usually have coagulation abnormalities, such as short or long partial thromboplastin time (PTT), increased fibrin split products, and reduced fibrinogen, that can evolve to fatal consumptive coagulopathy when treatment is initiated. Most APL demonstrates a t(15;17) translocation.

Chronic Myeloid Leukemia—Adult Type

Chronic myeloid leukemia (CML)–adult type involves erythroid, megakaryocytoid, and lymphoid cell lines, as well as the maturing myeloid cells that predominate in the marrow and account for the extreme leucocytosis in this disease. The t(9;22) Philadelphia chromosome translocation is noted in most cases along with the novel *BCR-ABL* gene transcript.

MONOCYTOID-HISTIOCYTOID CELLS

Malignant neoplasms of cells with morphologic and functional characteristics of monocytes and histiocytes are widely varied in clinical presentation. When they arise primarily in bone marrow, they usually present as monocytoid leukemia with a predominance of monocytoid cells in the peripheral blood. When they primarily involve lymph nodes, thymus, submucosa, and skin, they are considered histiocytoid or large cell lymphomas. When they diffusely infiltrate lungs, liver, spleen, and lymph nodes with or without partial marrow involvement and exhibit considerable phagocytic activity, the term *malignant histiocytosis* is likely to be applied.

Acute Monocytoid Leukemia (FAB M-5)

The morphology of acute monocytoid leukemia resembles monoblasts (M-5a), monocytes (M-5b), or histiocytes. The monoblasts tend to adhere to each other and to endothelium and to form intravascular aggregates that can result in hypoperfusion, ischemia, and infarction of brain and lungs and in the syndrome of disseminated intravascular coagulation. Elevated serum and urine lysozymes are the presumed cause of the renal insufficiency with hypokalemia that occurs in some cases. Hemolytic anemia and severe thrombocytopenia, neutropenia, and lymphopenia can result from cytophagocytosis by the neoplastic monocytes/histiocytes and hypoalbuminemia from their pinocytic activity. Gingival and cutaneous infiltrations are typical. The nonlymphoid leukemias of infants less than 1 year tend to be monoblastic.

In addition to typical morphology, the monocytoid leukemia cells demonstrate a positive reaction to alpha-naphthyl-acetate-esterase stain. Chromosome analysis usually reveals structural abnormalities, particularly involving chromosome 11 band q 23.

Acute Myelomonocytoid Leukemia (FAB M-4)

In acute myelomonocytoid leukemia, both myeloid and monocytoid cells are observed, with clinical and laboratory features of both types of leukemia. An inversion of chromosome 16 is often found and may be associated with eosinophilia and early onset of meningeal leukemia.

Infantile or Juvenile Subacute and Chronic Myelomonocytic Leukemia

Infantile or juvenile subacute and chronic myelomonocytic leukemia is observed in the first 3 years of life and is characterized by fever, massive splenomegaly, myclomonocytosis of marrow and peripheral blood, anemia, erythroblastosis, thrombocytopenia, and cutaneous infiltrates. Malnutrition and growth failure usually ensue. Fetal hemoglobin is increased and leukocyte alkaline phosphatase is reduced. There are no consistent chromosome abnormalities.

Several viral, protozoal, mycobacterial, and fungal infections of infants that can mimic juvenile chronic myelomonocytic leukemia must be ruled out before this diagnosis is made.

Diffuse Histiocytoid or Large Cell Lymphoma

Diffuse histiocytoid or large cell lymphoma arises from lymph nodes, thymus, submucosal, and cutaneous sites but can also occur in brain and bone. Although the neoplastic cells appear histiocytoid, they often demonstrate immunophenotypic properties of B-lymphoid and sometimes T-lymphoid lineage.

They are seen more often in older children and adolescents than in preschool children. Some patients develop bone marrow infiltration sufficient to qualify as acute leukemia.

Malignant Histiocytosis (Histiocytic Medullary Reticulosis)

Rare in infants and children and often bizarre in its presentation, the diagnosis of malignant histiocytosis is commonly missed or identified only at autopsy. The malignant histiocytes, often with phagocytic properties, infiltrate lungs, liver, spleen, lymph nodes, skin, and brain. Marrow infiltration may only be noted late in its hectic, febrile course.

Langerhan's Cell Histiocytosis (Histiocytosis X)

Although classified as a benign histiocytosis, the Letterer-Siwe disease form of Langerhan's cell histiocytosis, as seen in infants, can have an aggressive fatal course. The malignant-behaving cells are proliferating Langerhan's histiocytes with phagocytic properties. Electron microscopy features are diagnostic. Some of the clinical characteristics are fever, hepatosplenomegaly, large lymph nodes, pulmonary and cutaneous infiltrates, cranial bone lesions, pancytopenia, and monocytosis of bone marrow and peripheral blood.

ERYTHROID CELLS

Acute Erythroleukemia (FAB M-6)

Acute leukemia of erythroid cells is usually accompanied by acute myeloid leukemia (erythromyeloblastosis, Di Guglielmo's disease). Immature erythroid cells are identified by light microscopy and by electron microscopy using an iron stain. Massive splenomegaly, anemia, a slow course, and emergence of acute myeloid leukemia are typical. No consistent chromosomal abnormalities have been reported.

MEGAKARYOCYTOID CELLS

Acute Megakaryocytoid Leukemia (FAB M-7)

Acute megakaryocytoid leukemia has usually been misdiagnosed in the past as unclassified leukemia, myelodysplasia, or myelofibrosis. It is often associated with Down's syndrome and characterized by splenomegaly and severe thrombocytopenia. The bone marrow is usually difficult to aspirate, and marrow biopsy frequently demonstrates fibrosis. The neoplastic cells can vary from large anaplastic cells with cytoplasmic "buds" to multinucleated cells resembling megakaryocytes. Electron microscopy reveals platelet peroxidase activity. Chromosomal rearrangements are variable. Over-expression of *sis* oncogene has been reported.

MYELODYSPLASIA

The preleukemic state of myelodysplasia is rare in children. It is characterized by anemia, large red blood cells, abnormal hematopoiesis, and chromosome abnormalities.

TRANSIENT HEMATOPROLIFERATIVE SYNDROMES IN THE NEWBORN

Leukemia-like proliferations of myeloid, lymphoid, erythroid, or megakaryocytoid cells or a combination thereof can occur in the neonatal period, usually in newborns with trisomy 21. The babies generally behave and gain weight normally, do not experience significant anemia, neutropenia or thrombocytopenia, nor suffer from bleeding and infection. The proliferative disorder gradually resolves over three to four months. Such infants have a high risk of true leukemia in late infancy or during childhood.

2

Hodgkin's Disease

Kevin P. O'Brien, Robert A. Weisgrau, C. Thomas Black, and Joshua Halpern

PERSPECTIVE

The third most common malignancy in children is Hodgkin's disease. The male-female ratio ranges from 2 : 1 to 3 : 1; the ratio reverses in adolescence. Hodgkin's disease is uncommon in children younger than 5 years, but the incidence increases with age.

SIGNS AND SYMPTOMS

The patient with Hodgkin's disease usually exhibits painless, often cervical lymph node enlargement, anorexia, malaise, lassitude, weight loss, and fever (usually intermittent and low-grade).

EVALUATION

General Principles

1. History taking should focus on the duration of symptoms and prior infectious exposures.
2. A thorough physical examination is necessary to delineate the extent of nodal involvement.
3. Obtain a complete blood cell count, with differential and platelet counts, erythrocyte sedimentation rate, and coagulation profile.
4. Liver enzymes may reflect involvement by Hodgkin's disease and establish a baseline. Urinalysis should also be performed.
5. Serum copper should be evaluated as it is often elevated in Hodgkin's disease.
6. Throat culture should be performed if infection has not been ruled out as a cause of lymphadenopathy.
7. A tuberculin skin test may rule out mycobacterial lymphadenitis.
8. Evidence of immunity to varicella and cytomegalovirus should be sought on serologic testing. Antibodies to Epstein-Barr virus and *Toxoplasma* organisms may shed light on other causes of lymphadenopathy.
9. Diagnostic nodal biopsy should be done if it was not done before.
10. Chest radiography may reveal mediastinal involvement, which is common in Hodgkin's disease.
11. Evaluation of Hodgkin's disease patients for purposes of disease staging should include the following:

   Lymphangiography (see Radiology section).
   Computed tomography (CT) of the neck, axillae, chest, abdomen, and pelvis.
   Bone biopsy and marrow aspirate (sometimes done during staging laparotomy).
   Staging laparotomy: Because of the risks posed by splenectomy, this procedure is often reserved for evaluating children older than 12 years with stage I or II disease. The child with favorable stage I disease of a single node above the suprahyoid bone or in one single inguinal femoral region does not require stag-

ing laparotomy if an adequate examination by CT scan and lymphangiogram was negative. Laparotomy is also unnecessary in any patient with stage III or IV disease demonstrated by lymphangiogram.

Radiographic Evaluation

Lymphangiography is the best imaging technique for evaluating nodal size and architecture. However, it is painful and technically difficult because it requires patient cooperation and sedation. The contrast medium is retained for months, so that abdominal radiographs permit serial evaluation of the patient's response to therapy or detection of early disease recurrence. Routine chest radiography may detect thymic enlargement as well as mediastinal lymphadenopathy. Because mediastinal nodes are not consistently or completely opacified by lymphangiographic contrast, chest and neck involvement is best evaluated by CT with contrast. (Contrast enhances blood vessels and permits the radiologist to distinguish them from lymph nodes.) Although CT can detect nodal enlargement, size does not always correlate with disease: Unequivocally enlarged nodes may be due to inflammation, whereas normal-sized nodes may contain tumor. When it is important to determine the extent of disease (i.e., staging), biopsy of suspect nodes may be necessary. Visceral involvement by lymphoma is best evaluated by ultrasonography or CT.

Surgical Evaluation

Lymphoma is not a surgically treatable disease. Painless cervical adenopathy may, however, be the initial symptom, and a surgical consultation for diagnostic excisional lymph node biopsy may be indicated. Cervical nodes are preferable targets for biopsy, as opposed to axillary, submandibular, or inguinal nodes, which are more likely to harbor chronic inflammation. A repeat biopsy may occasionally be required. Involvement of bone marrow is patchy rather than diffuse, and false-negative aspirations may be misleading. The staging, and thereby the treatment, of Hodgkin's disease are based on determination of the extent of the disease. Specifically, it is necessary to establish whether one or both sides of the diaphragm are involved, altering a stage I or II diagnosis to a stage III diagnosis. For 25 years, staging laparotomy has been used to aid in this determination. The spleen is removed and examined for lymphoma. Abdominal nodes are sampled. In girls, the ovaries may be repositioned outside the radiation fields.

Because of the potential for developing overwhelming postsplenectomy sepsis, pneumococcal vaccine should be administered at least 2 weeks before removal of the spleen. When present within the spleen, Hodgkin's disease is usually also present in asymmetric nodules, so partial splenectomy, in an attempt to conserve splenic tissue, may not remove diagnostic tissue and is therefore not recommended.

Postoperatively, the patient should be given penicillin G. Long-term oral prophylaxis is often employed.

DISEASE STAGING

Stage I   One lymph node region (Fig. 2-1) positive
Stage II   Two or more lymph node regions, same side of diaphragm positive
Stage III Lymph node regions, both sides of diaphragm positive

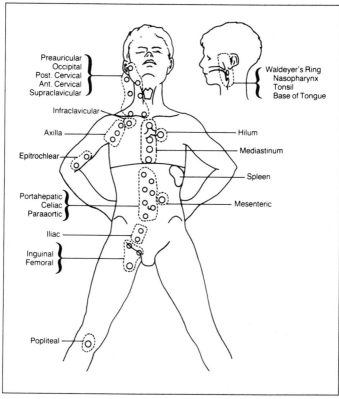

Fig. 2-1. Nodal regions used for defining Hodgkin's disease. Post. = posterior; Ant. = anterior. (Reproduced with permission from: M. P. Sullivan, L. M. Fuller, and J. J. Butler. Hodgkin's Disease. In W. W. Sutow, D. J. Fernbach, and T. J. Vietti (eds.), *Clinical Pediatric Oncology* [3rd ed.]. St. Louis, 1984, The C. V. Mosby Co.)

Stage IV   Involvement of liver, kidney, bone, and so forth

  Class A   No systemic symptoms

  Class B   Unexplained fever higher than 101.4°F (38.6°C), night sweats, or weight loss of 10 percent or more in 6 months (In children, poor weight gain may be a class B symptom.)

TREATMENT

Therapy is based on the clinical stage of disease at presentation and may include radiotherapy, combination chemotherapy, or both. Many different protocols exist. Stage I disease may be treated with radiotherapy or chemotherapy or limited chemotherapy in conjunction with low-dose radiation. Stage II or III disease may be treated with low-dose radiation to involved fields and combination chemotherapy. Radiotherapy is often sandwiched between chemotherapy courses. Stage IV disease (systemic involvement) is best managed with chemotherapy. Radiotherapy for bulky disease may be desirable. Because Hodgkin's disease is a curable disease, much is known about the late effects of radiotherapy and chemotherapeutic agents used in these patients.

Radiotherapy

Hodgkin's disease in children is not biologically different from Hodgkin's disease in adult patients. Early Hodgkin's disease (stages Ia, Ib, and IIa) is highly curable with irradiation only, which is currently the conventional treatment. The radiation fields consist of the so-called mantle field, which comprises the mediastinum, the supraclavicular and neck areas, and the axillae, and the "inverted Y," which is aimed at the paraaortic and pelvic fields. For patients with negative staging laparotomy, no radiotherapy is necessary below the diaphragm. Doses above 35 Gy every 3½ weeks are known to control Hodgkin's disease efficiently. For more advanced disease, involved-field radiotherapy of 15–25 Gy is added to the conventional chemotherapy regimen for better local control. In the very young, chemotherapy, which has less effect on growth and development than radiotherapy, is preferred.

Non-Hodgkin's lymphoma in children is different from that in adults in that it usually tends to disseminate early to bone marrow and the treatment is virtually always systemic. Radiotherapy may be administered for localized disease, reduction of bulky disease, and palliation.

Detailed discussion of radiotherapeutic management of Hodgkin's disease and non-Hodgkin's lymphoma is beyond the scope of this text.

Chemotherapy

Effective chemotherapeutic agents include prednisone, vincristine, doxorubicin, nitrogen mustard, lomustine, bleomycin, cyclophosphamide, procarbazine, dacarbazine, and methotrexate.

3

Neuroblastoma

Kevin P. O'Brien, Robert A. Weisgrau, C. Thomas Black, and Joshua Halpern

PERSPECTIVE

Neuroblastoma is a tumor of the sympathetic nervous system (Fig. 3-1) and is the most common solid tumor in children (not counting the heterogeneous class, central nervous system tumors). It comprises 25 to 50 percent of all malignant tumors in neonates, with an incidence of 1 per 10,000 live births. Fifty percent of neuroblastomas occur by 2 years of age; 75 to 80 percent occur by 5 years. The male-female incidence ratio is 1.2 : 1. The ratio of whites to blacks is 3:2.

Forty-five percent of neuroblastoma patients have distant bony metastases when first seen. The prognosis is highly dependent on the patient's age at the time diagnosis is made, with a high rate of spontaneous remission in the youngest age group (stage IV-S).

SIGNS AND SYMPTOMS

Children with neuroblastoma exhibit a variety of symptoms. Twenty-five percent are asymptomatic. Mediastinal tumors are often silent and therefore are detected only on a fortuitous chest radiograph. A mass, which is often tender, is usually the initial sign of tumors in locations other than the mediastinum. Weight loss, anorexia, diarrhea (from biogenic amines), and vomiting may occur. Fatigue, fever, or irritability may be present. Hypertension occurs frequently and may be due to tumor catecholamine production. Involvement of the stellate ganglion by a mediastinal or cervical tumor may produce an ipsilateral Horner's syndrome of ptosis, miosis, and anhidrosis. Orbital involvement may result in proptosis or orbital ecchymosis. Extension of a paraspinal tumor through an intervertebral foramen may produce spinal cord compression and paralysis. An unusual phenomenon of acute myoclonic encephalopathy, or the so-called dancing eye–dancing feet syndrome, may be the presenting symptom of an occult neuroblastoma. Metastatic disease may be indicated by bone pain, periorbital ecchymosis, lymphadenopathy, or liver enlargement.

EVALUATION

General Principles

1. Obtain a patient history and perform a physical examination.
2. A complete blood cell count, with differential and platelet counts, should be obtained.
3. A bone marrow aspirate and biopsy should be done to evaluate metastatic involvement.
4. Liver enzymes, a coagulation profile, and an imaging study of the liver may reveal tumor invasion.
5. Collect a 24-hour urine sample for catecholamine measurement, including vanillylmandelic acid (VMA), which may be normal in 15 to 20 percent of patients, vanil acetic acid (VAA), vanilglycolic acid (VGA), or homovanillic acid (HVA). In infants in whom 24-hour urine collection is difficult, a spot urine sample

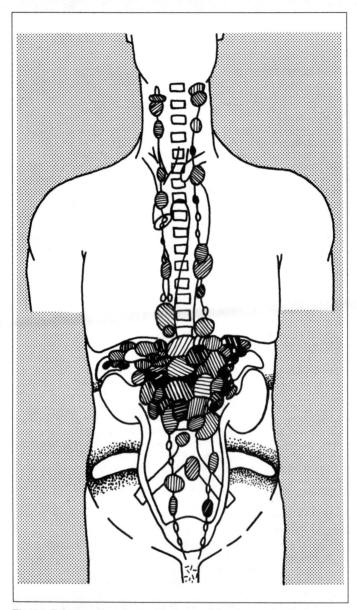

Fig. 3-1. Primary sites of neuroblastoma arising from sympathetic nervous system. (Reproduced with permission from: P. A. Voûte. Neuroblastoma. In W. W. Sutow, D. J. Fernbach and T. J. Vietti (eds.), *Clinical Pediatric Oncology* [3rd ed.]. St. Louis, 1984, The C. V. Mosby Co.)

for VMA and HVA is a helpful screening study. Other markers that correlate with prognosis are serum ferritin, neuron-specific enolase, N-*myc* copy number on tumor tissue, and DNA index by flow cytometry of tumor cells.

6. Computed tomography (CT) or magnetic resonance imaging (MRI) scans of the primary site should be obtained.
7. Chest radiography should be performed.
8. A skeletal survey and bone scan will aid in detecting bony invasion. MRI or CT with metrizamide is useful for spinal cord imaging.
9. Ultrasonography of the abdomen may reveal a mass.
10. Obtain a urinalysis and intravenous pyelogram (IVP).
11. An arteriogram may be requested by the surgeons for surgical guidance.

Radiographic Evaluation

Neuroblastoma may develop anywhere along the sympathetic chain, but it commonly arises from the adrenal medulla and presents as an abdominal mass. It is best evaluated by ultrasonography and excretory urography (IVP). CT scanning is also helpful in the initial evaluation.

Neuroblastoma has both cystic and solid components that are readily detected by ultrasonography. The abdominal mass may contain calcifications, best seen on a plain radiograph or CT scan, and often crosses the midline. Because of the extrarenal origin of neuroblastoma, IVP will show displacement of the entire kidney and collecting system, rather than the intrarenal distortion seen in Wilms' tumor. Evaluation for lymph node, liver, or vascular invasion may be accomplished by ultrasonography or CT scanning. Bony metastases are common and should be evaluated on a skeletal survey or radionuclide bone scan.

DISEASE STAGING

See Table 3-1 for the two independent staging systems in use.

TREATMENT

For stage I disease, complete surgical excision of the tumor is sufficient. No further therapy is needed.

With successful surgical removal of tumor in stage II disease, no further therapy is necessary if urinary VGA and VAA normalize postoperatively. If urinary VGA and VAA rise, chemotherapy should be started. If surgical removal is incomplete, radiotherapy and chemotherapy are instituted.

Radiotherapy, chemotherapy, or both are employed to treat stage III disease. Satisfactory therapy is still lacking.

Chemotherapy is the appropriate approach to stage IV disease, with radiotherapy applied to any residual tumor. Some institutions advocate autologous bone marrow transplantation after remission induction in stage III or IV disease. Stage IV-S disease is characterized by a high frequency of spontaneous remissions. Therefore, conservative therapy with short-term chemotherapy is recommended.

Chemotherapy

Although chemotherapy has not altered overall long-term survival, it has been shown to induce complete or partial responses in some patients. Effective agents include vincristine, cyclophosphamide,

Table 3-1. Two independent staging systems for neuroblastoma

Evans and D'Angio	Pediatric Oncology Group
Stage I Tumor confined to organ or structure of origin.	Stage A Complete gross resection of primary tumor, with or without microscopic residual. Intracavitary lymph nodes that are not adherent to the tumor and that are not removed with the tumor mass should be histologically free of tumor. (Nodes adherent to or within tumor resection may be positive without upstaging patient to stage C.) If primary in abdomen or pelvis, liver histologically free of tumor.
Stage II Tumor extending in continuity beyond organ or structure of origin but not crossing midline. Ipsilateral regional lymph nodes may be involved.	
Stage III Tumor extending in continuity beyond midline. Regional lymph nodes may be involved bilaterally.	Stage B Grossly unresected primary tumor. Nodes and liver same as stage A.
Stage IV Remote disease involving skeleton, bone marrow, soft tissue, and distant lymph node groups. N-*myc* expression is often elevated (see stage IV-S)	Stage C Complete or incomplete resection of primary tumor. Intracavitary nodes not adhered to histologically positive for tumor. Liver as in stage A.
Stage IV-S Patients who would otherwise be stage I or II, but who have remote disease confined to liver, skin, or bone marrow (without radiographic evidence of bone metastases on complete skeletal survey). N-*myc* amplification is uncommon.	Stage D Any dissemination of disease beyond intracavitary nodes, i.e., extracavitary nodes, liver, skin, bone marrow, bone.

doxorubicin, cisplatin, and teniposide. Studies of high-dose chemotherapy followed by autologous bone marrow transplantation for advanced disease are ongoing.

Radiotherapy

Radiotherapy does not improve the survival of children with stage II disease but did improve local control. Its role in stage III disease is undetermined [1]. However, neuroblastoma is a radiosensitive tumor, and radiotherapy may provide excellent palliation in the case of painful bony metastases, spinal cord compression, or tumor encroachment on vital structures.

Surgical Tumor Resection

A positive bone marrow aspiration in conjunction with elevated urinary catecholamine levels is diagnostic and precludes the necessity for a surgical biopsy. Unresectability is often due to involvement of adjacent vital structures such as major vessels. When no metastases are detected and the tumor appears resectable, surgical exploration should ordinarily be undertaken without delay.

The spinal canal adjacent to any paraspinal tumor should also be noninvasively examined for evidence of "dumbbell" extension. If evidence of cord compression is present, urgent myelography and chemotherapy or laminectomy should be performed, even if excision of the primary tumor must be postponed for a few days. Although complete excision is the goal, neuroblastoma is poorly encapsulated and residual tumor may easily be left behind. Radical procedures to attempt complete resection are usually more hazardous than beneficial. Rather, subtotal resection may allow a complete resection later if the tumor is responsive to adjuvant therapy.

REFERENCE

1. Evans, A. E., D'Angio, G. J., and Koop, C. E. The role of multinodal therapy in patients with local and regional neuroblastoma. *J. Pediatr. Surg.* 19:77, 1984.

SELECTED READINGS

Finkelstein, J. F. Neuroblastoma: The challenge and frustration. *Hematol. Oncol. Clin. North Am.* 1:675, 1987.

Levy, H. B., Sheldon, S. H., and Sulayman, R. F. *Diagnosis and Management of the Hospitalized Child.* New York: Raven, 1984.

Voûte, P. A. Neuroblastoma. In W. W. Sutow, D. J. Fernbach, and T. J. Vietti (eds.), *Clinical Pediatric Oncology* (3rd ed.). St. Louis: Mosby, 1984.

4

Wilms' Tumor

Kevin P. O'Brien, Robert A. Weisgrau, C. Thomas Black, and Joshua Halpern

PERSPECTIVE

Wilms' tumor, a congenital, embryonal renal cell neoplasm, is the most common abdominal malignancy in children. Nearly 450 new cases are seen annually in the United States. Eighty percent of cases occur before 5 years of age; the median age is 3½ years. The incidence is 7.8 per million children under the age of 14. There is no ethnic predisposition. Bilateral involvement is seen in 5 to 10 percent of patients.

The hereditary form of Wilms' tumor is characterized by autosomal dominant inheritance, earlier age at presentation, bilateral or multifocal tumor, and association with other anomalies, including nonfamilial aniridia, hemihypertrophy, Beckwith's syndrome, sexual ambiguity, genitourinary abnormalities, chromosomal abnormalities, microcephaly, and recurved otic pinnae.

SIGNS AND SYMPTOMS

Most children with Wilms' tumor will have an abdominal mass, but pain is unusual. It can reach an enormous size before being noticed by a parent or teacher. Hypertension or hematuria occurs in 25 percent of cases. Fever, hypotension, dyspnea, anemia, anorexia, and diarrhea may be present.

EVALUATION

General Principles

The finding of a flank mass in a child should be followed by prompt admission to the hospital and evaluation for possible surgical intervention within 48 hours.

1. Obtain a patient history and perform a physical examination.
2. Abdominal radiography and ultrasonography should be performed to delineate the mass, evaluate hydronephrosis, and detect bilateral disease and invasion of the inferior vena cava.
3. Chest radiographs or computed tomography (CT) scans of the chest are valuable, as metastatic disease most commonly involves the lungs.
4. A complete blood cell count, with platelet, differential, and reticulocyte counts, should be done.
5. A chemical survey will establish baseline renal function (since unilateral nephrectomy is likely to be performed), presence of liver disease, and tumor burden (elevated urates and phosphate).
6. Urinalysis may reveal hematuria, which is present in 25 percent of patients.
7. Bone marrow aspirate should be analyzed to detect metastatic involvement, which is rare.
8. A cytogenetic profile is useful, as deletion of the short arm of chromosome 11 is seen in many cases of aniridia and Wilms' tumor.

Radiographic Evaluation

The most common abdominal mass in children is hydronephrosis, which can be distinguished from Wilms' and other tumors by ultrasonography or excretory urography (IVP). A plain abdominal radiograph is indicated in any child with an abdominal mass. The presence of calcifications within the mass should suggest neuroblastoma, although in 10 percent of Wilms' tumors, peripheral cystic calcifications are noted. Because Wilms' tumor is bilateral in 5 to 10 percent of patients, attention must be paid to the opposite kidney. Ultrasonography, especially with the use of Doppler technique, may detect invasion of the renal veins or inferior vena cava and should be performed preoperatively. Pulmonary metastases should be sought on chest radiographs. If plain radiographs are negative, a chest CT scan is more sensitive for detecting metastatic disease.

DISEASE STAGING

Stage I   Tumor limited to kidney and completely resectable
Stage II   Tumor beyond kidney but completely resectable
Stage III   Tumor not completely resectable but confined to the abdomen
Stage IV   Hematogenous metastases (lung, liver, bone, and brain)
Stage V   Bilateral involvement at diagnosis

TREATMENT

Multimodal therapy has permitted successful treatment of most cases of Wilms' tumor. Excision of the primary tumor is attempted in most cases. Where there is bilateral involvement, unilateral nephrectomy and partial resection of the less involved kidney or presurgical chemotherapy and partial excision of both kidneys may be considered to preserve renal function. Chemotherapy commonly includes dactinomycin, vincristine, doxorubicin, and in some cases, cyclophosphamide. Radiotherapy may be included in the treatment regimen for higher stage disease or unfavorable histologic findings. Most institutions participate in the National Wilms' Tumor Study, which consists of randomized clinical trials of multimodal therapy stratified according to histologic characterization and disease stage at the time of diagnosis.

Radiotherapy

National Wilms' Tumor Studies I through IV evaluated the multimodal approach to therapy [1]. Currently, 10 Gy with an optional 10-Gy boost to the tumor is the recommended radiation dose for patients with stage III disease with favorable histologic findings and for those with disease in any stage but unfavorable histologic findings.

Surgical Evaluation

There is no pediatric tumor for which a multidisciplinary approach is more vital than for Wilms' tumor. From the time of diagnosis, the oncologist, surgeon, radiotherapist, and pathologist are integral partners in caring for the child with this tumor. Such cooperation has had a marked effect on survival.

Because, in most instances, this tumor is well encapsulated and unilateral, preoperative chemotherapy will not improve resectability. Unilateral nephrectomy is usually performed, and the contralateral kidney is visually examined, with biopsies taken if questionable areas are seen. Preoperative chemotherapy may transform an unresectable tumor into a resectable one.

The management of a child with contralateral disease must be individualized. Total resection of the kidney containing the largest tumor may be performed in conjunction with up to a heminephrectomy of the less affected kidney. Alternatively, a radical nephrectomy of the kidney affected by the largest tumor may be performed, followed by chemotherapy to reduce the size of the contralateral tumor and a later second-look procedure. Another alternative is to employ chemotherapy before any surgery is performed. Bilateral nephrectomy should be reserved for those situations in which there is clearly an insufficient amount of salvageable renal tissue. Because long-term postoperative chemotherapy is usually administered, a central venous catheter or subcutaneous port should be placed at the time of resection if one is not already in place.

REFERENCE

1. Green, D. M. The treatment of advanced or recurrent malignant genitourinary tumors in children. *Cancer* 60(Supp.):602, 1987.

SELECTED READINGS

Byrd, R. L. Wilms' Tumor—Medical Aspects. In B. H. Broecker and F. A. Klein (eds.), *Pediatric Tumors of the Genitourinary Tract.* New York: Liss, 1988.

Krummel, T. M. Wilms' Tumor—Surgical Aspects. In B. H. Broecker and F. A. Klein (eds.), *Pediatric Tumors of the Genitourinary Tract.* New York: Liss, 1988.

Levy, H. B., Sheldon, S. H., and Sulayman, R. F. *Diagnosis and Management of the Hospitalized Child.* New York: Raven, 1984. Pp. 574–576.

5

Liver Tumors

C. Thomas Black

PERSPECTIVE

The most common liver tumors in children are hepatoblastoma and hepatocellular carcinoma. Each has an annual incidence of approximately 1 in every million children. Fewer than 5 percent of all abdominal tumors are of liver origin. Hepatoblastoma nearly always occurs in children younger than 3 years, whereas hepatocellular carcinoma, although it affects a few children younger than 3, occurs most often in older children, with peak incidence at between 12 and 15 years of age. There is a slight predominance of occurrence in boys for both tumor types.

Although hepatoblastoma has been reported in conjunction with several inherited conditions, such as the Beckwith-Wiedemann syndrome and hemihypertrophy, and has occurred in siblings, it is as yet impossible to implicate a genetic basis for the tumor. Hepatocellular carcinoma, however, may be preceded by hepatitis B and by conditions leading to hepatic cirrhosis, such as biliary atresia and alpha$_1$-antitrypsin deficiency disease.

SIGNS AND SYMPTOMS

A tumor of the liver is usually first detected when a painless right-sided or midline upper abdominal mass is found by a parent or other caretaker. Anorexia or weight loss may be noted in the child but usually only in retrospect. Fifty to ninety percent of children with either hepatoblastoma or hepatocellular carcinoma will have an elevated serum alpha fetoprotein (AFP) level. Serum ferritin is another marker that is frequently elevated. Liver function studies are generally normal or nearly so, with one-third of patients having elevated transaminases and up to one-fourth having an elevated bilirubin level. Leukocytosis is occasionally present, and anemia, which is seen in approximately half of the cases of pediatric liver tumor, may be severe because of acute hemorrhage into the tumor. Definitive diagnosis may be made by percutaneous needle biopsy.

EVALUATION

General Principles

1. History taking and physical examination are primary.
2. Complete blood cell counts, with differential and platelet counts, and evaluation of liver enzymes, bilirubin, and AFP level should be performed.
3. The liver and abdomen may be evaluated by computed tomography (CT) or ultrasonography.
4. For detection of metastatic disease, obtain a chest CT scan and radionuclide bone scan.
5. Needle biopsy guided by CT or ultrasonography may be diagnostic.

Radiographic Evaluation

A plain film of the abdomen may show calcifications within a hepatoblastoma. CT, ultrasonography, and magnetic resonance imaging are complementary studies that may show the extent of the mass, its soft-tissue characteristics, and the relationship of the tumor to portal and hepatic venous structures. Preoperative hepatic arteriography is often unnecessary. If plain chest radiographs are negative, CT scanning of the lungs must be performed to search for pulmonary metastases, which are present in 10 percent of patients at the time of diagnosis. A bone scan is recommended for detecting osseous metastases.

DISEASE STAGING

Preoperative indication of metastases or of involvement of both hepatic lobes, the portal area, or all hepatic veins indicates unresectability—that is, complete surgical excision of the tumor is not possible. Such is the case for between one-third and one-half of all children at the time that hepatoblastoma or hepatocellular carcinoma is diagnosed.

HISTOLOGIC FEATURES

The hepatoblastoma consists of epithelial cells arranged in cords that are separated from the sinusoids. The better-differentiated type of tumor is termed *fetal cell* and the less differentiated type is *embryonal cell,* which has a poorer prognosis.

Hepatocellular carcinoma, which is much more similar to the adult form of liver cancer, is more often multicentric and more invasive. As a rule, the cells are more irregular and bizarre than those of hepatoblastoma, but occasionally differentiation between the two is difficult. In the past, ambiguous terminology has been used to identify these tumors, and careful distinction between them often was not made. Whereas terms such as *hepatoma, malignant hepatoma, embryonal hepatoma, carcinoma of the liver,* and *hepatocarcinoma* were once used somewhat interchangeably to identify the histologic diagnosis, these terms are rarely used now.

TREATMENT

It is generally agreed that complete gross surgical excision of either a hepatoblastoma or a hepatocellular carcinoma is necessary before any hope of cure can be entertained. Therefore, surgical intervention must be considered early in the therapeutic course. If the criteria for unresectability are met, chemotherapy should be started in an attempt to shrink the mass to a resectable status. Many oncologists and surgeons advise preoperative chemotherapy for all patients with hepatoblastoma or hepatocellular carcinoma to minimize the amount of liver tissue that must be resected when the child undergoes a delayed operation. Effective chemotherapeutic agents include cisplatin, either alone or with doxorubicin, dactinomycin, cyclophosphamide, and vincristine [1]. Tumor shrinkage in several patients, as evidenced by radiography and a decline in AFP levels, has been extraordinary. If an unresectable tumor fails to respond to chemotherapy, palliative surgery to resect the tumor mass should be considered. Debulking of hepatic tumors has been shown to prolong survival time and improve comfort but will not alter the ultimate outcome. Some children may be candidates for liver transplantation.

The young liver has an amazing regenerative capacity. Through hypertrophy and proliferation, the lost hepatic mass may be restored as early as 2 to 3 weeks after resection. Further chemotherapy must be delayed for at least 14 days postoperatively to allow for such recovery [2].

AFP levels, if elevated, should revert to normal within 10 days of complete tumor resection. A monthly AFP assay may detect an early recurrence long before it becomes clinically detectable [2].

Cures have followed second operations for recurrence and for metastatic disease. The presence of pulmonary metastases at the time of diagnosis is an ominous sign. If pulmonary metatases develop during treatment, tumor resection should be considered, because the prognosis without surgery is grave but cures have been reported following excision. Currently, approximately 60 percent of children with hepatoblastoma and 35 percent of those with hepatocellular carcinoma are cured by successful liver resection [3].

REFERENCES

1. Evans, H. E., et al. Combination chemotherapy in the treatment of children with malignant hepatoma. *Cancer* 50:821, 1982.
2. Lilly, J. R., Stellin, G. P., and Cheney, M. Right Trisegmentectomy for Pediatric Hepatic Malignancy. In B. F. Brooks (ed.), *Malignant Tumors in Childhood*. Austin: University of Texas Press, 1986.
3. Randolph, J. G., et al. Liver resection in children with hepatic neoplasms. *Ann. Surg.* 187:599, 1979.

6

Rhabdomyosarcoma

Melissa M. Hudson, C. Thomas Black, and
Joshua Halpern

PERSPECTIVE

Rhabdomyosarcoma is a malignant tumor of embryonic mesen-
chyme that gives rise to striated skeletal muscle. It is one of the
most common soft-tissue sarcomas of childhood, with 70 percent
being seen before the age of 10 years. The peak incidence is between
2 and 5 years of age, and boys are more commonly affected (1.4 : 1).
This embryonic tumor may arise anywhere in the body and tends to
disseminate early in the course of the disease. Primary sites are the
head and neck area (38% [10% of these being orbital]), the genitourinary region (21%), and the extremities (18%). A familial association of sarcomas has been reported (see Chaps. 29 and 30).

SIGNS AND SYMPTOMS

Signs and symptoms relate to the location of the primary tumor or
to areas of metastasis. Orbital tumor may be manifested by proptosis, chemosis, ocular paralysis, and eyelid or conjunctival masses. A
nasal voice, airway obstruction, epistaxis, pain, and dysphagia occur with a nasopharyngeal tumor. Sinus disease may result in sinus
swelling, pain, discharge, sinusitis, and epistaxis. Hoarseness and
dysphagia are associated with laryngeal tumor. Parameningeal
rhabdomyosarcoma may produce cranial nerve palsies, meningeal
symptoms, respiratory paralysis, or nerve root compression syndromes. An enlarging soft-tissue mass in the trunk or extremities
may signal local tumor. With rhabdomyosarcoma in the genitourinary system, urinary tract symptoms occur.

EVALUATION

1. A patient history should be obtained and a physical examination
   performed.
2. Computed tomography (CT) or magnetic resonance imaging of
   the primary tumor will establish the extent of the disease.
3. Open or needle biopsy of a primary tumor should be performed.
4. Obtain a complete blood cell count, with differential, platelet,
   and reticulocyte counts, which may reveal pancytopenia due to
   bone marrow involvement. Bone marrow aspirate and biopsy
   should also be performed.
5. Urinalysis may be abnormal if there is urinary tract invasion.
6. A chemistry panel is done to evaluate renal function (blood urea
   nitrogen, creatinine, phosphate, calcium, and urates) and liver
   function (bilirubin and enzyme profile).
7. Bone involvement may be detected by an elevated alkaline phosphatase level, abnormal bone scan, or skeletal survey.
8. Further metastatic workup may include a liver scan, chest radiograph, and CT scan of the chest (if the radiograph is negative), as
   well as a lumbar puncture if the tumor is parameningeal.

DISEASE STAGING

The Intergroup Rhabdomyosarcoma Study's clinical grouping classification, which follows, is the most widely employed scheme [1].

Group I: Localized disease, completely removed (as confirmed by
both gross impression of complete removal and microscopic evidence of complete removal), without regional node involvement
1. Confined to muscle or organ of origin
2. Contiguous involvement with infiltration outside the muscle or
organ of origin, as through fascial planes
Group II:
1. Grossly removed tumor with microscopic residual disease, no
evidence of gross residual tumor, and no evidence of regional
node involvement
2. Regional disease, completely removed (regional nodes involved
or extension of tumor into an adjacent organ, with no microscopic residual disease)
3. Regional disease with involved nodes, grossly removed but
with evidence of microscopic residual disease
Group III: Incomplete removal or biopsy with gross residual disease
Group IV: Distant metastatic disease present at onset

TREATMENT

The basic strategy for treating rhabdomyosarcoma is surgical excision of the primary tumor. For primary and metastatic tumor, 40 to
50 Gy doses of radiotherapy may be employed. The lung, kidney,
liver, and other vital structures must be protected. Chemotherapy
should be administered to all patients, with the goal of eradicating
microscopic metastases. Agents currently employed are dactinomycin, vincristine, cyclophosphamide, and doxorubicin in two, three,
and four-drug combinations. Intrathecal chemotherapy with cytosine arabinoside, hydrocortisone, and methotrexate is also important for parameningeal tumor. (See the procedure for administering
intrathecal chemotherapy in Chap. 1.)

Radiotherapy

The Intergroup Rhabdomyosarcoma Studies I through III consisted
of carefully designed clinical trials employing multimodal treatments. Age-adjusted radiation doses in the range of 35 to 55 Gy/3 to
6 weeks in conjunction with chemotherapy were shown to improve
survival.

Surgical Tumor Resection

A diagnosis of rhabdomyosarcoma may be established by needle biopsy, but classification into subtypes usually requires an open or
excisional biopsy. Before the institution of radiotherapy and chemotherapy, surgical excision alone resulted in only a 5 to 15 percent
survival rate, often with a long latent period before death occurred
from metastatic disease. It is clear that institution of the vincristine-
dactinomycin-cyclophosphamide chemotherapeutic regimen has had
a profound effect on expected survival. Currently most, if not all,
patients with rhabdomyosarcoma should receive chemotherapy or
combination chemotherapy and radiotherapy, followed by delayed
surgical excision.

Recommended surgical procedures vary with the diverse locations in which rhabdomyosarcoma may be found. For truncal or limb disease, complete en bloc excision of the tumor together with wide margins of surrounding tissue is the goal of surgical management. This must, of course, be weighed against the consequences of marked deformity or disability that might be created by such a procedure. For tumors involving internal organs where more than a limited resection is unrealistic, chemotherapy and radiotherapy assume an even greater importance as potentially curative rather than adjunctive modalities.

Second-look surgery may be considered in cases in which excision is deemed inadequate based on histologic examination of the initial specimen or recurrence at the primary tumor site. Relapse and failure of chemotherapy are associated with a particularly poor prognosis. However, successful control of the primary disease followed by the appearance, despite chemotherapy and radiotherapy, of a small number of resectable pulmonary nodules and no other evidence of metastatic spread may be an indication for thoracotomy and resection. The expected cure rate would be low.

REFERENCE

1. Maurer, H. M., et al. The Intergroup Rhabdomyosarcoma Study: A preliminary report. *Cancer* 40:2015, 1977.

SELECTED READINGS

Maurer, H. M. Pediatric Experience in Rhabdomyosarcoma. In J. R. Ryan and L. O. Baker (eds.), *Recent Concepts in Sarcoma Treatment.* Dordrecht, The Netherlands: Kluwer, 1988.

Sutow, W. W., Fernbach, D. J., and Vietti, T. J. (eds.). *Clinical Pediatric Oncology* (3rd ed.). St. Louis: Mosby, 1984.

7

Osteosarcoma

Kevin P. O'Brien and Robert A. Weisgrau

PERSPECTIVE

Osteosarcoma most commonly arises in the metaphysis of long bones, with peak incidence during the period of most rapid bone growth: age 15 in boys and age 14 in girls. Boys are more commonly affected (1.5 : 1). Osteosarcoma most commonly involves the distal femur, proximal tibia, and proximal humerus. Pelvic bone involvement is not rare. In patients who complete treatment for familial retinoblastoma, the incidence of osteosarcoma of the irradiated craniofacial bones is 1000 times that of the normal population (19% outside irradiated fields).

SIGNS AND SYMPTOMS

Pain is present, especially in the common sites for osteosarcoma, and there is occasional traumatic fracture with poor healing.

EVALUATION

General Principles

1. Obtain a patient history and perform a physical examination.
2. A complete blood cell count, with platelet and differential counts, should be obtained; a chemical survey to establish baseline parameters and a urinalysis should be performed.
3. Perform plain film anteroposterior, lateral, and oblique radiography of the involved site.
4. A computed tomography (CT) or magnetic resonance imaging (MRI) scan of the tumor-bearing bone is useful for determining the extent of disease.
5. Chest radiography is employed to detect pulmonary metastases, followed by chest CT if the radiograph is negative; this will permit detection of small metastases.
6. Perform a bone scan and skeletal survey to evaluate metastatic or multifocal disease.
7. Biopsy the tumor site (preferably by needle biopsy).

Radiologic Evaluation

Plain films are the initial approach to evaluation of a primary bone tumor. The tumor's location within the bone, border characteristics, matrix, and periosteal reaction allow the radiologist to distinguish osteosarcoma from other disease processes involving the bone. The radiographic features of osteosarcoma are often distinctive enough to allow the radiologist to make the diagnosis from plain films alone. CT or, better yet, MRI allows precise determination of the extent of disease in the affected limb. MRI may reveal intramedullary "skip lesions," which may alter surgical planning, particularly if limb salvage is being considered.

Pulmonary metastases are common and should be sought. Chest CT may reveal pulmonary nodules not evident on plain radiographs. Contrast enhancement is unnecessary for CT evaluation, because metastasis to lymph nodes is uncommon in osteosarcoma.

Interventional radiologic techniques permit the local infusion of intraarterial chemotherapeutic agents to reduce tumor bulk before surgical intervention is attempted.

Nuclear medicine bone scan may be useful for detecting bone or soft-tissue metastasis or for detecting local recurrence following treatment.

TUMOR CLASSIFICATION AND STAGING

Osteosarcomas are classified as osteoblastic, fibroblastic, chondro-blastic, telangiectatic, small round cell type, or mixed, based on the predominant structures seen on histologic examination. Osteoid must be present. Tumors are graded from I (low-grade) to IV (high-grade). Staging requires a search for metastatic involvement (particularly of the lungs).

TREATMENT

Preoperative and postoperative chemotherapy are necessary adjuncts to optimize surgical results in limb salvage. Studies investigating limb salvage combined with systemic chemotherapy, and chemotherapy without surgery, are ongoing [1–3]. Commonly used chemotherapeutic drugs include, among others, cisplatin, doxorubicin, methotrexate with folinic acid (Leucovorin) rescue, and cyclophosphamide.

REFERENCES

1. Jaffe, N., et al. Intra-arterial cis-Diamminedichloroplatinum-II in Pediatric Osteosarcoma: Relationship of Effect on Primary Tumors to Survival. In J. R. Ryan and L. O. Baker (eds.), *Recent Concepts in Sarcoma Treatment*. Dordrecht, The Netherlands: Kluwer Academic, 1988. Pp. 275–282.
2. Jaffe, N., et al. Osteosarcoma: Intra-arterial treatment of the primary tumor with cis-Diamminedichloroplatinum-II (CDP): Angiographic, pathologic, and pharmacologic studies. *Cancer* 51:402, 1983.
3. Link, M. P., et al. The effect of adjuvant chemotherapy on relapse free survival in patients with osteosarcoma of the extremity. *N. Engl. J. Med.* 314:1600, 1986.

SELECTED READING

Rosen, G. Spindle Cell Sarcoma—Osteogenic Sarcoma. In W. W. Sutow, D. J. Fernbach, and T. J. Vietti (eds.), *Clinical Pediatric Oncology* (3rd ed.). St. Louis: Mosby, 1984.

8

Ewing's Sarcoma

Keith F. Jorgenson, Robert A. Weisgrau, and Joshua Halpern

PERSPECTIVE

Ewing's sarcoma is a small round-cell sarcoma of the bone and is probably neural in origin. It is the second most common primary bone tumor in children and comprises approximately 1 percent of childhood malignancies; the annual incidence among whites is 2.7 per million, whereas it is rare in nonwhites. There is a male predominance in most studies. The peak incidence is in growth years (age 11–15 years, with a median of 13 years). In 75 percent of the cases, the patient is younger than 20 years, and Ewing's sarcoma is rare in very young children. Familial occurrence is reported, although no strong correlation to hereditary factors exists. Unlike osteosarcoma, there is no etiologic role of ionizing radiation.

Ewing's sarcoma may involve any bone and is occasionally extraosseous. It is often seen in the diaphysis of long bones and in flat bones. Of the long bones, the femur is affected in 22 percent of cases, the tibia in 11 percent, the fibula in 9 percent, and the humerus in 10 percent of cases. Of the flat bones, the ilium pubis is involved in 19 percent of cases, the ribs in 6 percent, and the scapula in 5 percent of cases. Multiple lesions are not uncommon. There is a high incidence of local recurrence and metastasis to lungs and bones; micrometastasis probably is present often at diagnosis. Local lymph nodes are involved in 10 percent of patients, and the presence of metastatic disease at diagnosis is reported in 14 to 35 percent of the cases [1].

SIGNS AND SYMPTOMS

Local involvement by Ewing's sarcoma leads to pain, swelling, warmth, and tenderness. Pathologic fractures are infrequent. Systemic signs and symptoms include malaise, pyrexia, weight loss, and anemia.

EVALUATION

General Principles

1. A patient history should be obtained and a physical examination performed.
2. A complete blood cell count, with differential and platelet counts, and determination of the erythrocyte sedimentation rate should be done to detect anemia and leukocytosis, which are common.
3. Liver enzymes should be measured. Although liver metastasis is rare, alkaline phosphatase often is elevated, and baseline liver enzyme levels are needed before chemotherapy may be instituted.
4. Urinalysis should be performed, as well as measurement of creatinine clearance and serum electrolytes.
5. Urinary vanillylmandelic acid (VMA) determination will aid in differentiating Ewing's sarcoma from neuroblastoma.
6. Obtain radiographs of the local lesion. These are valuable also for evaluation of metastastic disease. A CT of the chest should be performed.

7. Perform an open biopsy.
8. Bone marrow aspirate should be done.

Radiographic Evaluation

Ewing's sarcoma is suggested by plain film studies showing a moth-eaten pattern of bone destruction located in the diaphysis or, less commonly, extending throughout the entire bone, as well as the presence of a soft-tissue mass causing a scooped-out appearance of the bony cortex. As with all malignant bone tumors, sunburst periosteal reaction may be seen, reflecting rapid new bone formation. In the absence of a soft-tissue mass, the moth-eaten or permeative bone changes may suggest other round-cell neoplasms, such as leukemia or lymphoma, metastatic neuroblastoma, or eosinophilic granuloma. Osteomyelitis may also take on this appearance and so must be included in the differential diagnosis.

Because of the predilection for Ewing's sarcoma to metastasize to other bones and to the lungs, further radiologic evaluation should include a skeletal survey or radionuclide bone scan and chest radiographs. Chest computed tomography scanning may reveal metastases not apparent on the plain film radiographs. Thus, evaluation for metastasis involves obtaining a chest radiograph, CT scan or tomograms, and radionuclide bone scan.

PATHOLOGIC FEATURES

Small round cells, often in monotonous sheets, with very little background stroma are characteristic of Ewing's sarcoma. Frequently, there is evidence of necrosis and hemorrhage. There are no specific tumor features or markers that allow positive identification, except a characteristic cytogenetic reciprocal translocation (rcp 11;22). Without cytogenetics information, reaching a diagnosis tends to be an exercise of exclusion.

DIFFERENTIAL DIAGNOSIS

In the differential diagnosis of Ewing's sarcoma, chronic osteomyelitis, lymphoma, metastatic neuroblastoma, rhabdomyosarcoma, eosinophilic granuloma, and small-cell osteosarcoma must be considered.

PROGNOSIS

The prognosis is related to the location of the primary tumor, pelvic tumors having a worse prognosis than limb tumors. The prognosis improves with complete surgical removal of the tumor, independent of its primary site. An elevated lactate dehydrogenase level, erythrocyte sedimentation rate, and leukocyte count at the time of diagnosis are associated with a poor prognosis. Increased long-term survival can be expected if weight loss, paresthesias, and weakness are absent at the time the diagnosis is made. Overall long-term survival of more than 5 years occurs in approximately 50 percent of cases.

TREATMENT

Treatment for Ewing's sarcoma is multimodal, including surgery, radiotherapy, and chemotherapy. Surgical excision is recommended for localized lesions of relatively expendable bones, and amputation is indicated for (1) large destructive lesions, (2) lesions with extensive soft-tissue involvement, (3) patients with pathologic fractures, and (4) lesions of the distal femur, lower leg, or foot of a young child.

These tumors are fairly sensitive to radiotherapy, but the recurrence rate is high, owing to subclinical disseminated disease, if systemic multiagent chemotherapy is not used also. The Intergroup Ewing's Sarcoma Studies (IESS) I and II showed that irradiation of the primary tumor improves local control and may facilitate organ-sparing treatment [2]. Local control is achieved at doses ranging from 40 to 55 Gy/4 to 6 weeks.

Most chemotherapeutic regimens include vincristine, dactinomycin, doxorubicin, and cyclophosphamide. Chemotherapy is sometimes used for tumor reduction before surgical resection. Intrathecal chemotherapy may be employed if the neuraxis is involved.

REFERENCES

1. Nesbit, M. E., et al. Multimodal therapy for the management of primary non-metastatic Ewing's sarcoma of bone: An intergroup study. *Nat. Cancer Inst. Monogr.* 56:255, 1981.
2. Vietti, T. J., et al. Multimodal therapy in Ewing's sarcoma: An intergroup study. *Nat. Cancer Inst. Monogr.* 56:279, 1980.

SELECTED READINGS

Maletz, N., et al. Ewing's sarcoma: Pathology, tissue culture, and cytogenetics. *Cancer* 58:252, 1986.

Nesbit, M. E., Jr., Robison, L. L., and Dehner, L. P. Round Cell Sarcoma of Bone. In W. W. Sutow, D. J. Fernbach, and T. J. Vietti (eds.), *Clinical Pediatric Oncology* (3rd ed.). St. Louis: Mosby, 1984.

9

Brain Tumors

Joann L. Ater

PERSPECTIVE

Brain tumors, as a group, constitute the second most common cancer in children and the most common solid tumors of childhood. Fifty to 60 percent of childhood brain tumors are infratentorial, in contrast to the 25 percent seen in adults. The most common histologic types in childhood are primitive neuroectodermal tumor (PNET)/medulloblastoma, astrocytoma, and ependymoma.

SIGNS AND SYMPTOMS

The signs and symptoms at presentation of a pediatric brain tumor depend on the tumor's location rather than its histologic features. Nonetheless, the signs and symptoms may help the physician make an educated differential diagnosis based on the type of tumors that usually occur in specific locations.

Posterior Fossa (Infratentorial) Tumors

The most common types of posterior fossa tumors are PNET/medulloblastoma, astrocytoma, and ependymoma. Signs and symptoms of the posterior fossa tumors are related to obstruction of the cerebrospinal fluid pathways, leading to increased intracranial pressure, involvement of the cerebellum, and possible extension into the brainstem. With increased intracranial pressure, there may be vomiting, headache, changes in behavior, visual change, papilledema, diplopia secondary to nonspecific sixth nerve weakness, enlarging head, and splitting of sutures. Cerebellar signs include an unsteady wide-based gait, abnormal tandem gait, nystagmus, slow and halting speech, dysmetria, and hypotonia on the side of the tumor, such that the child may fall to that side. With brainstem involvement, other cranial nerve weakness and hemiparesis may occur.

Tumors of the Brainstem

Brainstem tumors may be intrinsic or within the brainstem, most commonly in the pons bulging into the floor of the fourth ventricle, or they may be exophytic, producing cerebellar signs. In children, 99 percent of brainstem tumors are astrocytomas or gliomas of various grades. Extremely rarely, an exophytic tumor may be a PNET. Involvement of the pons and upper medulla most commonly produces sixth nerve palsy (squint, head tilt), facial weakness (seventh nerve), hearing loss (eighth nerve), and dysarthria and dysphagia (ninth and tenth nerve), while altered sensation and spastic hemiparesis result on the contralateral side. Nonspecific symptoms are vomiting, lethargy, and headache.

Midline Tumors

Common types of midline tumors are chiasmal gliomas (optic glioma), suprasellar craniopharyngiomas and, in the pineal area, pinealomas, pinealoblastomas, and germ-cell tumors (germinoma, teratoma, embryonal carcinoma). Among the signs is increased intracranial pressure. Signs and symptoms specific to the pineal area include paralysis of upward gaze, impaired light reaction, and loss of convergence. With suprasellar tumors there may be endocrine disturbance (precocious puberty, diabetes insipidus, and the like). Chiasmal gliomas cause nystagmus, visual impairment, and visual field cuts.

Cerebral Tumors

Common types of cerebral tumors are low-grade and high-grade astrocytomas, glioblastoma multiforme, ependymomas (usually intraventricular), and PNETs.

The signs and symptoms include personality change; headache, vomiting, and increased intracranial pressure; lethargy; hemiparesis (contralateral to the side of the tumor); seizures (focal or focal with generalization); and others depending on the area of cortex involved.

Brain Tumors in Infants

In infants, brain tumors present differently because of open sutures and fontanelles and a supratentorial predominance in children younger than 1 year. The signs of increased intracranial pressure are an increasing head circumference, the "sunset sign" (paralysis of upward gaze), and vomiting. Other signs include focal deficit, progressive disuse of one hand, lethargy and hypotonia, developmental delay, failure to thrive, and diencephalic syndrome secondary to hypothalamic involvement. If the visual pathway is affected, nystagmus may occur.

EVALUATION

1. Obtain a thorough history and perform a physical examination with a detailed neurologic examination.
2. Computed tomography (CT) with and without contrast enhancement or magnetic resonance imaging (MRI) may delineate the extent of tumor growth.
3. Lumbar puncture should *not* be performed as part of the initial evaluation.
4. If signs of spinal compression are present on examination, MRI, especially with gadolinium contrast, is the best noninvasive approach to detect tumor metastasis to the spinal canal. Myelography provides similar information but may be risky in a patient with increased intracranial pressure.
5. If the child is stable, preoperative neuropsychologic testing and endocrine evaluation (L-thyroxine, triiodothyronine, thyroid-stimulating hormone, morning cortisol, somatomedin C, and urine specific gravity) are helpful for follow-up.

DIFFERENTIAL DIAGNOSIS

The following must be considered in the differential diagnosis of brain tumors:

Hydrocephalus secondary to occlusion of the foramina of Magendie and Luschka or aqueductal atresia
Encephalitis
Brain abscess
Hematoma
Pseudopapilledema and pseudotumor cerebri
Optic neuritis

Hemangioma
Venous sinus thrombosis
Gastrointestinal disorder (vomiting and failure to thrive)
Arteriovenous malformation
Metabolic disorder (lead poisoning, hypervitaminosis A, Addison's
    disease, hypoparathyroidism)
Guillain-Barré syndrome (ascending weakness and anorexia)
Central nervous system leukemia or lymphoma

DISEASE STAGING

For PNET/medulloblastoma, T and M staging has been found to be
prognostically significant. *T staging* defines the size and extent of
the tumor determined by preoperative and postoperative CT (within
48 hours) and a neurosurgeon's assessment. *M staging* relates to the
presence or absence of metastatic disease. Workup includes myelography or MRI of the spine with gadolinium enhancement, bone
marrow aspiration, cytologic evaluation of cerebrospinal fluid, and
bone scan.

TREATMENT

Emergency Treatment

1. Increased intracranial pressure (see Increased Intracranial Pressure in Chap. 24).
2. Spinal cord compression (see Spinal Cord Compression in Chap.
   24).
3. Seizures (see Seizures in Chap. 24).

Surgical Resection

Surgery is both diagnostic and therapeutic. When at all possible, in
the presence of increased intracranial pressure, rapid, neurosur-
gical intervention is indicated. To relieve pressure, dexamethasone
and furosemide can temporize, but tumor removal and sometimes
shunt procedures are the treatment of choice. Complete surgical
tumor excision is desirable, but debulking may help restore function
and reduce tumor burden, thus enhancing the patient's response to
other therapy (Table 9-1).

Radiotherapy, Chemotherapy, and Immunotherapy

The decision as to what type of therapy is indicated is determined by
age of the child, tumor type, disease staging, and the amount of
residual tumor. Studies on recurrent tumors over the last decade
have established that some pediatric brain tumors respond well to
chemotherapy and suggest that chemotherapy should be considered
as part of the multimodal therapy for certain brain tumors [1, 2].
Experimental protocols are underway to determine the efficacy of
adjuvant chemotherapy at diagnosis postoperatively. In addition,
experimental protocols including immunotherapy (interleukin-2,
lymphokine activated killer [LAK] cells) and interferon use are underway [3]. Because of the rapidly changing field, children with
brain tumors have the best results and survivals when they are
treated by or in consultation with physicians at pediatric cancer
centers. For example, children with medulloblastoma treated in university cancer centers had a 5-year survival rate of 74 percent as
opposed to 29 percent for those treated at community hospitals [4].
    In children younger than 4 years, the morbidity of radiotherapy

Table 9-1. Current treatment of brain tumors of childhood

Tumor and subgroup	Treatment	Five-year survival rate (% of patients)
Glioma		
Cerebellar astrocytoma		91
Type A	S	94
Type B	S, LR, (C)	24
Brainstem glioma	LR, (HFR), ± S	17
Supratentorial astrocytoma		
Low-grade (I and II)		69
Completely resected	S	
Partially resected	S, LR	
High-grade (III)	S, LR, C	35
Glioblastoma multiforme	S, LR, C, (HFR)	0
Medulloblastoma (PNET)		
Low-risk	S, LR + C/SR	65–70
High-risk	S, LR + C/SR, C	40
Infant (< 3 years)	(S,C), S, LR ± C/SR, C	15–30
Ependymoma		
Ependymoblastoma		33
Infratentorial	S, LR + C/SR, (C)	
Supratentorial	S, LR ± C/SR, (C)	
Low-grade	S, LR	60
Infant (< 3 years)	(S,C), S, LR	18
Pineal and suprasellar tumors		
Germinoma	S, LR or LR + C/SR, (C)	85
Teratoma, mature	S	78
Other malignant tumors	S, LR, (C)	33
Craniopharyngioma		70–90
Completely resected	S	
Partially resected	S, LR	
All tumors		50

Key: C/SR = craniospinal radiotherapy; C = chemotherapy; LR = local radiotherapy; HFR = hyperfractionated radiotherapy; S = surgical resection; ( ) = newer approach with unknown 5-year survival rate; ± = with or without; PNET = primitive neuroectodermal tumor.
Source: Five-year survival rate data are drawn from [3,7,8].

has led to trials of chemotherapy as the primary therapeutic modality postoperatively [5]. Results have been encouraging, especially with medulloblastoma, for which it was demonstrated that high survival rates and low morbidity could be obtained with surgical excision and chemotherapy, with omission or delay of radiotherapy [6]. Additional confirmatory studies are needed. Radiotherapy techniques have also advanced so as to make it possible to treat some tumors more optimally with less toxicity. A detailed discussion of treatment of individual tumor types is beyond the scope of this book.

CONDITIONS SIMULATING RELAPSE OF BRAIN TUMOR

Some conditions may occur that mimic brain tumor relapse. The physician must consider these in any patient who is seen after eradication of a brain tumor [9].

Edema, postoperative hemorrhage
Cerebrospinal fluid pleocytosis after metrizamide use
Cerebrospinal fluid flow obstruction (hydrocephalus)
Postradiation somnolence syndrome
Radiation necrosis
Pseudocyst
Seizures
Cerebral hemorrhage after chemotherapy
Infection

REFERENCES

1. Pendergrass, T. W., et al. Eight drugs in one day chemotherapy for brain tumors: Experience in 107 children and rationale for preradiation chemotherapy. *J. Clin. Oncol.* 5:1221, 1987.
2. van Eys, J., et al. Salvage chemotherapy for recurrent primary brain tumors in children. *J. Pediatr.* 113:601, 1988.
3. Kadota, R. P., et al. Brain tumors in children. *J. Pediatr.* 114:511, 1989.
4. Duffner, P., Cohen, M., and Flannery, J. Referral patterns of childhood brain tumors in the state of Connecticut. *Cancer* 50:1636, 1982.
5. van Eys, J., et al. MOPP regimen as primary chemotherapy for brain tumors in infants. *J. Neurol. Oncol.* 3:237, 1985.
6. Baram, T. Z., et al. Survival and neurologic outcome of infants with medulloblastoma treated with surgery and MOPP chemotherapy. *Cancer* 60:173, 1987.
7. Duffner, P. K., et al. Survival of children with brain tumors: SEER Programs, 1979–1980. *Neurology* (NY) 36:597, 1986.
8. Matsutani, M., Takakura, K., and Sano, K. Primary intracranial germ cell tumors: Pathology and treatment. *Prog. Exp. Tumor Res.* 30:307, 1987.
9. Zelzer, P. M., et al. Criteria and definitions for response and relapse in children with brain tumors. *Cancer* 56:1824, 1985.

Pathologic Evaluation

10

Pathologic Evaluation

Karen R. Cleary

The pathologist plays a vital role in the diagnostic evaluation of the cancer patient. The type of therapy employed will be determined on the basis of the type and stage of the neoplasm, but occasionally, histologic subtypes may also dictate alternate therapy regimens. This is particularly important, for example, in the treatment of leukemias, lymphomas, osteosarcomas, and Wilms' tumor.

The most important step in obtaining a histologic diagnosis is the acquisition of an adequate amount of representative tumor tissue. Many solid tumors incite a local inflammatory response, which may result in the presence of a large amount of benign fibrous tissue both in and around the tumor. Rapidly growing tumors may become extensively necrotic. These events can be the cause of serious sampling errors in which little of the actual diagnostic neoplastic tissue is obtained. Tissue sampling for suspected lymphoma, both Hodgkin's and non-Hodgkin's types, is especially problematic because not all the lymph nodes in one group may be involved. For this reason, the largest possible node should be removed intact. Physical distortion of the tissue during its removal can also lead to difficulties in establishing a diagnosis. The amount of tissue needed to establish a diagnosis depends on all these factors as well as on the type of tumor itself. Tumors in which architectural features are an important diagnostic characteristic (e.g., alveolar rhabdomyosarcoma) require more tissue than those that do not have such distinctive growth patterns.

Often, ancillary studies are needed in addition to the routine hematoxylin and eosin (H&E) sections to establish the diagnosis with certainty. These include electron microscopy, immunohistochemistry for antigenic markers (including lymphocyte markers), and enzyme histochemistry. Cytogenetic studies and, more recently, flow cytometry and molecular genetic studies also may provide valuable diagnostic and prognostic information. These procedures require advance planning so that the tissue specimen is handled appropriately as soon as it is received in the pathology laboratory. It is therefore very important that information about the forthcoming arrival of such a specimen be conveyed to the pathologist. The best way to achieve this is for the surgeon to speak directly with the pathologist in charge. Some hospitals may have a pathologist who is responsible for pediatric cases in general or for special types of neoplasms such as bone tumors or lymphoreticular neoplasms. Particularly in the case of patients referred to a tertiary care center, any previously excised tissue material, particularly tissue blocks and unstained slides, available at other hospitals also should be forwarded to the pathologist so that it may be reviewed in conjunction with the current material. All bone lesions must be interpreted in conjunction with the radiographic features, and both current and prior films must be available.

ROUTINE PROCESSING

Tissue taken for biopsy or removed at the time a tumor is resected is routinely fixed in 10% formalin for 6 to 12 hours. The tissue then undergoes a series of processing steps during which it is dehydrated and infused with paraffin. It is then sufficiently hardened so that thin slices of it may be cut from the paraffin blocks, placed on a glass slide, and stained. H&E is used as a general-purpose stain. The normal turnaround time for routine tissue processing, paraffin embedding, sectioning, and H&E staining is 1 to 2 days, depending on the time of day at which the specimen is received in the laboratory and the size of the specimen. Routine biopsy slides are usually available for review by the pathologist within 24 hours.

FINE-NEEDLE ASPIRATION

A technique that frequently provides diagnostic information within a shorter period of time is the fine-needle aspiration biopsy. A small-bore needle is inserted into the lesion and cells are aspirated from which smear, sedimentation, and cell block preparations are made. The first two types of preparations are available in less than 24 hours, but the cell block requires the same type of processing as a tissue biopsy. However, the cell block may provide important architectural information and should be prepared. The major advantage of fine-needle aspiration is the avoidance of a surgical procedure. Lesions involving intracavitary organs as well as superficial lesions may be biopsied in this manner, although aspiration of the former requires fluoroscopy or computed tomography guidance and will involve scheduling of those facilities as well as consultation with a diagnostic radiologist.

It should be pointed out that although fine-needle aspiration biopsies may save time, patient discomfort, and expense, there are some diagnostic limitations inherent in this technique. Classification of some tumors may be difficult owing to lack of diagnostic architectural or stromal features. This is particularly important in osteosarcomas, Hodgkin's and non-Hodgkin's lymphomas, and reactive, non-neoplastic processes. Sampling error may lead to a false negative diagnosis. In these instances, a tissue biopsy must be obtained to establish the diagnosis or subclassify the tumor. Despite the diagnostic limitations of fine-needle aspiration, all the ancillary diagnostic techniques that may be used on tissue specimens are also applicable to fine-needle aspiration material if a sufficient amount is obtained.

ELECTRON MICROSCOPY

Electron microscopy can be extremely valuable in the diagnosis of so-called small round-cell neoplasms of childhood, including neuroblastoma, rhabdomyosarcoma, lymphoma, and Ewing's sarcoma. When the tumor involves bone, the small-cell variant osteosarcoma is included in the differential diagnosis. Other tumors may be so poorly differentiated by light microscopy that only by ultrastructural examination are features revealed that suggest cell type. It is essential that material for this examination be well fixed. Special fixatives, usually glutaraldehyde, are used, and the tissue is divided into very small pieces (1 μl) to ensure rapid complete penetration. Some examples of diagnostic ultrastructural features are neurosecretory granules in neuroblastomas, actin and myosin filaments in rhabdomyosarcoma, and large pools of glycogen in Ewing's sarcoma.

IMMUNOHISTOCHEMISTRY

Immunohistochemistry studies often furnish important information about the presence of certain characteristic antigenic substances that are on the surface or within the cytoplasm of tumor cells. An antibody (monoclonal or polyclonal) that has been generated against such an antigen is allowed to react with the tumor cells on the glass slide. The presence of attached antibody is detected by adding a peroxidase-conjugated antibody that has been generated against the first antibody to the tissue on the slide after appropriate washings to remove the nonreacted antibody.

Although there are significant problems with cross reactivity, certain antibodies (markers) are very useful. Again, special handling procedures must be used. Many markers, especially lymphocyte markers, are reactive only in fresh (unfixed) tissue (i.e., on frozen sections or cytologic preparations). Others require certain fixatives such as B-5 or methacarn for optimum results. Such decisions regarding handling must be made at the time that the tissue is received.

Examples of tumors and associated markers are as follows:

Rhabdomyosarcoma	Desmin, an intermediate filament found in smooth muscle, and, occasionally, fibroblastic tumors Myoglobin, which is very specific for skeletal muscle but much less sensitive than desmin Myosin, which is muscle specific but, again, not as sensitive as desmin
Lymphoma	Pan-leukocyte markers such as leukocyte common antigen (LCA) in frozen tissue and smears and T-200 in paraffin sections (these are also positive in cells of granulocytic or monocytic lineage) Markers specific for certain types of lymphocytes (B cells versus T cells, immature versus mature), most of which must be used on frozen sections, aspiration smears, or cell suspensions

Because of lack of sensitivity or specificity, several antibodies are generally used in evaluating each tumor. Several different antibodies generated against the same or a related antigen may be commercially available. This sometimes accounts for the differences in antigenic properties for the same tumor as reported by different laboratories and is, in part, a result of variations in tissue fixation and processing. The field of immunohistochemistry is rapidly changing, and new antibodies are continuously being developed and tested for tumor specificity. Nevertheless, it must be borne in mind that results of electron microscopy and immunoperoxidase studies must always be interpreted in conjunction with histologic or cytologic features.

ENZYME HISTOCHEMISTRY

Enzyme histochemistry studies are of limited value in surgical pathology although they are very useful to the hematopathologist in classifying leukemias, especially acute leukemias. Most stains require unfixed smear preparations. Extramedullary granulocytic proliferations (e.g., chloroma) are diagnosed with the aid of a positive naphtha-ASD-chloracetate esterase (NASD) stain in paraffin sections. However, cells that are differentiated toward the monocytic line may be negative for this enzyme. Leukemic infiltrates of lymphocytic lineage may be identified with the aid of immunoperoxidase markers on frozen sections or aspirated material.

CYTOGENETICS, MOLECULAR GENETICS, AND FLOW CYTOMETRY

Cytogenetic abnormalities have been associated with hematopoietic and lymphoreticular neoplasm as well as other tumors such as retinoblastoma, Wilms' tumor, and Ewing's sarcoma. The prognostic significance of these findings is becoming increasingly important. *Sterile* fresh tissue in sufficient quantity to obtain an adequate number of cells in metaphase (approximately 1 million cells or 0.5 gm of tissue) is required for this study. Because cytogenetic evaluation is not a routine diagnostic technique, advance notice must be given to the pathologist, and the cytogeneticist must be consulted before the tissue is obtained (except in the case of Hodgkin's and non-Hodgkin's lymphomas, which are always sent for cytogenetic study if sufficient sterile material is available).

More recently, molecular genetic studies, particularly those utilizing recombinant DNA techniques to detect gene rearrangements, have been useful in detecting clonal cell populations. The existence of clonal cell populations is considered strong supporting evidence for the presence of a neoplastic cell population. In lymphoreticular neoplasms, the existence of clonal cell populations serves as supportive evidence of cell lineage (B cell versus T cell) depending on which genetic locus is rearranged (immunoglobulin versus T-cell receptor). These studies are performed on fresh tissues or cell suspensions (5–10 million cells or 0.5 gm of tissue), which must be processed immediately or snap-frozen and stored at subzero temperatures.

Analysis by flow cytometry of cellular DNA and RNA content and the S-phase fraction in tumor cell suspensions has been shown to be of some prognostic value in lymphomas as well as other tumors such as neuroblastoma. Again, fresh tissue (approximately 0.1 gm) is required.

SELECTED READING

Finegold, M. (ed.). *Major Problems in Pathology: Vol. 18. Pathology of Neoplasia in Children and Adolescents.* Philadelphia: Saunders, 1986.

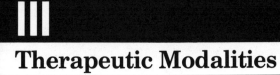

III

Therapeutic Modalities

11

Cancer Chemotherapeutic Agents

Principles
J. Arly Nelson

Theoretically, cancer results from the malignant transformation of one or very few cells. In experimental models, the implantation of a single tumor cell can lead to death of the host. Therefore, a conservative goal for cancer therapy is eradication of the total tumor cell population (i.e., total cell kill).

Most available anticancer agents are cytotoxic. Cytotoxicity is a quantal response characterized by the killing of a constant fraction of the cell population by a given dose rather than the killing of a constant number of cells (i.e., the log cell kill concept). If cure is the objective, a major consequence of this phenomenon is the principle that the same dose of a given anticancer agent (or a given combination of agents) required to treat large, clinically evident tumor cell populations (i.e., 10^9 cells or greater) must be used also to treat nonsymptomatic patients in whom the tumor cell population is small and unknown. This is perhaps the most critical principle of cytotoxic chemotherapy, which wreaks havoc with both the patient and the physician.

Cytotoxic anticancer agents are toxic to normal cells as well as tumor cells. In general, rapidly dividing cells, whether normal or malignant, are more sensitive to the available drugs. As far as is known, the mechanisms for cytotoxicity toward normal and tumor cells are the same; consequently, the characteristic steep dose-response curves for therapeutic and toxic effect are parallel. The difference between the dose that cures and the dose that is toxic or lethal is generally small: That is, these drugs possess narrow therapeutic indexes, and patients must often be treated to the point of toxicity to achieve maximum therapeutic response.

With few exceptions, available cytotoxic anticancer agents appear limited in their log cell kill capacity, and combinations of agents are generally necessary to achieve total tumor cell kill. Consequently, combination chemotherapy is the rule rather than the exception in the use of cancer chemotherapeutic agents. The goal of combination cancer chemotherapy is to achieve a greater tumor cell kill by the drug combination than is otherwise possible, at the same or reduced cost (toxicity) to the host. Thus, agents with different dose-limiting toxicities often are combined so that each agent may be administered near its maximally effective dose. In recent years, the inability of a given agent or combination of agents to eradicate the total tumor cell population has been attributed to the selection of resistant mutants. Like bacteria, these drug-resistant mutants arise both spontaneously and randomly during the growth of the tumor cell population. Cancer patients almost invariably present with a body burden in excess of 10^9 tumor cells. Therefore, given a reasonable mutation frequency of 10^{-5} to 10^{-7}, it is not surprising that considerable numbers of tumor cells will have mutated to drug resistance before the initiation of drug therapy. Another major consideration in the design of drug combinations, therefore, is to select agents with different mechanisms of action so that several mutations will be required for a given cell to become resistant to all the drugs in the combination.

List of Chemotherapeutic Drugs
Kevin P. O'Brien

The dosages that follow should be regarded as general recommendations only. For actual prescriptions, pediatric oncologists should consult more detailed literature. In almost all cases, doses are normalized to body surface area (sq m).

L-Asparaginase

Synonyms:	L-Asp, amidohydrolase, Elspar
Class:	Miscellaneous cytotoxic agent
Action:	Hydrolyzes L-asparagine to L-aspartic acid. Leukemic cells that are unable to synthesize L-asparagine will be unable to carry out protein synthesis. Hepatocytes are affected as well.
Metabolism:	Absorbed from the intramuscular site to intravascular space; cleared in slow, erratic fashion.
Side effects:	Hypersensititivity may occur with any dose during the course of therapy.
	Pancreatitis or sialadenitis are common: monitor amylase, blood and urine glucose (glucose intolerance exacerbated by concomitant use of steroids and may be delayed).
	Prerenal azotemia
	Hepatotoxicity with decreased synthesis of both clotting and inhibitory factors (protein C and antithrombin III) rarely may precipitate disseminated intravascular coagulation.
	Hyperammonemia
	Central nervous system symptoms of somnolence, lethargy, and confusion
	Death caused by anaphylaxis, cerebral infarct, or necrotizing pancreatitis
Comments:	May interfere with cytotoxic action of methotrexate
	Risk of severe anaphylactoid reactions. Therefore, observe for 1 to 2 hours postinjection; have epinephrine available.
	Fewer severe reactions with intramuscular versus intravenous route
	If hypersensitivity to *Escherichia coli* L-asparaginase occurs, switch to *Erwinia* L-asparaginase (no cross reactivity).
Formulation and route:	Injection vials (10,000 U/vial) intramuscularly or, less commonly, intravenously

Commonly
used dosage: 6000 U/sq m intramuscularly 3 times weekly

5-Azacytidine

Synonyms: 5-AZA, azacytidine, 5-aza-C
Class: Antimetabolite
Action: Analog of cytidine that becomes incorporated into nucleic
                acids to block DNA and RNA synthesis; S phase–specific.
Metabolism: Converted intracellularly to nucleotide; most is excreted
                unchanged in the urine.
Side effects: Nausea and vomiting, minimized with slower infusion
                Severe diarrhea (occasional)
                Myelosuppression: leukopenia and thrombocytopenia 4 to
                    17 days postinfusion
                Hepatotoxicity
                Hypomagnesemia
Comments: Dose-limiting toxicity is myelosuppression.
                Decomposes in alkaline fluids; stable in 5% dextrose in
                    water at 2 mg/ml for up to 4 to 6 hours. Investigational
                    drug.
Formulation
and route: Injection vials (100 mg); slow or continuous intravenous
                infusion. Solution is unstable and should be changed ev-
                ery 3 hours.
Commonly
used dosage: 150 to 200 mg/sq m/day continuous infusion for 5 days or
                100 mg/sq m intravenous push every 8 hours for 5 days

Bleomycin

Synonyms: BLM, Blenoxane
Class: DNA-binding agent
Action: Cytotoxic glycopeptides from *Streptomyces* that bind DNA,
                leading to strand scission; cell cycle–specific.
Metabolism: Distributed in intravascular and extravascular space; ex-
                creted in urine.
Side effects: Mild nausea, vomiting, anorexia, fever and chills
                Skin changes: mouth ulcers, hair loss, pigmentation, ery-
                    thema, hyperkeratosis, vesiculation, pruritus, striae,
                    bleeding, nail changes
                Pulmonary toxicity in 10 percent of patients; increased
                    risk of pulmonary toxicity with radiotherapy; age- and
                    dose-related; monitor pulmonary function.
                Avoid high inspired F_iO_2
Comments: Dose-limiting toxicities include skin changes and pulmo-
                    nary fibrosis.
                Fever and chills may be averted with prophylactic acet-
                    aminophen given for 12 hours with each of the first two
                    doses.

A test dose of 2 U or less intramuscularly may be desired in patients with lymphoma, who have increased risk of anaphylactoid, acute pulmonary, or hyperpyretic response within 4 hours of the dose.

Formulation
and route: Injection ampules (15 U/ampule); dissolve in 5 ml normal saline or 5% dextrose in water and inject slowly over 10 minutes. May be given intramuscularly, intravenously, subcutaneously, intraarterially, or instilled into pleural space for treatment of malignant effusions.

Commonly
used dosage: 10 to 20 U/sq m intravenously or intramuscularly twice weekly

Cisplatin

Synonyms: CDDP, cisplatinum, *cis*-diamminedichloroplatinum (II), Platinol
Class: Alkylating agent
Action: Binds DNA and cross-links complementary strands to inhibit replication and, to a lesser extent, RNA transcription and translation
Metabolism: Eliminated in urine
Side effects: Nausea and vomiting during infusion may last 4 to 12 hours after infusion, and occasionally up to 1 week.
                Occasional hypersensitivity (wheezing, tachycardia, hypotension) in those with prior exposure to the drug
                Renal tubular dysfunction with hypomagnesemia and hypocalcemia may require chronic oral supplementation; follow electrolytes, calcium, and magnesium levels.
                Uremia and hyperuricemia are late findings.
                Myelosuppression 2 weeks after infusion, with recovery in approximately 1 week
                Ototoxicity (tinnitus, high-frequency hearing loss); follow with audiometry.
                Color blindness may develop; monitor at intervals.
                Neurotoxicity (peripheral neuropathy, hypogeusia, seizures)
                Hepatotoxicity; monitor liver enzymes.
Comments: Dose-limiting toxicity is cumulative renal tubular injury.
                Mannitol diuresis and fluid loading decrease nephrotoxicity.
                Do not use aluminum needle (platinum reacts with aluminum).
Formulation
and route: Injection vials (10 mg or 25 mg/vial) intravenously or intraarterially. Can be given as rapid intravenous infusion over 3 to 5 minutes or as 1 mg/kg/hour.
Commonly
used dosage: 50 to 100 mg/sq m over 6 hours every 3 to 4 weeks or 20 mg/sq m over 1 hour every day for 5 days
                20 to 120 mg/sq m for intraarterial administration

Corticosteroids

Specific agents:	Prednisone, prednisolone, hydrocortisone, dexamethasone
Class:	Antimetabolite
Action:	Interacts with DNA to modify transcription; lysis caused by release of stores of free fatty acids.
Metabolism:	Rate of clearance depends on specific agent; dexamethasone crosses the blood-brain barrier easily.
Side effects:	Sodium and water retention with hypertension
	Glucose intolerance, glycosuria, and polyphagia
	Immunosuppression
	Growth suppression
	Osteoporosis, aseptic necrosis of bone
	Iatrogenic Cushing's syndrome
	Glaucoma, cataracts
	Neurologic disorders (myalgias, weakness, psychiatric symptoms, irritability)
	Adrenal suppression
Comments:	Use appropriate dose equivalencies; be aware of mineralocorticoid activity. Taper gradually if steroid use is long-standing.
	Effective intrathecal agent

Dose equivalencies: (mg of drug needed to equal 100 mg of cortisone for glucocorticoid or mineralocorticoid effect)

	Glucocorticoid	Mineralocorticoid
Cortisone	100	100
Dexamethasone	2	No effect
Hydrocortisone	80	80
Prednisolone	20	100
Prednisone	20	100
Methylprednisolone	16	Small effect

Formulation and route:	Prednisone: 1 mg/ml, or 1-, 5-, 10- or 25-mg tablets orally
	Prednisolone: 1 mg/ml orally or 20 mg/ml intravenously
	Hydrocortisone: 5-mg tablets, or 10 mg/5 ml oral suspension, or 5 or 10 mg/ml intravenously
	Dexamethasone: 0.5 mg/5 ml oral elixir or 10 mg/ml intravenously
Commonly used dosage:	Prednisone or prednisolone: 40 mg/sq m/day in two to three divided doses, orally or intravenously; maximum dose 60 mg/day

Cyclophosphamide

Synonyms:	CTX, Cytoxan, Neosar
Class:	Alkylating agent
Action:	Cyclic nitrogen mustard (mechlorethamine) is converted

	to phosphoramide mustard, which interacts with nucleic acids and proteins; non–cell cycle–specific.
Metabolism:	Inert until converted to active form by liver microsomal enzymes; active metabolites are excreted in urine.
Side effects:	Mild nausea, vomiting, and anorexia 6 hours after dose may last a few hours.
	Sensation of sinus congestion experienced with intravenous infusion
	Myelosuppression apparent 7 to 10 days after dose; nadir is dose-related.
	Hemorrhagic cystitis: ensure good hydration; give oral dose in the morning so that metabolites are largely cleared from urine by bedtime.
	Temporary hair loss 2 to 3 weeks after treatment
	Syndrome of inappropriate antidiuretic hormone secretion seen with doses in excess of 40 mg/kg
	Gonadal suppression, sterility, amenorrhea
	Potent immunosuppression
Comments:	Dose-limiting toxicity is myelosuppression.
	Cardiotoxicity is seen with doses at 200–400 mg/kg; potentiates anthracycline cardiotoxicity.
	Hemorrhagic cystitis risk may be reduced with good hydration.
	Pelvic irradiation increases risk of hemorrhagic cystitis.
Formulation and route:	Tablets (25 mg, 50 mg)
	Injection vials (100 mg, 200 mg, 500 mg); dissolves slowly
Commonly used dosage:	50 to 150 mg/sq m/day orally for 7 to 14 days, or 400 mg/sq m/day intravenously for 5 days, or 300 to 600 mg/sq m/week intravenously

Cytosine Arabinoside

Synonyms:	ARA-C, Cytosar-U, cytarabine
Class:	Antimetabolite
Action:	Analog of deoxycytidine that (1) becomes incorporated into DNA to prevent replication and (2) acts as a competitive inhibitor of DNA polymerase; S phase–specific.
Metabolism:	Converted intracellularly to active form, ara-C triphosphate; rapidly deaminated by liver and kidney; excreted in urine. Diffuses into cerebrospinal fluid with prolonged infusion.
Side effects:	Nausea, vomiting, and anorexia
	Phlebitis during infusion
	"Cytarabine syndrome" of chest pain, fever, arthralgias, headache, malaise, diarrhea
	Erythroderma, photosensitivity
	Mucositis 2 to 7 days after treatment
	Myelosuppression is dose- and duration-related: onset 8 to 10 days posttreatment; megaloblastosis of erythroid precursors, reticulocytopenia, leukopenia (notably granulocytes), and thrombocytopenia occur; recovery in 2 to 3 weeks.

Cerebellar toxicity at high doses

Temporary hair loss or thinning within weeks after treatment

Comments: Dose-limiting toxicity is myelosuppression

Effective intrathecal agent

Radiation recall phenomenon

Formulation
and route: Injection vials (100 mg, 500 mg) for continuous intravenous infusion or intrathecal injection (preservative-free diluent)

Commonly
used dosage: 100 mg/sq m intravenously every 12 hours for 6 days, or 100 to 200 mg/sq m/day (continuous infusion) for 3 to 10 days, or 1 gm/sq m over 24 hours

Dacarbazine

Synonyms: DTIC, dimethyl-triazeno-imidazole-carboxamide
Class: Alkylating agent
Action: Alkylates nucleic acids and proteins, interferes with purine synthesis, interacts with sulfhydryl groups; non–cell cycle–specific.
Metabolism: Converted to active form in liver; excreted in urine.
Side effects: Nausea and vomiting within 1 to 3 hours of administration, lasting up to 12 to 24 hours

Pain at injection site

Flushed face or skin

Flu-like syndrome (aching, fatigue, low-grade fever)

Myelosuppression: leukopenia followed by thrombocytopenia 10 to 15 days after dose, continuing up to 2 to 4 weeks after last dose

Elevation of hepatic enzyme levels

Temporary alopecia weeks after treatment

Comments: Dose-limiting toxicities are nausea, vomiting, and myelosuppression.

Use carefully in patients with renal damage.

Formulation
and route: Injection vials (100 mg, 200 mg) for intravenous rapid infusion (10 to 15 minutes). Note drug is light-sensitive, stable up to 8 hours; pink indicates decomposition.

Commonly
used dosage: 375 mg/sq m intravenously every 14 to 28 days

Dactinomycin

Synonyms: actinomycin D, Act D, Cosmegen
Class: DNA-binding agent
Action: Tricyclic agent that intercalates with DNA and complexes with guanine residues to block RNA transcription
Metabolism: Phase-specific agent. Excreted by the liver; cleared slowly.
Side effects: Nausea, vomiting, anorexia

Myelosuppression may become apparent 2 to 4 days after

dose with nadir in 1 to 2 weeks; marked thrombocytopenia.

Stomatitis, cheilitis, glossitis, and proctitis, worse in previously irradiated areas.

Erythroderma, desquamation, and hyperpigmentation,
worse in previously irradiated areas

Temporary alopecia

Comments: Dose-limiting toxicities are nausea, vomiting, and diarrhea, as well as severe myelosuppression.

Extravasation causes skin necrosis.

Used in very small doses; do not confuse micrograms (μg)
with milligrams (mg).

Reduce dose in presence of liver damage.

Dactinomycin intensifies toxic effects of radiation.

Radiation recall phenomenon

Formulation
and route: Injection vial (500 μg), administered by intravenous push

Commonly
used dosage: 0.6 mg/sq m/day (= 600 μg/sq m/day) for 5 days

Doxorubicin and Daunorubicin

Synonyms: Doxorubicin: Adriamycin, ADR

Daunorubicin: DNR, daunomycin, Cerubidine, rubidomycin

Class: DNA-binding anthracyclines

Action: Bind DNA to inhibit replication.

Metabolism: Doxorubicin: eliminated by liver via glucuronidation or
sulfation.

Daunorubicin: Must be metabolized to daunorubicinol for
activation; excreted by liver.

Side effects: Nausea and vomiting for 24 to 48 hours

Fever, chills, and urticaria are encountered infrequently.

Febrile reaction may also accompany stomatitis and
leukopenia.

Myelosuppression with nadir at 10 to 12 days, rapid
recovery

Mucositis less common with daunorubicin.

Cumulative toxicity leads to cardiomyopathy; current recommendations limit total dose to 380 mg/sq m. Cardiomyopathy may be irreversible; monitor for toxicity
with serial electrocardiography (QTc) and echocardiography although these are not very sensitive or predictive. Slower infusions may be associated with less
cardiotoxicity (see Chap. 17).

Hair changes: color bands; reversible alopecia.

Nail changes: white streaks, softening, loosening, or loss.

Hepatic injury

Comments: Dose-limiting toxicity is myelosuppression.

Extravasation causes tissue necrosis.

Doxorubicin causes reddish discoloration of urine after
administration.

Reduce dose in patients with liver impairment; if bilirubin level is 1.2 to 3 mg/dl, reduce dose by 50 percent;

if bilirubin level is greater than 3 mg/dl, reduce dose by 75 percent.

Radiation recall phenomenon (may be marked)

Formulation
and route: Injection vials (10 mg, 50 mg) for intravenous administration

Commonly
used dosage: Doxorubicin: 75 mg/sq m intravenously every 3 weeks or 20 mg/sq m/week

Daunorubicin: 30 mg/sq m/day intravenously for 3 days or weekly

5-Fluorouracil

Synonym: 5-FU, Adrucil
Class: Antimetabolite
Action: Fluorinated pyrimidine that (1) inhibits thymidylate synthetase thus preventing DNA synthesis, and (2) is incorporated into RNA, blocking translation.
Metabolism: Rapidly inactivated by liver
Side effects: Nausea, vomiting, and anorexia

Stomatitis within several days of treatment

Diarrhea may be severe and dose-limiting.

Myelosuppression with nadir 1 to 3 weeks after treatment; thrombocytopenia follows leukopenia.

Reversible alopecia

In 1 percent of patients, reversible cerebellar ataxia may occur at any time after therapy, usually after several months.
Comments: Dose-limiting toxic effects are esophagitis and myelosuppression.

Reduce dose in presence of hepatic damage.

Stomatitis is an early and reliable sign of toxicity.

Not compatible with diazepam, doxorubicin, methotrexate, or cytosine arabinoside.
Formulation
and route: Injection vials (500 mg) for intravenous administration or by intracavitary route to control malignant effusions. Intrathecal use is contraindicated.

Commonly
used dosage: 500 mg/sq m/day intravenously for 5 days every 4 weeks or 500 mg/sq m/week intravenously

Ifosfamide

Synonym: IFF
Class: Alkylating agent similar to cyclophosphamide
Action: Chloroethyl nitrogen mustard is converted by microsomal enzymes to active form, which interacts with nucleic acids and proteins; non–cell cycle–specific.
Metabolism: Liver microsomal enzymes convert ifosfamide to several metabolites that are excreted in urine.

Side effects:	Central nervous system symptoms of altered mental status, cerebellar dysfunction, cranial nerve dysfunction, and seizures.
	Hemorrhagic cystitis; monitor urine output.
	Myelosuppression; monitor blood counts; rarely, inhibition of antidiuretic hormone; monitor electrolytes.
Comments:	Associated with more hemorrhagic cystitis than cyclophosphamide
	Mesna, a sulfhydryl uroprotector, is given to reduce hemorrhagic cystitis and does not appear to affect systemic antitumor action.
	Hydration and diuretic use reduce hemorrhagic cystitis severity and incidence.
	Myelosuppression is less severe than that seen with cyclophosphamide.
Formulation and route:	Injection vials (1 gm) for intravenous administration
Commonly used dosage:	2400 mg/sq m intravenously over 1 hour. Mesna, 480 mg/sq m, is administered intravenously with ifosfamide and every 3 hours thereafter.

Lomustine and Carmustine

Synonyms:	Lomustine: CCNU (chloroethyl-cyclohexyl-nitrosourea)
	Carmustine: BCNU (bis-chloroethyl-nitrosourea)
Class:	Alkylating agents
Action:	Nitrosourea, non-phase-specific, lipid-soluble; alkylate DNA and RNA; inhibit several key enzymatic processes.
Metabolism:	Lomustine: absorbed rapidly from stomach, diffuses into cerebrospinal fluid (CSF).
	Carmustine: rapidly cleared; good penetration into CSF.
Side effects:	Nausea and vomiting 2 to 6 hours after administration; resolves within 24 hours.
	Stomatitis
	Myelosuppression with delayed nadir (4 to 6 weeks after dose).
	Renal and hepatic toxicity may occur (reversible).
	Reversible alopecia
	Possible disorientation, lethargy, ataxia, dysarthria
	Possible delayed leukemia, pulmonary fibrosis
Comments:	Dose-limiting toxicity is myelosuppression.
	Lomustine: well-absorbed on empty stomach
	Carmustine: extravasation causes local ulcerations; phlebitis common.
Formulation and route	Lomustine: oral capsules (10 mg, 40 mg, 100 mg); different-colored capsules (different strengths) are taken in combination to achieve desired dose. Must be taken on an empty stomach (no food 2 hours before or after dose)
	Carmustine: injection vials (100 mg) for intravenous administration

Commonly
used dosage: Lomustine: 80 to 500 mg/sq m orally every 6 weeks
                Carmustine: 100 to 225 mg/sq m intravenously every 6
                weeks.

6-Mercaptopurine

Synonym: 6-MP
Class: Antimetabolite
Action: Guanine analog that inhibits de novo synthesis of purines
                and DNA synthesis.
Metabolism: Absorbed erratically from gastrointestinal tract; con-
                verted intracellularly to active form; catabolized within
                hours and excreted in urine.
Side effects: Nausea, vomiting, and anorexia; lower abdominal pain.
                Myelosuppression apparent 7 to 14 days after treatment;
                    depending on protocol, dose should be halved if abso-
                    lute granulocyte count is lower than 1000.
                Oral ulceration rare
                Hepatotoxicity uncommon and reversible; cholestasis.
Comments: Allopurinol inhibits metabolism of 6-MP, necessitating a
                    dose reduction (one-third to one-fourth usual dose).
                Typically given orally on daily basis
Formulation
and route: Oral tablets (50 mg)
Commonly
used dosage: 100 mg/sq m/day orally for 5 days or 50 to 75 mg/sq m/day
                orally. High-dose: 1 gm/sq m every 8 hours intravenously.

Methotrexate

Synonym: MTX, Mexate, Folex
Class: Antimetabolite
Action: Suicide substrate for dihydrofolate reductase; prevents
                synthesis of tetrahydrofolic acid, a necessary cofactor for
                pyrimidine synthesis and a precursor for DNA, RNA, and
                protein synthesis.
Metabolism: Binds to plasma proteins, accumulates in effusions or
                ascites; metabolized in liver, excreted in urine.
Side effects: Mild nausea, vomiting, and anorexia
                Mucositis possible within 2 to 7 days
                Myelosuppression with nadir occurring 4 to 10 days after
                    treatment
                Skin rash, erythema within 1 to 3 days; reversible
                    alopecia, photosensitivity.
                Reversible hepatic injury may be followed by hepatic fi-
                    brosis with prolonged therapy.
                Kidney damage possible with high doses.
                Central nervous system toxicity with high-dose or in-
                    trathecal methotrexate, including meningismus with
                    headache, fever, nausea, pleocytosis, myalgias; hemi-

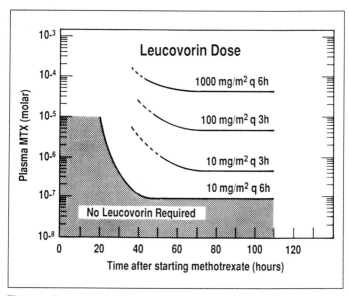

Fig. 11-1. Recommended Leucovorin dosage at various methotrexate (MTX) levels. (Reprinted from A. Bleyer. *The Clinical Oncologist* 2:1, 1988.)

paresis (transient or permanent); convulsions; dementia; and death. May be ameliorated with concomitant administration of intrathecal hydrocortisone.

Comments: Toxic effects can be reversed by folinic acid (Leucovorin), thymidine, or L-asparaginase. Leucovorin rescue usually initiated 6 to 24 hours after MTX and continued every 6 hours for 24 to 28 hours. Oral absorption of Leucovorin in the MTX-toxic patient is unknown, so the intravenous route is preferred. If Leucovorin rescue is to follow intrathecal MTX, it should be started 12 to 24 hours posttreatment (Fig. 11-1).

Dose-limiting toxic effects are mucositis and myelosuppression.

Highly protein bound; displaced by aspirin, sulfonamides, phenytoin, and tetracycline.

Good renal function and aggressive hydration are prerequisites.

Urine alkalinization prevents intranephric precipitation of high concentrations of methotrexate.

Sequestration of methotrexate in ascites, edema, or effusions may result in prolonged toxicity.

Formulation
and route: Injection vials (2.5 mg/ml, 25 mg/ml, and 100 mg/vial)
Oral tablets (2.5 mg)

Commonly
used dosage: 20 to 30 mg/sq m intramuscularly, orally, or intravenously twice weekly, or 1.5 gm/sq m intravenously (with Leucovorin rescue) every 3 weeks

Thioguanine

Synonyms:	6-Thioguanine, 6-TG
Class:	Antimetabolite
Action:	Purine analog that becomes incorporated into DNA and RNA
Metabolism:	Absorbed slowly from gastrointestinal tract; converted intracellularly to active ribonucleotide; subsequently detoxified and excreted in urine.
Side effects:	Nausea and vomiting uncommon except with overdosage
	Leukopenia and thrombocytopenia
	Hepatotoxicity
Comments:	Dose-limiting toxicity is myelosuppression.
	Dose should be reduced if renal or hepatic dysfunction occurs.
	Dose reduction *not* necessary when used with allopurinol.
Formulation and route:	Oral tablets (40 mg) (give between meals to facilitate absorption)
Commonly used dosage:	100 mg/sq m/day intravenously for 5 days or 40 to 60 mg/sq m/day orally. IV preparation investigational.

Vinblastine

Synonyms:	VLB, Velban
Class:	Tubulin-binding drug; cell cycle-specific.
Action:	Vinca alkaloid binds to microtubules, interfering with mitotic spindle formation and maintenance of cytoskeletal microtubules, as well as neuronal microtubules.
Metabolism:	Eliminated by liver over several hours
Side effects:	Mild nausea, vomiting, and anorexia
	Leukopenia with nadir at 4 to 10 days, recovery at 7 to 21 days; thrombocytopenia and anemia uncommon.
	Neurotoxicity (nerve axons are supported by microtubules), including paresthesias, peripheral neuritis; loss of deep tendon reflexes, jaw pain; weakness or loss of fine motor control, which may be indication for withholding dose.
	Headaches and transient depression within 2 to 3 days after dose
	Constipation and abdominal cramping within 14 days; treat prophylactically with bulk-adding agents and mineral oil or lactulose.
Comments:	Extravasation causes skin necrosis; local injection of hyaluronidase and warm compresses may help to disperse drug and may decrease cellulitis.
Formulation and route:	Injection vial (10 mg) for intravenous administration over 1 minute; avoid extravasation

*ommonly
used dosage:* m/week intravenously, or first dose 2.5 mg/sq m; 4.0 mg weekly by 1.25 mg/sq m to a maximum of 12.5 mg/sq m. Strict adherence to dosage interval is important.

Vincristine

Synonyms:	Oncovin, VCR
Class:	Tubulin-binding drug
Action:	*Vinca* alkaloid binds microtubules to cause mitotic arrest, as well as disruption of cytoskeletal and neuronal microtubules.
Metabolism:	Eliminated rapidly by liver
Side effects:	Mild nausea, vomiting, or anorexia
	Mild myelosuppression
	Obstipation, abdominal pain, and cramping. Paralytic ileus may develop, necessitating nasogastric suction and monitoring for possible intestinal perforation; peritoneal signs, tenderness, fever, and leukocytosis merit prompt surgical consultation.
	Jaw and bone pain common
	Syndrome of inappropriate antidiuretic hormone secretion more commonly seen in infants; watch for it.
	Neurotoxicity (gradually reversible on cessation of treatment); paresthesias, occasionally severe; loss of deep tendon reflexes (first: Achilles tendon), ataxia, foot drop, slapping gait, cranial nerve palsies, muscle wasting (hand dorsiflexors, foot extensors); severe jaw pain (more common in adolescents). May be dose-limiting. Convulsions are seen rarely.
	Reversible alopecia.
	Ineffective erythropoiesis with resultant anemia
Comments:	Extravasation causes skin necrosis; therefore it should be administered through a freshly placed intravenous catheter.
	Use with caution in presence of liver damage.
	Never to be used intrathecally nor to be anywhere nearby when intrathecal medications are being prepared or administered.
Formulation and route:	Injection vials (1 mg, 5 mg) for intravenous push
Commonly used dosage:	1.0 to 1.5 mg/sq m/week intravenously (maximum 2 mg) For infants < 10 kg, start at 0.05 mg/kg/week.

VM-26 and VP-16

Synonyms:	VM-26: Teniposide
	VP-16: Etoposide
Class:	Tubulin-binding drugs, DNA intercalating drugs, plant alkaloids

Action: Podophyllotoxin derivatives that (1) inhibit DNA sy sis by binding topoisomerase II; (2) produce mitotic ar at metaphase, perhaps by interfering with spindle form. tion; and (3) alkylate nucleic acids and proteins.

Metabolism: Bound to plasma proteins; excreted in bile and, to a lesser extent, in urine.

Side effects: Nausea, vomiting, cramping, and diarrhea

Hypotension, especially during rapid infusion; stop infusion and give fluids.

Hypertension occasionally in children

Allergic reactions may occur; consider premedicating with diphenhydramine.

Myelosuppression with nadir occurring at 7 to 14 days

Reversible alopecia

Peripheral neuropathy (uncommon)

Comments: Dose-limiting toxicity is myelosuppression.

Formulation
and route: Injection ampules (VM-26, 50 mg; VP-16, 100 mg/5 ml) infused over 1 hour; monitor heart rate and blood pressure

Commonly
used dosage: VM-26: 100 to 200 mg/sq m intravenously once or twice weekly

VP-16: 150 to 300 mg/sq m intravenously once or twice weekly, or 100 mg/sq m/day for 5 days, or 200 mg/sq m/day for 2 to 3 weeks

SELECTED READINGS

Bleyer, W. A. Antineoplastic Agents. In J. Yaffe (ed.), *Pediatric Pharmacology: Therapeutic Principles in Practice.* New York: Grune & Stratton, 1980. Pp. 349–377.

DeVita, V. T., Jr. The relationship between tumor mass and resistance to chemotherapy. *Cancer* 51:1209, 1983.

Goldie, J. H., and Coldman, A. J. The genetic origin of drug resistance in neoplasms: Implications for systemic therapy. *Cancer Res.* 44:3643, 1984.

Schabel, F. M., Jr., et al. Increasing therapeutic response rates to anticancer drugs by applying the basic principles of pharmacology. *Pharmacol. Ther.* 20:283, 1983.

Radiotherapy in the Pediatric Oncology Patient

Joshua Halpern and Moshe H. Maor

Radiotherapy is the administration of electromagnetic waves or particulate rays to a target volume, in order to kill tumor cells in that area. Radiotherapy is therefore a local or regional treatment. In contrast to surgery, however, irradiation may be administered to large fields that include vital organs not amenable to surgical resection or even to the whole body, in which case it may be considered systemic therapy.

TYPES OF RADIOTHERAPY

Teletherapy (External Beam Irradiation)

Photon Beam (Electromagnetic) Irradiation
Gamma radiation originates in a radioactive isotope (e.g., cobalt 60 or cesium 137). *X radiation* originates in an electron acceleration device. X rays are produced by bombardment of a heavy metal anode with accelerated electrons, similar to the diagnostic x-ray machine.

Particulate Irradiation
Beta radiation is equivalent to *electron beam radiation* and is the most commonly employed particle. It is obtained from an electron acceleration device with direct release of accelerated electrons. *Other particles,* including protons, neutrons, alpha-particles and Pi-mesons, are used experimentally. Currently, clinical studies explore these beams for possible treatment benefit in appropriate situations.

Brachytherapy (Contact Irradiation)

Intracavitary irradiation involves the placement of a radioactive source (radium 226, cesium 137, iridium 192) in an anatomic cavity (e.g., vagina, uterus, esophagus) for irradiation of a tumor that is located in appropriate proximity. For interstitial irradiation, radioactive sources are placed in needles or plastic tubes that are then inserted in the tumor and surrounding tissues as necessary, when an anatomic cavity is not available. *Surface irradiation* is the application of radioactive sources in a surface mold and is feasible for superficial skin or mucosal tumors.

INDICATIONS FOR EMPLOYMENT OF SPECIFIC TYPES OF RADIOTHERAPY

Photon Beam Irradiation

Photon beam irradiation (with x or gamma rays) has a high degree of penetration when obtained from the megavoltage machines available today. It is used for deeply located tumors and for treatment of large fields that require a homogeneous dose, such as in adjuvant treatments and irradiation of lymphatic drainage areas when a specific tumor volume cannot be assessed. The distribution of the radiation may be improved in a treatment volume area by means of field shaping using shielding, multiple fields, rotational techniques, appropriate beam energies, and the like. Photon beam irradiation is the most commonly used modality.

Electron Beam Irradiation

Electrons are negatively charged particles that have much shallower penetration than photons. Their advantage in irradiation lies in a sharp drop in the dose at a certain depth, which is a function of the electron beam energy. Electron beam irradiation is very useful for treating superficial lesions without damaging deeply located structures. (For example, a chest wall lesion may be irradiated with electrons without harming lung tissue, heart muscle, spinal cord, or the like, all of which are located at some depth.)

Implants

With implant irradiation (brachytherapy) the radiation dose drops with the square of the distance from the source. Radioactive implants, which are placed in the tumor itself, thus have the advantage of treating the adjacent volume without damaging distant normal tissues (as opposed to external beams, which have to travel through the skin and all the tissues overlying the tumor before reaching the target). Intracavitary treatments are useful for lesions that are anatomically adjacent to normal body cavities, such as carcinoma of the uterine cervix and endometrium in adult women. Interstitial irradiation will be required for lesions that cannot be reached through normal cavities or that are too big for such treatment. Surface mold irradiation is useful for superficial lesions of the skin and mucosa. Radioactive implants are rarely used in pediatric patients.

PRESCRIPTION, SIMULATION, AND ADMINISTRATION OF RADIOTHERAPY*

Treatment Prescription

Target Volume

The radiation oncologist has to define the volume to be irradiated, which usually includes the whole tumor and a margin of surrounding normal tissue. This process usually is supported with all the available imaging modalities. For example, the initial target volume may include the tumor and the first echelon of lymphatic drainage. This field will be prescribed a dose derived from the known radiosensitivity of the tumor and the tolerance of the normal tissue in the irradiated area. A booster dose, aimed at the tumor volume itself, may then be added.

Prescription of Irradiation Technique

The radiation treatment prescription has to include the size, shape, number, and angles of the fields, as well as beam characteristics, dose, and fractionation. Simple treatment designs or treatments with predictable features may be prescribed by the experienced radiotherapist without computer analysis. More complicated treatments or circumstances will require sophisticated three-dimensional analysis. This is done by interfacing dedicated radiotherapy

---

*Doses and fractionations mentioned in this text should be regarded as general recommendations only. For actual prescriptions of radiotherapy, radiation oncologists are advised to consult more detailed literature.

planning computers with computed tomography (CT) or magnetic resonance imaging (MRI) spatial scans. (For further details, refer to Selected Readings.)

The radiation dose is currently prescribed in grays (Gy), which is defined as the radiation unit that deposits 1 joule of energy in 1 kg of tissue. The previously used unit, the rad (radiation absorbed dose), is equivalent to 0.01 Gy (100 rad = 1 Gy).

Treatment Simulation

Following the initial prescription of external radiation treatment parameters, diagnostic x-ray films of the designated treatment fields are obtained. This is done with a simulator, which uses diagnostic (not therapeutic) doses of radiation to simulate the treatment fields in terms of size, shape, and angle. The diagnostic radiographs obtained during the simulation process are used to demonstrate coverage of the tumor volume and to ascertain reproducibility of the treatment fields (see the next section). The radiographs are kept as a permanent record for documentation of the field location.

Administration of Radiotherapy

The external beam treatment itself is carried out with machines that radiate photons or particles, as indicated in the treatment prescription. Young children may find it difficult to cooperate with positioning and immobilization during treatment, necessitating sedation and, in rare circumstances, anesthesia. Most children can learn to cooperate with treatment if appropriate behavior modification techniques are employed. Radiographs are obtained during treatment to assess reproducibility of treatment fields. These radiographs, or portal films, have poor resolution because of the high penetrating energy of the beams. The experienced radiotherapist, however, can compare them with the radiographs obtained during treatment simulation and thereby confirm proper positioning of the patient and shields with respect to the photon beams.

INDICATIONS FOR IRRADIATION IN PEDIATRIC CANCER PATIENTS

Radiotherapy should be administered with extreme care in children because of a high potential for harmful effects (see Radiation Toxicity in Children). There are conditions, however, for which irradiation is the only curative modality. Indications for radiotherapy vary among institutions and also according to the tumor type and stage of disease. Specific recommendations are beyond the scope of this book.

A number of situations can arise that require emergency initiation of radiotherapy in children. These are listed below and are discussed in greater detail in Chaps. 16–28.

Central Nervous System Emergencies

The following central nervous system disorders constitute emergencies and should be treated with radiotherapy in the pediatric cancer patient:

Brain tumors with increased intracranial pressure (see Increased Intracranial Pressure in Chap. 24).

Spinal cord compression (see Spinal Cord Compression in Chap. 24).

Meningeal carcinomatosis (see Meningeal Carcinomatosis in Chap. 24).

Impending Pathologic Fractures of Weight-Bearing Bones

Large osteolytic lesions around the acetabulum, in the femur, and in the tibia may result in disabling pathologic fractures. Prophylactic irradiation of such lesions prevents collapse of these bony structures in a high proportion of treated patients. Irradiation is indicated in these locations even after the pathologic fracture has occurred, with internal fixation whenever feasible, for both alleviating the pain and securing the internal nailing. The prescribed dose is usually 30 Gy in 10 daily fractions.

Pericardial Effusion and Cardiac Tamponade

Pericardial effusion with cardiac tamponade is rare in pediatric solid tumors but is encountered in hematologic malignancies. Electrocardiogram-directed pericardiocentesis and permanent opening of a pericardial window are effective treatments. Chemotherapy-responsive malignancies may be treated systemically when appropriate. A viable alternative is low-dose irradiation of the cardiac silhouette. Doses up to 24 Gy/2½ weeks have been tolerated well. Radiotherapy to the heart muscle should be avoided whenever possible in children receiving doxorubicin.

Superior Vena Cava Syndrome

Radiotherapy may be required in pediatric cases of superior vena cava syndrome of neoplastic origin (see Superior Vena Cava Syndrome in Chap. 18).

Paraneoplastic Syndromes

When hypercalcemia, disseminated intravascular coagulation, syndrome of inappropriate antidiuretic hormone secretion, and other potentially life-threatening conditions are suspected to have a paraneoplastic origin, irradiation of the tumor may ablate the secretion of the humoral factor involved. Radiotherapy, when feasible in these conditions, may provide better and longer palliation than continuously administered medication(s) needed to control the metabolic derangement.

RADIATION TOXICITY IN CHILDREN

Any tissue encompassed in a radiation treatment field will be potentially affected. The damage to normal tissues is determined by many factors related to both the sensitivity of the tissues involved (radiosensitivity) and the irradiation parameters. Generally, tissues with a high rate of turnover of the cell population will be affected earlier than tissues with a low cellular turnover. The radiation damage to normal tissues may appear during and immediately after the irradiation (acute toxicity) or months to many years after radiotherapy (late toxicity). The acute affects are usually reversible and may be minimized by means of conservative management, sparing of normal tissues whenever possible and, eventually, rest periods during radiation treatment. Late effects are of longer duration, sometimes irreversible, and often difficult to treat. The use of lower doses per fraction and more fractions per treatment may reduce long-term toxicity. Mathematical calculations have been developed for optimizing the fractionation of radiation treatments.

Acute Radiation Toxicity

The skin, mucosal linings, and bone marrow are examples of tissues with high cellular turnover, and as such they are highly susceptible to acute radiation damage. The skin may develop a sunburnlike condition, ranging from (1) mild erythema, to (2) dry desquamation, (3) wet desquamation, and (4) necrosis. Damage to the oral and gastrointestinal mucosae may produce difficulty in swallowing, nausea and vomiting, abdominal cramps, and diarrhea, depending on the involved field. Irradiation of the mucosa in the head and neck areas results in dryness of the mouth, sore throat, and loss of the senses of taste and smell. When the radiation fields cover large portions of bone marrow, myelosuppression and pancytopenia may ensue. Rarely, other conditions may emerge, such as acute radiation pneumonitis, pleuritis, and pericarditis. Brain irradiation may acutely produce severe headaches and lethargy. The radiation oncologist is familiar with these conditions and their management and should be responsible for their treatment.

Chronic Radiation Toxicity

Any irradiated organ may suffer from chronic radiation toxicity. Whenever such a condition is suspected, a radiotherapist should be consulted; treatment is often carried out by a multidisciplinary team. Before a diagnosis of chronic radiation toxicity is made, other conditions or primary tumor recurrence must be ruled out.

Skin and Soft Tissues

The skin and subcutaneous tissues may exhibit changes varying from telangiectasia, skin discoloration, and mild fibrosis to severe fibrosis and deep ulcerations. These conditions were more common when low-energy (orthovoltage) treatment machines were used. The orthovoltage beams had no skin-sparing effect, and the dose to the skin and subcutaneous tissues was much higher than to the deeper target volume. Treatment of large areas of ulceration is difficult and may require surgical debridement and skin grafting. The compromised vascular supply and severe fibrosis produced by irradiation in these areas may cause severe healing problems.

Gastrointestinal Tract

Late radiation damage to the gastrointestinal tract may result in fibrosis, strictures, and fistulas. The small intestine is more sensitive, with effects seen at doses of 45 Gy/4½ weeks. The esophagus may withstand doses of up to 70 Gy/7 weeks, and the colon doses in excess of 50 Gy/5 weeks. The symptoms in the lower gastrointestinal tract may vary from tenesmus, diarrhea, and rectal bleeding to fistulas and intestinal obstruction. Treatment ranges from dietary adjustments and steroid enemas to surgical correction. Irradiation of the esophagus and the stomach may result in dysphagia, nausea, and vomiting due to fibrosis, stenosis, and fistulization. The treatment may be symptomatic or surgical as necessary.

Bone and Bone Marrow

The epiphyseal plate is the critical area in the growing bone. Doses of 25 Gy/2½ weeks and higher may affect subsequent growth. The bone absorption of radiation is higher at the lower energies generated by orthovoltage machines. Modern megavoltage machines produce a better dose distribution and produce less bone damage.

Doses in excess of 30 Gy/3 weeks to a bone marrow area are believed to ablate hematopoiesis permanently in the irradiated field. When a patient is considered for chemotherapy, an estimation of the potentially compromised bone marrow should be made before radiotherapy is undertaken; often, a realistic compromise is feasible.

Central Nervous System

The central nervous system consists of cellular compartments with slow or no renewal potential. The acute toxicity to neurons is therefore fairly low but, in the long run, a damaged neuron will never be replaced and toxicity will accumulate.

BRAIN Disorders of intellectual function were described for doses as low as 24 Gy/2½ weeks. This occurred mostly in young children with leukemia who also received intrathecal chemotherapy [1]. The most recent study of children treated with cranial irradiation versus intrathecal chemotherapy does not show a difference in intellectual function between the groups [2]. The brain tissue may be affected in a patchy manner called multifocal leukoencephalopathy, which has a characteristic appearance on CT scanning. Frank brain necrosis may occur at doses above 55 Gy/5 weeks.

A special entity is the so-called central nervous system syndrome, which consists of lethargy, nausea, occasional vomiting, and dizziness. It may appear 2 to 3 months after treatment and may last 2 to 4 weeks.

SPINAL CORD Doses in excess of 50 Gy/5 weeks may result in transverse myelitis with consequences similar to a transection of the spinal cord. Extreme care must be taken by radiotherapists when matching radiation fields, so that overlap of the spinal cord is avoided.

A syndrome probably related to the central nervous system syndrome that follows brain irradiation is the Lhermitte's sign. It may appear 1 to 3 months after radiation treatment and last 1 to 9 months. Symptoms are episodes of severe paresthesias triggered by flexion of the cervical spine.

Gonads

Because of a high cellular turnover in the gonads, irradiation of these organs should be avoided whenever possible.

OVARIES The ovaries of prepubertal girls appear to be less radiosensitive than those of adults. Doses of more than 30 Gy, however, produce gonadal failure in most patients.

TESTES The adult testis may be sterilized with only 5 Gy. Although the prepuberal testis is less radiosensitive, testicular irradiation should be avoided whenever possible. Production of testosterone in the Leydig cells is unaffected by low to moderate doses of radiation.

Lungs

Any amount of lung tissue irradiated with more than 25 Gy/2½ weeks becomes fibrotic and loses respiratory function. A special caution should be made against administering steroids during or after radiotherapy because a severe form of radiation pneumonitis may be precipitated on withdrawal of these agents. Recall phenomenon is the emergence of radiation pneumonitis after administration and withdrawal of steroids long after the radiation treatment. Whenever possible, care should be taken to shield lung tissue.

Other Organs

KIDNEYS Doses of more than 25 Gy/2½ weeks for a whole kidney or 30 Gy/3 weeks for a portion of a kidney will decrease renal function in the irradiated area.

URINARY BLADDER Doses of more than 50 Gy/5 weeks to the urinary bladder may produce bladder fibrosis and contraction. Doses of more than 70 Gy/5 weeks to portions of the bladder may cause perforation and fistulization.

LIVER Doses of more than 30 Gy/3 weeks to the liver produce fibrosis of the liver parenchyma and loss of function in the irradiated area. In certain conditions, such as irradiation for a right-sided Wilms' tumor or neuroblastoma, shielding of the liver is a difficult technical problem.

HEART The heart muscle, especially the left ventricle, should be shielded at a maximum dose of 30 Gy/3 weeks. Special caution is required when doxorubicin is given systemically because the two treatments may produce synergistic myocardiotoxicity. This is a special concern in multimodal treatment for Hodgkin's and non-Hodgkin's lymphoma with mediastinal involvement.

ENDOCRINE GLANDS Hypothyroidism was reported especially after irradiation for Hodgkin's disease with a mantle field without shielding the thyroid gland [3]. Currently, shielding of the larynx and the thyroid area is the rule whenever possible. Doses in excess of 45 Gy/4½ weeks to brain fields that include the pituitary gland have been reported to produce chronic pituitary insufficiency [4] (see Chap. 23).

EYE The globe of the eye is irradiated primarily in cases of retinoblastoma, rhabdomyosarcoma of the orbit, malignant melanoma, lymphoma, and intraorbital metastases. The whole eye and the retina may withstand high doses, up to 50 Gy/5 weeks, but the lens is much more sensitive. Cataract formation may be seen with doses in excess of 4 Gy/week; it may be treated by extraction of the lens. For irradiation of the anterior portion of the brain, the beam is usually angled posteriorly to avoid divergence into the contralateral eye.

Radiation-Induced Secondary Tumors

The pediatric cancer patient population suffers from a significant incidence of radiation-induced cancers. Four contributing factors may be implicated: (1) the critical growth and development period; (2) longer expected survival in cured children; (3) frequent concomitantly administered chemotherapy; and (4) predisposition to cancer. On retrospective analysis, a 17 percent cumulative incidence of cancers secondary to radiotherapy was found [5], although some investigators consider this figure to be inflated.

Bone Tumors

The overall incidence of radiation-induced osteosarcomas is estimated at 0.03 percent [6]. Diagnosis of radiation-induced osteosarcoma should follow the criteria of Cahan [7], which generally require the following:

The tumor should develop in the irradiation field.
The total dose should exceed 50 Gy.
A latent period of more than 3 years should elapse between radiotherapy and development of the secondary tumor.

The second tumor should not develop in the bed of the previous tumor.

The second tumor should be proved to be histologically different from the initial tumor

Many of the reported cases of radiation-induced secondary cancers (approximately 250 are reported in the literature) do not fulfill all these criteria. Second malignancies, most of which occurred at the site of the initial tumor, have been reported in patients irradiated for Ewing's sarcoma [6]. In most of these cases, orthovoltage radiotherapy had been administered. The modern megavoltage irradiation is expected to produce fewer secondary bone tumors (see Chaps. 26, 29, and 30).

Thyroid Neoplasms

It has been stated that approximately 7% percent of patients whose thyroid glands were irradiated developed thyroid cancers [8]. Today, the thyroid gland is shielded during neck irradiation whenever possible. Three to four decades ago, children received radiation indiscriminately for a variety of benign and malignant conditions, with the consequence that the thyroid gland was exposed to radiation. This and the inherent sensitivity of the gland explain the fact that the thyroid is the most common site of tumors induced by radiation during childhood.

Other Sites

Irradiation to other sites may give rise to radiation-induced cancers. However, because of the sporadic nature of such events, this will not be discussed further.

TOTAL BODY IRRADIATION

Total body irradiation (TBI) may be administered by itself or with high-dose chemotherapy when it is followed by bone marrow transplantation. TBI can rarely be administered at very low doses without bone marrow transplantation (e.g., 0.3 Gy/week in three fractions for a total of 1.5 Gy), as in radiosensitive lymphomas. The dose with bone marrow transplantation is higher and, when delivered with high-dose chemotherapy, the radiation dose is modified accordingly. It was found that fractionated TBI produces less toxicity than when it is administered in a single dose [9]. TBI in one fraction will usually be in the range of 5 to 10 Gy. The fractionated TBI is usually delivered in the range of 9 to 14 Gy in 3 to 10 fractions over 3 to 6 days.

Clinical experience with TBI has been gained predominantly with hematologic tumors. In solid tumors, the use of TBI followed by bone marrow transplantation has been reported in patients with neuroblastoma or Ewing's sarcoma, when systemic chemotherapy failed.

Lung toxicity is the limiting factor. Acute toxic effects of TBI include gastroenteritis, mucositis, myelosuppression, and alopecia. Chronic effects may manifest as impairment of growth and development, gonadal failure, cataracts, and possibly, second malignancies. TBI should be administered only in institutions where there are dedicated and experienced radiotherapy teams and where multidisciplinary treatments are available for severe complications.

REFERENCES

1. Eiser, C. Intellectual abilities among survivors of childhood leukemia as a function of CNS irradiation. *Arch. Dis. Child.* 53:391, 1978.
2. Ochs, J., et al. Prospective evaluation of CNS changes in children with ALL treated with prophylactic cranial irradiation or IV methotrexate. Proceedings of the American Society of Clinical Oncology 1989, A824.
3. Gladstein, E., et al. Alterations in serum thyrotropin (TSH) and thyroid function following radiotherapy in patients with malignant lymphomas. *J. Clin. Endocrinol.* 32:833, 1971.
4. Samaan, N. A., et al. Hypothalamic, pituitary, and thyroid dysfunction after radiotherapy to the head and neck. *Int. J. Radiat. Oncol. Biol. Phys.* 8:1857, 1982.
5. Li, F. P., Cassady, J. R., and Jaffe, N. Risk of second tumors in survivors of childhood cancer. *Cancer* 35:1230, 1975.
6. Jaffe, N. Late Sequelae of Cancer Therapy. In W. W. Sutow, D. J. Fernbach, and T. J. Vietti (eds.), *Clinical Pediatric Oncology* (3rd ed.). St. Louis: Mosby, 1984. Pp. 810–832.
7. Cahan, W. G., Woodward, H. Q., and Higginbotham, N. L. Sarcoma arising in an irradiated bone: Report of eleven cases. *Cancer* 1:3, 1948.
8. Refetoff, S., et al. Continuing occurrence of thyroid carcinoma after irradiation to the neck in infancy and childhood. *N. Engl. J. Med.* 292:171, 1975.
9. Peters, L. J., et al. Radiobiological considerations in the use of total body irradiation for bone marrow transplantation. *Radiology* 131:243, 1979.

SELECTED READINGS

Bleehen, M. M., Glatstein, E., and Haybittle, J. L., (eds.). *Radiation Therapy Planning.* New York: Marcel Dekker, 1983.

Fletcher, G. H. (ed.). *Textbook of Radiotherapy.* Philadelphia: Lea & Febiger, 1980.

Parsons, J. T. The Effect of Radiation on Tissues of the Head and Neck. In R. R. Million and N. J. Cassisi (eds.), *Management of Head and Neck Cancer.* Philadelphia: Lippincott, 1984. Pp. 173–207.

Perez, C. A., and Brady, L.H. (eds.). *Principles and Practice of Radiation Oncology.* Philadelphia: Lippincott, 1987.

Perez, C., and Thomas, P. R. N. Radiation Therapy: Basic Concepts and Clinical Applications. In W. W. Sutow, D. J. Fernbach, and T. J. Vietti (eds.), *Clinical Pediatric Oncology* (3rd ed.). St. Louis: Mosby, 1984. Pp. 167–209.

13

Bone Marrow Transplantation

Steven J. Culbert

BONE MARROW TRANSPLANTATION VERSUS CHEMOTHERAPY

Bone marrow transplantation and chemotherapy represent different modalities for treating disease in the same patient population. The best candidates for either therapy are those patients who are relatively healthy with little accumulated toxic injury and who are in an early phase of treatment (less resistant disease, so that they are more likely to respond to therapy). These are the patients who are more likely to survive and complete aggressive therapy successfully. Controversy exists over specific indications for transplantation versus chemotherapy in a variety of disorders. Transplantation is associated with greater morbidity and mortality initially; however, late relapses are fewer than with chemotherapy, which results in similar long-term survival. Transplantation may offer long-term survival in later-stage disease, when chemotherapy is less successful. As treatment-related mortality due to infection and graft-versus-host disease (GVHD) continues to decline, bone marrow transplantation may be utilized for broader indications.

PURPOSE OF BONE MARROW (STEM-CELL) TRANSPLANTATION

The purpose of bone marrow (stem-cell) transplantation is to restore normal hematopoietic and immunologic functions in the host recipient by donor stem cells. In the classic transplant situations of severe combined immunodeficiency disease and aplastic anemia, donor marrow permits the establishment of a permanent stable chimera (both donor and recipient stem cells functioning). In cancer therapy, marrow transplantation represents both a rescue from lethal-dose chemotherapy and radiotherapy, aimed at killing all tumor cells, as well as a means of restoring normal hematopoietic and immunologic functions [1, 2]. In transplantations for genetic disorders, the goal is to restore to near-heterozygous levels previously absent gene products; this has been referred to as displacement transplantation [3, 4].

Autologous bone marrow transplantation is a misnomer for a stem-cell rescue procedure employing techniques developed for allogeneic stem-cell transplantation. Strictly speaking, there are no hematopoietic or immunologic transplantation barriers to be overcome. Function following stem-cell rescue approximates that of the marrow before the procedure (excepting residual effects of conditioning on the marrow microenvironment) [5, 6].

INDICATIONS FOR BONE MARROW TRANSPLANTATION [1]

Allogeneic Transplantation

Transplantation is generally accepted as the potentially curative treatment of choice in the following conditions:

Severe combined immunodeficiency disease syndrome, Wiskott-Aldrich syndrome, adenosine deaminase deficiency

Chronic myelogenous leukemia (chronic or early accelerated phase)
Juvenile chronic (monomyelocytic) leukemia
Aplastic anemia
Thalassemia major
Osteopetrosis

In the following conditions, the results of transplantation are considered to be better than those of chemotherapy alone, although this remains controversial:

Acute nonlymphocytic leukemia in first or subsequent remission
Acute lymphocytic leukemia in second or subsequent remission
Burkitt's lymphoma, stage IIIA or IV
Hodgkin's disease, third or subsequent relapse
Neuroblastoma (Evans stage III or IV, age over 1 year) in complete
    remission

Transplantation is controversial in these conditions; but there is a small number of patients reported in the literature:

Malignant histiocytosis
Malignant histiocytoma
Sickle cell anemia
High-risk acute lymphocytic leukemia, first remission
Hunter's, Hurler's, Morquio's, and Sanfilippo's syndromes
Gaucher's disease
Metachromatic leukodystrophy

Autologous Transplantation

Early results suggest that transplantation may be curative in the following conditions:

Acute nonlymphocytic leukemia (as consolidation of first or second
    remission)
Burkitt's lymphoma, stage III or IV, relapsed or as consolidation
Non-Hodgkin's lymphoma in second or subsequent remission
Neuroblastoma (Evans stage III or IV, or over 2 years of age) in
    complete remission
Hodgkin's disease (in third or subsequent relapse)

The published results of transplantation in these conditions are debatable:

Acute lymphocytic leukemia in second or subsequent hematologic
    remission
Neuroblastoma with active abdominal disease [7]
Non-Hodgkin's lymphoma with history of marrow involvement

**TYPES OF BONE MARROW (STEM-CELL)
TRANSPLANT [8]**

The various types of bone marrow transplants are listed here in order of increasing immunologic incompatibility based on the source of donor marrow (stem cells).

Autologous   Recipient's own marrow or harvested peripheral blood
              stem cells are usually cryopreserved in anticipation of
              rescue (generally used as part of cancer therapy). In the
              near future, in vitro genetic manipulation may permit
              this marrow source to be used in displacement transplan-
              tation for genetic disorders.

| Syngeneic | The recipient is an identical twin (genetically identical to the donor). |
| Allogeneic: | The recipient is genetically nonidentical to the donor. The possibilities for such transplants are: (1) related donor (generally sibling) human leukocyte antigen (HLA) and mixed lymphocyte culture (MLC) are compatible; (2) related haplotype is nonidentical and MLC is compatible; (3) unrelated but HLA and MLC are compatible; and (4) related HLA is nonidentical, and MLC is incompatible. |

DONOR SELECTION

The technical aspects of donor screening and testing are beyond the scope of this book. A laboratory experienced in routine HLA and MLC testing, with the capability of restriction fragment-length polymorphism confirmation, is an absolute necessity in allogeneic transplant donor selection. In general, the tissue-typing laboratory should be one dedicated to marrow transplantation only. An immunologist or blood banker with specialized experience in donor testing should be responsible for interpretation of all donor testing.

The donor should not be jeopardized physically or psychologically from marrow donation. As a rule, age should not be a factor in selecting the donor.

SOURCES OF STEM CELLS FOR TRANSPLANTATION [6]

There are basically two sources of donor stem cells: bone marrow and peripheral blood. Bone marrow is a better source (10^3–10^4 more stem cells) and is generally preferred for allogeneic bone marrow transplantation and most autologous procedures.

In autologous situations in which tumor cell contamination of marrow space is possible or documented, peripheral blood pheresis can be carried out. In most centers, this is tedious and expensive and requires expertise in cryopreservation. Innovative programs, however, have reduced the number of pheresis procedures to obtain sufficient cells for engraftment to one or two. Peripheral blood stem-cell collection may be best employed in patients receiving aggressive chemotherapy; the concentrations of stem cells after rebound from chemotherapy are 10^2 to 10^3 times higher than under normal circumstances. Careful planning and skilled organization are required to maximize efficacy. One advantage of this procedure is the availability of small pheresis bowls, permitting collection in very young children with more efficiency and less trauma than marrow collection. The utilization of various recombinant hematopoietic growth factors in conjunction with peripheral blood is expected to alter autologous transplantation greatly. A number of studies indicate that many of the adverse hematologic effects created by conditioning regimens can be alleviated to some degree by the use of available hematopoietic growth factors [9].

PRETRANSPLANTATION (CONDITIONING) REGIMENS

In cases of allogeneic transplantation, the original purpose of conditioning regimens is to bring about sufficient immunosuppression to permit engraftment of the transplanted marrow. The standard has been to use cyclophosphamide in total dosages of 3000 mg/sq m to 6000 mg/sq m in two to four daily intravenous infusions. Further attempts to increase immunosuppression involve adding a combination of total lymphoid irradiation, and other chemotherapeutic agents.

In autologous and allogeneic transplantations performed for treating malignancies, total tumor ablation is attempted with combinations of chemotherapeutic agents (generally including cyclophosphamide) and/or total body irradiation. Conceptually, the more aggressive therapy is necessary to carry out total tumor cell kill; the marrow is administered as a rescue from the lethal-dose therapy.

In displacement transplantations performed for correction of genetic disorders, the standard regimen for conditioning incorporates cyclophosphamide for immunosuppression and busulfan for stem-cell ablation. This combination is also used in a wide variety of schedules for transplantation in malignant disorders as well [3].

Individual institutions or study groups tend to have standard conditioning regimens. There are some disease-specific conditioning regimens, such as high-dose cytosine arabinoside for transplantation in leukemics and melphalan for transplantation in neuroblastoma [7]. Dosages, routes, and schedules are highly variable and generally institution specific.

COLLECTION AND PREPARATION OF STEM CELLS FOR TRANSPLANTATION

In allogeneic situations, once a suitable donor is identified and informed consent is obtained, the transplantation is scheduled. In general, donor blood for autotransfusion is collected weeks before marrow is collected. Blood bank expertise and patient tolerance determine the minimum size of the donor permitted to donate his or her own blood. Marrow collection is an outpatient procedure involving hundreds of small-volume marrow aspirations from the iliac crests and elsewhere as needed; general or spinal anesthesia is required. During marrow collection, the donor red blood cells and colloid are infused. An ongoing cell count is maintained to ensure that adequate numbers of cells are collected. The aspirated marrow is sieved through a series of screens to remove bone and other debris. Approximately 3×10^8 mononuclear cells/kg recipient body weight is believed to be the lower limit of adequate cells for successful transplantation.

For autologous bone marrow transplantation, the marrow or stem cells, once collected, are frequently manipulated to remove residual malignant cells. For allogeneic transplantation, the manipulations are aimed at reducing the risk of severity of GVHD by removing T lymphocytes. A wide variety of pharmacologic, physical, and immunologic methods to remove undesirable cells can be employed, either singly or in combination. In many institutions, these manipulations are the main focus of experimentation in transplantation. In transplantations for genetic disorders, major breakthroughs are now permitting planned insertion of various DNA segments into transplantable cells in small mammals [4].

GRAFT-VERSUS-HOST DISEASE [10, 11]

GVHD accounts for much of the morbidity and mortality associated with allogeneic marrow transplants. In optimum conditions (HLA-identical, MLC-compatible sibling donor) and with an unmanipulated marrow, 25 percent of marrow recipients will die of GVHD; 40 to 70 percent of recipients will experience morbidity of a mild to severe degree. In similar conditions with lymphocyte-depleted marrow, GVHD is less severe and less frequent, but failure of engraftment results in similar mortality. In leukemia, the relapse rate is statistically higher [12]. GVHD is on occasion seen with autologous or syngeneic transplants. The disease is mediated by mature donor thymic T lymphocytes with reaction against recipient non-HLA antigens or minor determinants in the HLA system.

Acute and Chronic GVHD

The principal target tissues of GVHD are the skin, liver, and gut. Specific classification by clinical staging is shown in Table 13-1. Simplistically, GVHD comes in two forms, acute and chronic. *Acute GVHD* occurs before day 100 and is often the first sign of marrow engraftment. If it extends past or arises de novo after day 100, it is conventionally called chronic GVHD. The clinical grading is that for acute GVHD (Table 13-2). Acute GVHD, in general, presents with cutaneous involvement that progresses to the liver and intestinal tract. *Chronic GVHD* is a multisystem syndrome resembling a diffuse collagen vascular disease. Skin involvement (from erythema to severe scleroderma), esophagitis, ocular sicca, oral mucositis and sicca, myositis, hepatitis, polyserositis, and intestinal disorders have been described. Chronic GVHD exhibits similarities to scleroderma, systemic lupus erythematosus, lichen planus, and primary biliary cirrhosis.

Both acute and chronic GVHD are profoundly immunosuppressive, with residual long-term immunodeficiency being characteristic. Acute and, to some extent, chronic GVHD are myelosuppressive and can mimic graft failure, particularly when supervening cytomegalovirus (CMV) infection is present.

Prevention of GVHD

The problem of GVHD has been addressed in several ways, the most important of which is selection of the most appropriate (i.e., most immunologically compatible) donor. Prevention and treatment of GVHD are the subject of a variety of protocols. Preventive measures include prophylactic pretransplantation and posttransplantation immunosuppression, methotrexate and cyclosporine being the agents considered most often. Pretransplantation marrow lymphocyte depletion or posttransplantation intravenous infusions of monoclonal antilymphocytic antibodies (CD-4 and CD-8) are also popular. The posttransplantation methotrexate schedule pioneered in Seattle remains the standard, although cyclosporine combined with methotrexate is now in more general use. The technologic development of stem-cell concentration (lymphocyte depletion) employing monoclonal antibodies (with or without complement), or immunomagnetic beads, or immunotoxin conjugates is being used in a number of transplantation centers. A major result of the lymphocyte-depletion technology is an increased rate of leukemic relapse, 10- to 30-percent graft failure rate, and a substantial risk of B-cell lymphoma development [14]. Believing there is insufficient evidence to warrant prophylaxis when potential toxicity is considered, some centers actually employ no prophylactic measures for GVHD.

Diagnosis and Treatment of GVHD

GVHD is a great mimic. Diagnosis and treatment of the disease often is delayed because of confusion arising from the large number

Table 13-1. Clinical and histopathologic staging of graft-versus-host disease

Stage	Skin	Liver	Intestinal tract
Clinical stage			
+	Maculopapular rash over < 25% of body surface	Bilirubin 2–3 mg/dl	> 500 ml diarrhea/day
+ +	Maculopapular rash over 25–50% of body surface	Bilirubin 3–6 mg/dl	> 1000 ml diarrhea/day
+ + +	Generalized erythroderma	Bilirubin 6–15 mg/dl	> 1500 ml diarrhea/day
+ + + +	Generalized erythroderma with bullous formation and desquamation	Bilirubin > 15 mg/dl	Severe abdominal pain, with or without ileus
Histopathologic stage			
+	Basal vacuolar degeneration or necrosis (or both)	< 25% Abnormal atypical degenerated or necrotic (or both) small interlobular bile ducts	Dilatation of glands; single-cell necrosis of epithelial cells
+ +	+ findings and spongiosis, dyskeratosis, eosinophilic necrosis, and epidermal cells	25–50%	Stage I findings and necrosis and dropout of entire glands
+ + +	Stage II findings and focal epidermal-dermal separation	50–75%	Stage II findings and focal microscopic mucosal denudation
+ + + +	Frank epidermal loss	> 75%	Diffuse microscopic mucosal denudation

Source: E.D. Thomas, et al. Bone marrow transplantation. Reproduced with permission from *The New England Journal of Medicine.* 292:896, 1975.

of confounding variables during early disease. Features and staging of GVHD are summarized in Tables 13-1 and 13-2. The treatment of established acute GVHD is not highly successful, particularly when it occurs after cyclosporine prophylaxis. The frontline agents are corticosteroids with dosages ranging from the conventional 2 mg/kg of prednisone to 50 to 100 mg/kg of methylprednisolone. Antithymocyte globulin, cyclophosphamide, continuous-infusion cyclosporine, monoclonal antibodies to T-cell subsets, and thalidomide, among others, have been used with variable success in acute GVHD. Chronic GVHD is managed with steroids in combination

Table 13-2. Clinical grading of graft-versus-host disease

Grade	Signs and symptoms*
I	Stage I–II skin rash; no gut involvement; no liver involvement; no decrease in clinical performance
II	Stage I–III skin rash; stage I gut involvement or stage I liver involvement (or both); mild decrease in clinical performance
III	Stage II–III skin rash; stage II–III gut involvement or stage II–III liver involvement (or both); marked decrease in clinical performance
IV	Similar to grade III with stage II–IV organ involvement and extreme decrease in clinical performance

*See Table 13-1 for explanation of clinical staging.
Source: From E. D. Thomas, et al. Bone marrow transplantation. Reproduced with permission from *The New England Journal of Medicine* 292:896, 1975.

with either azathioprine or cyclosporine; there is no universally accepted regimen. Thalidomide has shown impressive responses in chronic cutaneous disease. Unfortunately, even in the setting of allogeneic bone marrow transplantation, the diagnosis of GVHD can be extremely difficult. The skin rash of early GVHD may be mimicked by a variety of drug-induced rashes (those caused by trimethoprim plus sulfamethoxazole and vancomycin, commonly), postirradiation skin changes, and a variety of viral rashes (CMV and adenoviruses). A skin biopsy with appropriate histochemical stains is essential if one plans to employ some of the newer agents (i.e., immunotoxin conjugates or intravenous monoclonal antibodies) in the early treatment of GVHD. Similar considerations apply to the evaluation of abnormalities associated with the other major target organs for GVHD. As a general rule, the earlier the diagnosis of GVHD is made, the more likely it is that GVHD will be controlled. Be aware that the treatments for established or early GVHD are highly immunosuppressive; they must be to be effective. Large-volume diarrhea may be due to a variety of infectious agents including cytomegalovirus; in this setting, one would want to avoid further immunosuppression in the patient. *When in doubt, perform a biopsy* [12].

DENTAL CARE
The oral cavity is a common site for complications during bone marrow transplantation. Appropriate dental care can reduce the potential for infection during periods of bone marrow suppression. Irradiation, cytotoxic drugs, and GVHD are known to induce a breakdown of structures in the oral cavity as well as mucosal atrophy, ulceration, mucositis, and xerostomia. Involvement of a knowledgeable pediatric dentist is of extreme importance. Oral management during bone marrow transplantation can be separated into four phases. Phase 1 occurs before transplantation, phase 2 is the first 100 days, phase 3 is the follow-up year after transplantation, and phase 4 covers the long period after the first year. During phase 1, clinical and radiologic dental examinations are carried out; if possible, defects are corrected, loose primary teeth are extracted, and instruction in oral hygiene is given. During phase 2, a preven-

tive program of 0.1% isotonic chlorhexidine solution and 1-ml nystatin (100,00 IU/ml) rinses is carried out 4 to 6 times daily, at least over the first 2 months, to control oropharyngeal candidiasis. Toothbrushing with a sponge toothbrush can be resumed once circulating phagocytes are present. The patient with pretransplantation herpes simplex virus titers should receive acyclovir, 250 mg/sq m intravenously 3 times daily, until granulocytes exceed 1000 per microliter; acyclovir is then administered orally for 4 to 6 months. Close observation, particularly for xerostomia, is continued in phase 3. Artificial saliva and topical fluoride are used to preserve enamel.

VENOOCCLUSIVE DISEASE OF THE LIVER [13]

Although venoocclusive disease (VOD) is not unique to marrow transplantation, it is one of the more dramatic complications. There is obstruction of blood flow by the nonthrombotic narrowing or fibrinous obliteration of the terminal hepatic venules or sublobular veins. Depending on the degree and rapidity of onset of obstruction, hepatic enlargement, ascites, encephalopathy, and hepatocellular necrosis may occur; the onset may be gradual or breathtaking. Patients at high risk for VOD include those with previous hepatic function abnormalities, leukemia, a second or subsequent transplant, and GVHD. The clinical diagnosis must be entertained when two of the following three conditions occur within the first 30 days after transplantation: (1) jaundice, (2) hepatomegaly and right upper quadrant pain, and (3) ascites, unexplained weight gain, or both. It is ultimately a pathologic diagnosis, with biopsy necessary to differentiate between GVHD, viral hepatitis (particularly CMV), and other causes of similar nonspecific findings.

Clinical management of VOD is the same as that for acute onset of hepatic failure, with restriction of fluids, vigorous use of furosemide or other loop diuretics, and exclusion of all but essential amino acids from hyperalimentation fluids.

The clinical course typically begins with sudden weight gain (15–20% over the basal value) and an associated drop in urinary sodium excretion. Jaundice and hepatomegaly are almost universal, with abdominal pain and ascites in more than 70 percent of the cases. There are direct bilirubin increases. Elevation of liver enzymes is variable, with no universal pattern. Mild abnormalities of coagulation may occur. VOD may be associated with rapid development of hematologic aplasia; disease is expected to be refractory to platelet transfusion because of splenic sequestration. Renal dysfunction is seen in more than half of the patients and is more common in the most severe cases of VOD. In some patients, renal failure is the underlying cause of death from VOD.

CYTOMEGALOVIRUS

CMV infection remains a major obstacle to the successful outcome of allogeneic bone marrow transplantation. It has been claimed that with newer techniques of GVHD prevention, CMV is now the leading cause of death after transplantation. Such infections must be due to (1) acquisition of exogenous virus, causing either primary infection or reinfection, or (2) reactivation of latent endogenous virus. The clinical manifestations of CMV-induced disease are many and may mimic other disease processes commonly seen after bone marrow transplantation, particularly GVHD. The risk of developing an infection is related to serologic status of the recipient before transplantation and to the serologic status of the donors of marrow and blood products. Prevention of CMV infection is complicated by the ease with which CMV can be transmitted via blood products. The risk of CMV infection is directly related to the number of units of blood products infused; the large number of units necessary for support in the period following conditioning creates a considerable risk. Granulocyte transfusions are of particular concern. Seronegative patients transfused only with seronegative products do not develop CMV infections. Unfortunately, it is difficult to maintain a large enough catalog of blood donors to supply neonatal nurseries as well as bone marrow transplant units. Patients who are seropositive for CMV need not receive precious CMV-negative units of blood products since CMV appears not to be transmitted as a latent virus.

Diagnosis of CMV

Atypical lymphocytosis and thrombocytopenia are hallmarks of CMV infection; unfortunately, GVHD, drug toxicity, and infections of other origins may have similar associated findings. Until recently, CMV infections of the gastrointestinal tract were frequently mistaken for GVHD. The importance of a rectal biopsy in differentiating the two cannot be overemphasized.

As serologic responses are unreliable in bone marrow transplant recipients, the diagnosis of CMV infection should be made by the detection of the virus itself. Molecular biological techniques employing cDNA probes for CMV DNA or messenger RNA are preferred over culture because of the rapidity of the results and ability for direct detection in tissue sections.

Clinical Sequelae of CMV

The clinical sequelae of CMV infections are many and varied. The manifestations range from a short-lasting febrile illness to cystitis, retinitis, hepatitis, esophagitis, gastritis, pancreatitis, colitis, and encephalitis. Particularly troublesome is pneumonitis. Graft failure has been associated with active CMV infection.

CMV pneumonitis classically occurs during the second and third month after allogeneic bone marrow transplantation. There are basically two forms. In the miliary form, multiple focal lesions are present; patients develop rapid pulmonary failure (over 3–7 days), necessitating mechanical ventilation, which is almost universally fatal. The other form, diffuse interstitial pneumonitis, is associated with a more insidious presentation and may require ventilation, with complete recovery expected. The major risk factors are high-grade (grade II or greater) GVHD, total body irradiation, older patient age, and poor nutritional status. A recently acquired CMV infection is probably associated with more rapid onset of pulmonary failure.

Prevention and Treatment of CMV

Currently available antiviral agents have shown little or no activity in established advanced CMV infections. Investigational agents are the only available treatment. Until active agents are available, meticulous attention should be paid to the prevention of primary infection.

REFERENCES

1. Vega, R. A., et al. Bone marrow transplantation in the treatment of children with cancer. *Hematol. Oncol. Clin. North Am.* 1:777, 1988.

2. Thomas, E. D., et al. Bone marrow transplantation. *N. Engl. J. Med.* 292:895, 1975.

3. Bone marrow transplantation for neurovisceral disorders (editorial). *Lancet* 2:788, 1986.

4. Kantoff, P. W., et al. In utero gene transfer and expression: A sheep transplantation model. *Blood* 73:1066, 1989.

5. Appelbaum, F. R., and Buckner, C. D. Overview of the clinical relevance of autologous bone marrow transplantation. *Clin. Hematol.* 15:1, 1986.

6. Gorin, N. C. Collection, manipulation, and freezing of haemopoietic stem cells. *Clin. Hematol.* 15:19, 1986.

7. August, C. S., et al. Treatment of advanced neuroblastoma with supralethal chemotherapy, radiation, and allogeneic or autologous marrow reconstitution. *J. Clin. Oncol.* 2:609, 1984.

8. Fefer, A. Current status of syngeneic marrow transplantation and its relevance to autografting. *Clin. Hematol.* 15:49, 1986.

9. Brandt, T., et al. Effect of recombinant human granulocyte-macrophage colony-stimulating factor on hematopoietic reconstitution after high-dose chemotherapy and autologous bone marrow transplantation. *N. Engl. J. Med.* 318:869, 1988.

10. Sullivan, K. M., et al. Late complications after marrow transplantation. *Semin. Hematol.* 21:53, 1984.

11. Sullivan, K. M., et al. Influence of acute and chronic graft-versus-host disease on relapse and survival after bone marrow transplantation from HLA-identical siblings as treatment of acute and chronic leukemia. *Blood* 73:1720, 1989.

12. Sale, G. E., et al. Gastrointestinal graft versus host disease in man: A clinicopathologic study of the rectal biopsy. *Am. J. Surg. Pathol.* 3:291, 1979.

13. McDonald, G. B., et al. Venocclusive disease of the liver after bone marrow transplantation: Diagnosis, incidence, and predisposing factors. *Hepatology* 4:116, 1984.

14. Martin, P. J., et al. Effects of in vitro depletion of T cells in HLA-identical allogeneic marrow grafts. *Blood* 66:664, 1985.

14

Surgical Intervention in the Child with Cancer

C. Thomas Black

INDICATIONS FOR SURGERY

When caring for children in an oncology ward, a number of clinical situations warrant a surgical consultation. Some of these are: (1) diagnosis of suspected malignancy, (2) resection of a primary tumor, (3) resection of metastases, (4) debulking of tumor mass, (5) palliation, (6) second-look procedure, (7) vascular access, (8) complications of the disease or treatment, and (9) coincident surgical conditions. Even if a surgical procedure is not imminent, early consultation with the surgeon who will eventually be involved in a particular child's care is of great importance. The surgeon's input will aid in planning the proper timing of the procedure, and establishing early contact with the family will give the family time to accept and prepare for a major operation.

Diagnosis of Suspected Malignancy

When a child is suspected of having a particular type of cancer, a tissue diagnosis is usually desirable before instituting treatment. Such tissue is obtained by means of a biopsy and, in many instances, this does not involve a trip to the operating room. Bone marrow aspiration is adequately performed under local anesthesia in the ward treatment room, although it is ideally done under general anesthesia if the child is to undergo a concomitant procedure in the operating room. A fine needle aspiration biopsy of a visible or palpable lesion may also be performed under similar conditions by one familiar with the procedure. Internal masses may be biopsied using the fine-needle technique and computed tomographic or ultrasonographic guidance. Needle biopsy is not advisable (1) when surgical resection is planned to follow immediately a biopsy with abnormal results; (2) for small masses such as lymph nodes that are firm and mobile and therefore difficult to enter with a needle; (3) for lesions in risky areas or those difficult to access because of surrounding vital structures; and (4) for masses that may have local areas of disease mingled with areas of normal tissue. In the latter case, normal biopsy results cannot be relied on to represent the entire mass.

A surgical biopsy is either *excisional,* in which the entire mass is removed, or *incisional,* in which only a portion of the mass is resected. Excisional biopsy is preferred unless a tumor believed to be resectable proves otherwise or safety dictates that an incisional rather than a needle biopsy be performed.

The definitive treatment of Hodgkin's disease is not surgical, but the manner in which chemotherapy and radiotherapy are administered depends on the extent of the disease. The staging laparotomy is used to define this extent by providing tissue samples from several abdominal organs for microscopic examination.

Another staging procedure may be lymph node dissection, which comprises surgical excision and microscopic examination of a group of lymph nodes draining the area in which a malignant tumor has been found. A finding of tumor cells in any of the nodes worsens the prognosis.

Resection of a Primary Tumor

Despite the dramatic advances in chemotherapy for pediatric malignancies over the past few decades, the majority of solid tumors in children must be completely resected if a cure is to be anticipated. Although preoperative assessment varies with tumor type, abdominal and extremity masses require at least computed tomography (CT), ultrasonography, or magnetic resonance imaging (MRI) for delineation of the tumor's extent. Factors to be considered when determining resectability include evidence of wide dissemination, evidence of spread into unresectable areas, and the necessity of leaving sufficient residual tumor-free tissue for preservation of life.

A considerable number of tumors are judged to be unresectable before or during surgical exploration. In such cases, reconsideration for definitive resection is delayed until the tumor has been rendered as resectable as possible by chemotherapy or radiotherapy. At that time, successful resection may occasionally be performed.

If a resectable tumor is not expected to decrease in size with preoperative chemotherapy or radiotherapy, resection should be performed as soon as preoperative assessment has been completed. If, however, resection of normal tissue can be minimized, adjuvant treatment should be considered before resection is undertaken. Risks and side effects of such therapy and the fact that the use of some therapeutic modalities preoperatively may limit their usage subsequently must be weighed against the benefits of potential tissue salvage in each situation.

Resection of Metastases

Patterns of metastatic spread are known for each individual tumor, and so following resection of the primary lesion, frequent evaluation should be made of the primary organs potentially affected by metastases. Generally, the detection of metastatic disease in a patient removes him or her from consideration for further surgical intervention, with a few exceptions. If only regional lymph nodes are believed to be affected, a lymph node dissection should be performed, both for potential cure and for staging purposes. The most common site for distant metastatic spread is the lung, and pulmonary nodules have been resected with subsequent cure for patients with Wilms' tumor, osteosarcoma, and hepatoblastoma. Surgery is usually contemplated when such nodules fail to respond to chemotherapy and radiotherapy, as evidenced by increasing size on plain radiography or CT scans, or by increasing levels of serum-borne tumor markers. Multiple resections and multiple thoracotomies are limited only by the necessity of sparing sufficient pulmonary tissue for survival. The possibility of resection should be given careful consideration in each case, since the survival of a patient with unresected metastases is usually nil.

Debulking of Tumor Mass

When a tumor is found to be unresectable, consideration should be given to debulking that tumor if this can be performed with minimal anticipated morbidity or mortality. Survival time can often be prolonged, and the patient can be made more comfortable by reducing the tumor burden. The benefits of chemotherapy and radiotherapy may also be potentiated, both by a reduction of the tumor size and by the application of radiopaque clips that allow radiation to be directed with greater precision.

Palliation

When the goal is not cure but an improvement in the quality of remaining life, palliative surgery should be considered. Obstructed organs may be bypassed, sensation to painful areas ablated, pressure on surrounding organs relieved, or enteral feeding routes established for nutritional support by gastrostomy or jejunostomy.

Second-Look Procedures

After the primary resection of certain types of malignancies, an earlier detection of recurrence than that afforded by less invasive modalities may be afforded by a second-look operation. This is usually performed 3 to 6 months after the initial procedure. Visual inspection of the site of resection, surrounding tissues, and other internal organs can then be carried out, and biopsies of suspicious areas can be performed to exclude recurrence. Decisions regarding continuation or cessation of chemotherapy may then be made based on the findings.

Vascular Access

The need for vascular access is perhaps the most frequent impetus for a pediatric oncologist to obtain a surgical consultation. A lack of peripherally accessible veins; the need for infusion of certain caustic agents into central rather than peripheral veins, frequent intravenous infusions of chemotherapeutic agents, frequent blood sampling, and administration of central intravenous hyperalimentation; and the desire to limit the pain of repeated attempts for venipunctures are all valid reasons for considering placement of a long-term indwelling catheter.

Forms of Central Venous Access

Several forms of central venous access are available. Most catheter tubing is made of Silastic, which is flexible, inert, and relatively resistant to infection. Some catheters have subcutaneous injection ports, which must be percutaneously accessed each time they are used. Other catheters are brought through and anchored to the skin and are accessed through external ports. Although subcutaneous ports require a skin puncture for usage, when not in use they require no upkeep or limitation of activity and are unnoticeable. Catheters with external ports are more easily accessed but are also more easily damaged and infected. Most long-term external catheters (Broviac or Hickman variety) have a Dacron cuff that is implanted just under the skin and acts both as an anchor and as a barrier against infection. Long-term percutaneous catheters and subcutaneous ports come in both single-lumen and double-lumen varieties, and temporary (less than 2 weeks of anticipated usage) percutaneous catheters are noncuffed and come in single-, double-, or triple-lumen varieties.

Central Venous Catheter Placement

Catheters are usually inserted into large veins of the upper body (i.e., the subclavian or the external or internal jugular veins). They are then directed toward the heart so that the tip comes to rest at the junction of the superior vena cava and the right atrium. Some prefer the tip to be located within the right atrium itself. Insertion may be by subclavian puncture or by direct cutdown onto a jugular vein. Most or all children should undergo placement of any of these catheters under general anesthesia because of the long period during which the patient must remain motionless to avoid hazards of insertion. It is imperative that the prothrombin and partial thromboplastin times be normalized before insertion, and the platelet count should exceed 50,000 per microliter. Catheters with external ports may be used immediately after correct placement has been verified radiographically. In contrast, catheters with subcutaneous ports should be used only after 72 hours have elapsed to allow a fibrous pocket to form around them. This protects against infection and problems associated with extravasation of infusion fluid.

*Central Venous Catheter Occlusion**

With the increasingly widespread use of central venous catheters (CVCs) for chemotherapy, a number of complications are encountered, notably central line sepsis (see Chap. 22), and central line thrombosis. CVC obstruction may be safely reversed with the following procedure:[†]

1. CVC occlusion is recognized when it is difficult or impossible to infuse fluids through the catheter. Failure to obtain a blood return in the face of easy infusion of fluids may signify a normally positioned catheter in a small child, hypotension, narrow tubing, a malpositioned or extravascular catheter, or a ball valve type obstruction.
2. *Do not* attempt to force fluids through the catheter line; syringes smaller than 10 ml can generate excessive pressures. Forceful flushing can introduce thrombotic material into the bloodstream, which has the potential for instigating pulmonary embolus.
3. Check for blood return with the patient sitting and leaning forward or in the right or left lateral decubitus position.
4. Confirm intravascular location and occlusion with a radiographic contrast study, after first having ruled out extravascular obstruction (tight sutures, crimped tubing).
5. With the infusion site at or below the level of the heart, the physician or specially trained intravenous therapist, using aseptic technique, should infuse a volume of urokinase (5000 U/ml) to fill the lumen of the tubing (usually < 1 ml; see Table 14-1).
6. Allow the urokinase to dwell for 10 to 15 minutes, and then check for blood return.
7. If there is no blood return, allow the urokinase to dwell 30 to 60 minutes and recheck for blood return.
8. When blood return is obtained, withdraw and discard 3 to 5 ml of blood and urokinase; then flush gently with 10 ml of normal saline.

---

*This section was written by the University of Texas M.D. Anderson Cancer Center IV therapy team.
[†]Additional information may be obtained from the following manufacturers: Pharmacia, Piscataway, NJ; Infusaid Corporation, Norwood, MA; Cormed, Medina, NY; Cook Medical Inc., Bloomington, IN; Arrow International Inc., Reading, PA; Evermed Inc., Kirkland, WA; and Deseret Medical Inc., Sandy, UT.

9. If no blood return is obtained after 1 to 2 hours with this procedure, the catheter should be removed. *Do not* attempt to exchange it over a wire as this is liable to release a blood clot into the bloodstream.

Intraarterial Access

Rarely, an intraarterial catheter is placed surgically into the hepatic artery and attached to an intracorporeal pump. This pump periodically may be refilled percutaneously, and it slowly infuses chemotherapeutic agents into the hepatic circulation for the treatment of unresectable malignant disease within the liver parenchyma.

Complications of the Disease or Treatment

Certain chemotherapeutic agents, such as doxorubicin, are highly caustic, and if extravasation occurs at the site of peripheral infusion, serious tissue damage may result. Debridement and skin grafting may be necessary in severe cases.

Strict aseptic technique is essential in preventing central line sepsis when indwelling catheters are in place. Aseptic technique requires those changing dressings or opening the infusion pathway to wash their hands, wear gloves, and use antiseptic agents. Most infections are due to gram-positive organisms and may be eradicated by antibiotic therapy. If the patient is severely neutropenic, or the infection is unresponsive to antibiotic treatment, or the line is infected by fungus, the catheter may require surgical removal (see Chap. 22).

The superior vena cava syndrome may develop as a complication of the presence of an indwelling catheter within the superior vena cava. It is causally unrelated to but may be complicated by infection. Upper body plethora, venous distention, and edema are signs of this condition. Removal of the catheter is generally recommended to attempt reinstitution of flow, but complete occlusion may yet occur. Recanalization following lysis of the thrombosis or organization and fibrous occlusion are possible ultimate consequences. Superior vena cava syndrome may also arise as a result of a bulky tumor and is best managed with chemotherapy or radiotherapy (see Chap. 18).

Many chemotherapeutic agents cause nausea and vomiting and are sometimes accompanied by abdominal pain, which causes concern about the development of an acute abdomen. L-Asparaginase is known occasionally to cause acute hemorrhagic pancreatitis, which may truly appear to be an acute abdomen. Right lower quadrant pain in a child with leukemia, particularly acute myelogenous leukemia, has been associated with typhlitis or neutropenic colitis—inflammation of the cecum accompanied by an extremely depressed absolute neutrophil count. The cause is unknown, but typical ulceration of the mucosa is present with thickening of the cecal wall, which may be detected on an abdominal radiograph or CT scan. The differential diagnosis includes acute appendicitis which, compared with the general population, is known to accompany leukemia with a frequency that is disproportionately high. Symptoms are often subdued because of neutropenia and absence of the usual inflammatory response to developing infection. Occasionally, steroids are being administered as part of a chemotherapeutic regimen, the effect of which is further suppression of the normal immune response. While the optimum treatment of appendicitis is appendectomy, treatment of typhlitis is controversial, with some advocating surgi-

Table 14-1. Lumenal volume of central venous catheters (CVC)

| Type | Size | | Volume (ml) | | |
	Gauge	Length (inches)	Port	Catheter	Total
Percutaneously placed CVC					
Brachial	16	20			0.65
Subclavian	16	6			0.35
Cutdown	18	9			0.15
Cutdown	20	9			0.10
Deseret or Bard (Teflon)[a]	16				0.30
Cook double-lumen[b]					
Large	16	8			0.25
Small	18	8			0.20
Arrow double-lumen[c]					
Large	14				0.60
Small	18				0.40
Arrow triple-lumen[c]					
Distal	16				0.5
Medial	18				0.4
Proximal	18				0.4

Surgically placed catheters

Hickman catheter No. 10 Fr[d]				1.8
Broviac catheter No. 6.5 Fr[d]				0.7

Implantable vascular access devices

Port-a-Cath[e]	10	0.4	0.2	0.6
Infuse-a-Port[f]	10	0.2	0.2	0.4
Mediport[g]	10	0.6	0.2	0.8

[a]Deseret Medical Inc., Sandy, UT.
[b]Cook Medical Inc., Bloomington, IN.
[c]Arrow International Inc., Reading, PA.
[d]Evermed Inc., Kirkland, WA.
[e]Pharmacia, Piscataway, NJ.
[f]Infusaid Corporation, Norwood, MA.
[g]Cormed, Medina, NY.

cal resection and others advocating medical management only. Despite therapy, mortality due to either of these conditions is high (See Chaps. 20 and 22).

Enlarged lymph nodes of abdominal lymphoma or secondary spread of known tumors may cause intestinal obstruction and require resection, bypass, or creation of an ostomy. The development of an idiopathic and unresponsive pulmonary infiltrate may necessitate a diagnostic open-lung biopsy, and the development of progressive respiratory insufficiency, whether due to infection, tumor involvement, or damage from chemotherapy, may be grounds for consideration of a tracheostomy.

Coincident Surgical Problems

Of course, a child afflicted with cancer may also develop an unrelated surgical problem, from a case of appendicitis to an inguinal hernia. Because the oncologist is the child's primary physician and because the assumption is made that any problem the child develops is related to his or her cancer, the child is usually brought first to the oncologist who must recognize the problem for what it is and make the appropriate disposition for further treatment.

POSTOPERATIVE COMPLICATIONS

Infection

The body has several mechanisms for resisting its invasion by microorganisms. Mechanical barriers include the skin, mucous membranes, and intestinal epithelium. Whenever one of these barriers is broken, infection is possible. Although stringent measures are taken during a surgical procedure to cleanse any such site that will or may possibly be disrupted during the procedure, complete sterility is impossible to achieve. A wound over which the skin has been reapproximated becomes epithelialized after 24 to 48 hours, but before then, clean conditions such as maintaining a sterile dressing must be observed.

Should microorganisms breach this barrier, phagocytic cells in and around the site will ingest and kill them. These phagocytes are attracted to the area by chemotaxins, breakdown products, and complement. Phagocytosis is aided by opsonins, a heterogeneous group of specific and nonspecific proteins that bind to the intruder's cell membrane. Local application of warmth to an area believed to be infected aids the process of phagocytosis by creating vasodilatation, which allows phagocytes easier access to the site.

Humoral and cell-mediated immunities are based on cell destruction by lymphocytes or their immunoactive products. Humoral or B-cell immunity involves the production of antibodies that will specifically inactivate a particular antigen or foreign substance. Cell-mediated or T-cell immunity consists of the production by T lymphocytes of nonspecific factors or lymphokines, which ultimately promote the death of an invading organism.

Soft-tissue infection may be classified as involving superficial tissues, fascia, or muscles. Superficial infections are generally called cellulitis and have an erythematous appearance, usually surrounding a break in the skin barrier. *Staphylococcus aureus, Haemophilus influenzae,* and some species of streptococci are the most common causes of postoperative cellulitis. The vast majority of these cases will be adequately treated by systemic antibiotics, local wound cleansing, and local application of heat. Deeper infections may involve the superficial fascia and are thus called fasciitis. These are highly lethal infections that have a rapid onset and progress quickly. They are due to two or more organisms, usually an aerobe and an anaerobe, acting in synergy to digest fascial tissues and secrete toxins. Pain and edema with a rapidly advancing border around an incision site, watery brownish wound discharge, and signs of systemic toxicity, such as high fever and occasionally altered sensorium, are signs of fasciitis and typically occur within the first few postoperative hours. Immediate recognition is difficult but essential, and wide debridement of affected tissue with institution of potent antibiotics is necessary for survival of the child. Involvement of the muscle and muscle fascia constitutes myositis, the classic example of which is gas gangrene caused by *Clostridium perfringens*. Rapid spread along muscle fascia and toxin production causes edema, myonecrosis, and severe systemic toxicity. Prevention is much more satisfactory than treatment.

Complications Specific to Children

Children are markedly less prone to postoperative complications than are adults. They are more compliant regarding early ambulation, pulmonary toilet, and pain management. Deep venous thrombosis of the lower extremities because of inactivity is uncommon in children. The effects of aging and pollution, tobacco, alcohol, and other ingested substances are not generally seen in children undergoing cancer surgery. The cardiopulmonary status is therefore usually excellent if unimpaired by chemotherapeutic agents.

Overwhelming sepsis after splenectomy for the staging of Hodgkin's disease was once believed to be confined to the pediatric age group. However, numerous cases have now been reported in adults as well.

Although not specific to children, the first suspicion of an inherited clotting disability might come about as a result of surgical intervention for a malignant condition. Obtaining a careful history regarding easy bruisability and a familial tendency toward bleeding are more precise and cost-effective than are blood tests.

A child may display signs of previously unsuspected malignant hyperthermia up to 24 hours after receiving a general anesthetic agent. Arrhythmias, hypercapnia, and hyperkalemia are fairly early signs; hyperthermia is a dangerously late finding.

Complications Specific to a Particular Tumor

Neuroblastoma and Wilms' Tumor

Complications of surgery may occur intraoperatively or they may first develop postoperatively. Because of the extent of some adrenal neuroblastomas, injury to the spleen or surrounding organs may occur. If the pancreas was traumatized during the procedure, a postoperative amylase level would be warranted. Because of the proximity to the diaphragm and occasional partial resection required for removal of a neuroblastoma or Wilms' tumor, a postoperative chest radiograph to exclude a pneumothorax is wise. Diaphragmatic and rib pain may cause a child to "splint" the affected thorax, resulting in basilar atelectasis. Early mobilization and encouragement for deep breathing will assist in early resolution. Because of the lymphatics transected during excision of the usual Wilms' tumor, a chylous ascites may occasionally result. This is self-limited and no specific treatment is ordinarily required. Approximately 10 percent of children with Wilms' tumor develop a transient period of hypertension postoperatively. This is due to increased renin, which is probably a result of either vascular impairment or tumor manipulation during resection.

Rhabdomyosarcoma

Adequate resection of a rhabdomyosarcoma may result in temporary or permanent limb disability. In many cases, physical therapy may help in compensating for the loss. Such an outcome should be considered preoperatively, and the potential disability should be weighed against the anticipated benefits.

Hepatoblastoma

Resection of a hepatic lobe for hepatoblastoma is a formidable surgical procedure. The potential for substantial loss of blood with ensuing hypotension, hypocoagulation, and hypothermia makes this procedure acutely life-threatening. Hypoglycemia, hypoalbuminemia, infection, and liver failure threaten the patient postoperatively. Complications are frequent but may be lessened by careful preoperative preparation. Hematologic and coagulation studies should be performed and abnormalities corrected, and the patient must be well-hydrated. Vitamin K may be administered. A total blood volume (80 ml/kg) of packed red blood cells and the same amount of fresh-frozen plasma should be available for intraoperative and postoperative use. An additional 10 to 20 ml/kg of fresh whole blood or cryoprecipitate and platelets, should be available for treating a possible dilutional coagulopathy. Air embolism is also a serious threat. Although bowel contamination is not expected, a broad-spectrum antibiotic is given preoperatively because the incision is large, the operation is relatively long, and the child is severely immunologically compromised for a period of time afterward. The possibility of a perihepatic abscess is present because of the large "dead space" left after removing a significant portion of the liver mass, much of which was enlarged by the tumor. Antibiotics should be maintained until abdominal drains are removed. An enema administered immediately preoperatively makes the procedure less difficult for the surgeon and more comfortable for the child postoperatively.

Afterward in the intensive care unit, intravenous fluids containing 10 to 20% glucose should be given at maintenance rates to prevent hypoglycemia. A large amount of intravascular plasma is expected to be lost as third-space fluid, accumulating as ascites and edema. Hypoalbuminemia is caused by decreased synthesis as well as increased losses. Failure to replace these losses with sufficient amounts of similar fluids will lead to decreased urine output, hypoproteinemia, and fluid and electrolyte imbalances. Fresh-frozen plasma or 5% albumin is administered in amounts sufficient to maintain normal urine output. A prolonged prothrombin time is secondary to decreased manufacture of vitamin K–dependent coagulation factors by the traumatized liver, and fresh-frozen plasma will be needed to offset this deficiency until the prothrombin time has returned to normal.

Pheochromocytoma

Pheochromocytoma is an unusual tumor in the pediatric population but accompanies several familial syndromes including the multiple endocrine adenomatosis (MEA) type II syndrome (Sipple's syndrome). Intraoperative hypertension may be avoided by alpha-adrenergic blockade, gentle manipulation of the tumor, and early ligation of the venous drainage. Following resection, rebound hypotension may be avoided by previous alpha-adrenergic blockade or by adequate volume replacement.

SELECTED READING

Lawson, M., et al. The use of urokinase to restore patency of occluded central venous catheters. *Am. J. IV Ther. Clin. Nutr.* 9:29, 1982.

15

Immunotherapy and Colony-Stimulating Factors

Sima Jeha

LYMPHOKINES

Perspective

In 1969, a new term, *lymphokines,* was used to describe a family of glycoproteins generated by activated lymphocytes that participates in a variety of cellular responses. Lymphokines are released in response to antigen (Ag). However, in contrast to antibodies (Ab), the specificity and action are not determined by the stimulating Ag. Induced lymphokines function to amplify the response to Ag in a nonspecific fashion. They are independent of the specific Ag initiating the immune response.

In 1970, it became clear that lymphokines could be derived from a number of cell sources. Neither their production nor their effects were restricted to lymphoid cells. They were ascribed the names of the activities they affected (Table 15-1), and the term *interleukin* (meaning "between leukocytes") was adopted for the most well-characterized factors determined initially by conventional biochemical methods and subsequently by recombinant DNA technology.

Neither approach to classification is truly satisfactory because interleukins influence cells other than leukocytes and most factors have multiple activities. Also, the ability of one lymphokine to induce the synthesis of others introduces a further level of complexity that must be taken into account when considering their biology (Fig. 15-1).

Many authors recently have suggested using the word *cytokine.* For the purpose of this review, the reader should bear in mind that the terms *lymphokines, interleukins,* and *cytokines* may be used interchangeably.

The sole source of lymphokines used to be cell supernatant. With recent advances in genetic engineering, the cloning of several lymphokines has been accomplished, and large amounts of pure material are available for studies in animals and humans. With some exceptions, notably studies of viral infections and autoimmune diseases, clinical investigations with lymphokine therapy have focused on malignant and hematologic diseases.

Biological Roles of Lymphokines

Lymphokines have important roles in five major areas of immunology: T-cell activation, B-cell activation, hematopoiesis, inflammation, and toxicity. In both experimental and clinical studies [1], mixing recombinant lymphokines has frequently produced synergistic effects, suggesting that lymphokines work in concert or in cascade. They amplify the interaction between sensitizing Ag and sensitized lymphocytes. Many lymphokines mobilize, attract, and activate a variety of cells that participate in inflammation. The growth factors, colony-stimulating factors, can stimulate the proliferation of specific types of hematopoietic progenitor cells. Some lymphokines,

Table 15-1. Summary of prominent biological properties of human lymphokines

Lymphokine	Biological properties
Interferon (alpha and beta)	Exerts antiviral activity; induces class I antigen expression; augments natural killer cell activity; has fever-inducing and antiproliferative properites
Interleukin-2	Is growth factor for activated T cells; induces synthesis of other lymphokines; activates cytotoxic lymphocytes
Colony-stimulating factor (CSF)	
Granulocyte-macrophage CSF	Promotes neutrophilic, eosinophilic, and macrophagic bone marrow colonies; activates mature granulocytes
Granulocyte CSF	Promotes neutrophilic colonies
Macrophage CSF	Promotes macrophagic colonies
Interleukin-1 (alpha and beta)	Activates resting T cells; is cofactor for hematopoietic growth factors; induces fever, sleep, adrenocorticotropic hormone release, neutrophilia, and other systemic acute-phase responses; stimulates synthesis of lymphokines, collagen, and collagenases; activates endothelial cells and macrophages; mediates inflammation, catabolic processes, and nonspecific resistance to infection
Interleukin-3	Supports growth of pluripotent (multilineage) bone marrow stem cells; is growth factor for mast cells
Interleukin-4 (B-cell-stimulating factor 1)	Is growth factor for activated B cells; induces HLA-DR expression on B cells; is growth factor for resting T cells; enchances cytolytic activity of cytotoxic cells; is mast-cell growth factor
B-cell-stimulating factor 2 (B-cell-differentiating factor)	Induces differentiation of activated B cells into immunoglobulin-secreting plasma cells; is identical to beta-2-interferon, plasmacytoma growth factor, and hepatocyte-stimulating factor, interleukin-6
Gamma-interferon	Induces class I, class II (HLA-Dr), and other surface antigens on a variety of cells; activates macrophages and endothelial cells; augments or inhibits other lymphokine activities; augments natural killer cell activity; exerts antiviral activity
Tumor necrosis factor (alpha and beta)	Is direct cytotoxin for some tumor cells; induces fever, sleep, and other systemic acute-phase responses; stimulates synthesis of lymphokines, collagen, and collagenases; activates endothelial cells and macrophages; mediates inflammation, catabolic processes, and septic shock

Source: C. A. Dinarello and J. W. Mier, Lymphokines. Reprinted with permission from *The New England Journal of Medicine* 317:941, 1987.

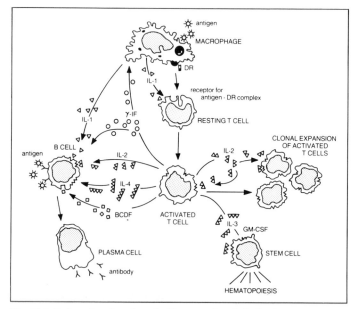

Fig. 15-1. Roles of various lymphokines produced during immune activation by antigen. The macrophage takes up, processes, and presents antigen to the resting T cell with the histocompatibility molecule (DR) and interleukin-1 (IL-1). T cell becomes activated and produces gamma-interferon (γ-IF), interleukin-2 (IL-2), interleukin-3 (IL-3), interleukin-4 (IL-4), and B-cell differentiating factor (BCDF). B cell is activated by antigen through surface antibodies and, under the influence of the cytokines γ-IF, IL-2, IL-3, IL-4, and BCDF, differentiates to become an antibody-secreting plasma cell. Activated T cells are induced by IL-2 to undergo clonal expansion. Activated T cell secretes IL-3 and granulocyte-macrophage colony-stimulating factor (GM-CSF), which stimulates hematopoietic progenitor cells. (From C. A. Dinarello and J. W. Mier, Lymphokines. Reprinted with permission from *The New England Journal of Medicine* 317:942, 1987.)

such as interferon and tumor necrosis factor, antagonize colony-stimulating factors and may contribute to aplastic anemia.

Lymphokines—particularly the interferons (IFs), interleukin-1 (IL-1), and tumor necrosis factor—may gain access to the circulation during infection, injury, and Ag challenge, causing a variety of systemic effects including tissue damage, metabolic abnormalities, and neuroendocrine changes. The vascular endothelium, several endocrine organs, and liver are prominent target tissues for these and other lymphokines.

Inadequate production of lymphokines has been observed in several disease states, which raises important questions about the therapeutic use of these substances in the management of human illness. There is decreased interleukin-2 (IL-2) production in the acquired immunodeficiency syndrome (AIDS), autoimmune diseases, type 1 diabetes mellitus, burns, and cancer. Gamma-interferon (γ-IF) production is decreased in lepromatous leprosy, systemic lupus erythematosus, and rheumatoid arthritis, as well as in normal newborns. Alpha-interferon (α-IF) levels are low in immunoproliferative diseases and in chronic hepatitis B. IL-1 production is decreased in patients with large tumor burden.

The decreased lymphocyte response associated with reduced lymphokine production can often be corrected in vitro by the addition of exogenous lymphokines [2]. It remains to be seen whether these defects could be corrected in vivo by the systemic administration of lymphokines or lymphokine inducers and whether such treatment would result in regression of disease. On the other hand, several disorders, such as graft rejection and septic shock, are due to an undesired immune response in which lymphokines may play a part.

Failure to achieve biological effect may be due to end organ resistance (e.g., absence of progenitor cells in the bone marrow in the case of colony-stimulating factors). The potential development of antibodies and serum-neutralizing factors should also be kept in mind.

INTERFERONS

IF was first described by Isaacs and Lindenman in 1957 as a naturally occurring antiviral substance [3]. Shortly thereafter, it was associated with antineoplastic properties. It was not until 1981 when large amounts of highly purified α-IF produced by recombinant DNA technology became available that large-scale phase 1 and 2 trials could be initiated [4]. In June 1986, IF was approved for use in the United States. Phase 1 through 3 trials have now been conducted in more than 5000 individuals.

IF Subtypes

IF is classified into three subtypes—alpha, beta, and gamma—according to its antigenicity. α-IF and β-IF are both referred to as type I IF because they are similar in many ways and apparently bind to the same receptor with high affinity. γ-IF (type II) differs from type I IF in its biochemical and biological properties. Also, the receptor for γ-IF is distinct from the type I IF receptor and is encoded for by a separate gene.

Type I IF (α-IF and β-IF)

Both α-IF and β-IF are synthesized in response to viral infection and correspond to leukocyte and fibroblast IF in the old nomenclature. They are structurally related and possess potent antiviral, antiproliferative, and immunomodulatory properties. They induce major histocompatibility complex (MHC) class I antigen expression and augment natural killer (NK) cell activity. They can be immunosuppressive secondary to their antiproliferative properties.

Type II IF (γ-IF or Immune IF)

Produced by NK cells and T lymphocytes following mitogenic or antigenic stimulation, γ-IF differs from α-IF and β-IF not only structurally but also biochemically and in its biological properties. γ-IF is associated with various malignant and autoimmune diseases, particularly rheumatoid arthritis and multiple sclerosis. It induces MHC class I and II Ag expression and other surface antigen expression, augments NK cell activity, activates macrophages, exerts antiviral activity, and augments or inhibits other lymphokine activities.

γ-IF appears to have more potent antiproliferative activity than either α-IF or β-IF. Mixed β-IF and γ-IF interact synergistically to cause even greater antiviral and antiproliferative activity.

Production and Action

IF can be produced by virtually all eukaryotic cells in response to a wide range of stimuli and is capable of acting on a range of homologous and heterologous cells with relative species specificity in these actions. Cells activated to produce IF secrete it into the extracellular space. It then diffuses to other cells and binds to specific receptors (a single receptor for α-IF and β-IF and a separate receptor for γ-IF). Subsequent to this binding, a number of genes are activated, which results in the production of proteins responsible for the action of IF. The IF receptor complexes are then internalized and degraded within a few hours. This *receptor down-regulation* is believed to be responsible for the reduced IF binding observed shortly after the exposure of cells to IF and might represent an autoregulatory feedback loop for IF activity in vivo. However, it did not preclude clinical efficacy in patients with chronic myeloid leukemia (CML) [5]. IF has many of the properties of classic hormones in that its release can influence the functioning of cells of distant and unrelated tissues.

Biological Activities

IF is capable of influencing cellular physiology and behavior in a number of ways, including the following.

Antiviral Effect

Cells treated with IF become refractory to infection with viruses. Viral protein synthesis is a major target for inhibition, but later stages of viral replication are also affected (the mechanism is unknown but might involve alteration of the membrane metabolism). Another mechanism is the activation of immunocompetent host cells.

Activation of Nonspecific Cytotoxicity of Lymphocytes

IF activates NK cells. It seems likely that NK cells are precursors to the lymphokine-activated killer (LAK) cells. However, the induction of LAK cell activity is complex, with probably several cell types and lymphokines (particularly IL-2) being involved.

Modulation of MHC Ag Expression by IF

Up-regulation of MHC Ag expression is one of the most interesting effects of IF because it is required for T-lymphocyte recognition of foreign antigen. α-IF and β-IF up-regulate class I MHC Ag. γ-IF up-regulates class I and II MHC Ag, thus enhancing T-cell recognition and cytotoxicity.

Regulation of Cell Growth and Antiproliferative Activity

IF inhibits the division of tumor cells grown in monolayers as well as in suspension cultures [6]. Usually the killing is indirect and is completed within 48 hours. Many investigators have observed IF-induced down-regulation of different oncogenes (c-*myc*, c-*fos*, and others). The growth of normal cells is restricted as well.

Modulation of Cell Differentiation

IF affects the phenotype of malignant cells by inducing or enhancing the expression of tumor-associated antigens. Increased cellular adhesion and decreased cellular motility are observed after IF treatment, which can reverse the ability of cultured tumor cells to overcome contact inhibition and to grow to high cell densities.

ALPHA-INTERFERON

α-IF will be considered separately because at present it is the IF of most clinical importance. Recombinant α-IF was one of the first recombinant human proteins to be administered in vivo. The role of γ-IF, which has only more recently become available in recombinant sources, has been limited, although it appears to have some efficacy in hematologic malignancies.

In humans, there are 20 species of α-IF, all of which exhibit rather similar activities, although some subtypes differ markedly in their potency. They are not all produced under the same inducing conditions.

Pharmacokinetics

α-IF can be administered intravenously, intramuscularly, or subcutaneously. There is full absorption from an intramuscular injection site, and the bioavailability of α-IF given intramuscularly is similar to that of α-IF given intravenously. The half-life of α-IF is 6 hours. It shows initial rapid and then slower clearance, allowing fairly constant serum levels to be maintained by administering interferon intramuscularly once or twice daily.

The median time for tumor response is long, averaging 10 weeks in some diseases, such as hairy-cell leukemia. In CML, peripheral counts have improved within 2 to 3 months, but improvement in bone marrow cytology has required 6 to 12 months.

The maximum tolerated dose of α-IF appears to be 20×10^6 U/sq m 3 times weekly.

Clinical Activity

The mechanism by which IF exerts its activity is unknown. Postulated mechanisms include a direct antiproliferative effect on the tumor, augmentation of induction of host-effector mechanisms such as NK cell activation, and induction of membrane antigens on the tumor cells, allowing subsequent immune recognition.

α-IF is used with some success in chronic hepatitis B, various neurologic diseases, and topically for herpes keratitis, genital warts, rhinovirus, and cytomegalovirus (CMV) infection. α-IF gives a response rate of 30 to 50 percent in AIDS-related Kaposi's sarcoma, which occurs in approximately one-third of AIDS patients [7]. However, there is no demonstrable effect against the underlying immunodeficiency in patients with advanced clinical AIDS. α-IF inhibits human immunodeficiency virus (HIV) retrovirus replication in vitro, but this has not been demonstrated in vivo.

Response to IF has been most notable in certain hematologic malignancies. The most dramatic results of α-IF therapy to date have been in hairy-cell leukemia, with a durable objective response in 75 percent of patients [4].

CML also appears to have unique sensitivity to α-IF. Like the available alkylating agents, α-IF is capable of reducing the leukocyte and platelet counts for a sustained period in 80 to 90 percent of patients. However, as a unique feature of the response, some patients have also shown decreased numbers of Philadelphia chromosome positivity in the bone marrow [5]. Studies are under way to determine whether this will translate into a long time delay or elimination of blast cell crisis.

α-IF is effective in B-cell non-Hodgkin's lymphomas, for which the response rate approaches 50 percent in some reports. It has a 15 to 20-percent response rate in multiple myeloma [8]. Other leukemias were not studied comprehensively; however, it seems that α-IF has a relative lack of activity in chronic lymphoid leukemia and acute myeloid leukemia, whereas childhood acute lymphoid leukemia and cutaneous T-cell lymphomas show some responsiveness.

The results of α-IF treatment in most adult solid tumors have not been encouraging. Since the majority of trials have focused on patients with advanced disease, this may denote lack of activity in large bulky tumors. The most encouraging results were obtained in melanoma and hypernephroma, with a response rate of 20 to 25 percent in advanced disease.

There has been growing interest lately in the administration of α-IF locoregionally: intravesically in bladder cancer [9] and intraperitoneally in ovarian cancer. α-IF seems to be effective when given by such routes and there is no systemic absorption or side effects. Further studies are required in this area. Also, more studies are needed to define the role of α-IF therapy in acute lymphocytic leukemia, Hodgkin's disease, osteosarcomas, and brain tumors. α-IF appears to be ineffective in tumors of the breast, colon, lung, or prostate. Currently, there is interest in using IF in combination with established chemotherapy and radiotherapy.

Toxicity

Virtually all patients experience some toxic effects at some time during α-IF therapy. All side effects are dose-related and rapidly reversible on discontinuation of treatment or dose modification [10].

Flulike Symptoms

Flulike symptoms consisting of fever, chills, fatigue, malaise, rigors, anorexia, myalgias, and arthralgias occur in 95 percent of patients and are severe in 35 percent. They are usually experienced 30 to 120 minutes after treatment and last several hours. Usually, these symptoms are most severe at initiation of therapy and improve with time as IF is continued. Treatment is supportive (antipyretics and analgesics). Dose reduction or discontinuation of treatment may be required in extreme cases. Toxicity should be weighed against the therapeutic response.

Myelosuppression

Myelosuppression can occur but is rarely dose-limiting. It is mainly reflected by granulocytopenia. However, thrombocytopenia is not uncommon. The hemoglobin is usually affected minimally.

Gastrointestinal Effects

Gastrointestinal side effects include nausea and vomiting in 40 percent of patients, diarrhea in 20 percent, and abdominal pain in 3 percent. There is an asymptomatic reversible increase in hepatic transaminases, alkaline phosphatase, and lactic dehydrogenase in approximately 60 percent of patients.

Central Nervous System Toxicity

Central nervous system toxic effects occur in approximately one-third of the patients. These consist of somnolence (11%) and confusion (10%). In general, these symptoms are mild, dose-related, and prevalent in the elderly. There are reports of seizures associated with fever in children.

Cardiovascular Effects

Cardiovascular toxic effects include asymptomatic hypotension, which occurs in 6 percent of patients, and tachycardia, which occurs in 3 percent. Most of the reported cases of cardiovascular toxicity involve elderly patients.

Metabolic Disturbances

Hypocalcemia, hypokalemia, elevated blood urea nitrogen, and prolonged partial thromboplastin time have been reported at high doses.

Skin Disorders

Skin disorders occur in 13 percent of the patients on α-IF. They consist of transient rash, pruritus, dry skin, or nonspecific dermatitis. The rashes are usually intermittent, do not progress to more serious manifestations, and do not require dose adjustment or discontinuation of treatment. Skin testing in affected patients failed to yield evidence of true hypersensitivity reaction.

Other Side Effects

Alopecia may occur in up to 15 percent of patients being treated with α-IF. There is no appreciable evidence of either renal toxicity or cumulative toxicity in any organ system. In fact, during long-term treatment, patients develop increasing tolerance to some symptoms. This tachyphylaxis is seen in most patients after an initial period of maximum subjective symptoms during the first 2 weeks of therapy. IF is usually well tolerated at low doses, with very few side effects.

INTERLEUKIN-2

Perspective [11, 12]

In 1976, IL-2 was first described as the T-cell growth factor. A human IL-2 complementary DNA (cDNA) clone was isolated and the complete nucleotide sequence determined in 1983. One year later, cDNA clones of genes for IL-2 were expressed in large-scale in *Escherichia coli*. Finally, purification to homogeneity and biological characterization were accomplished.

Production and Action

IL-2 is exclusively produced by helper T lymphocytes (OKT4-positive or Leu3-positive in humans) stimulated by antigen or mitogen. It can maintain the proliferation of activated T lymphocytes, induce and augment the proliferation of cytotoxic T lymphocytes, and increase the number and activity of NK cells in vitro. The action of IL-2 is mainly on T cells and closely related lymphocytes (NK and LAK cells), although IL-2 also exerts effects on B cells (B-cell growth) and macrophages (increased macrophage cytotoxicity). In contrast to other biological agents, such as IF, that have direct antiproliferative effects, IL-2 appears to act solely by modulating the host's immune response. IL-2 can react across species.

IL-2 Receptors

Resting T cells do not produce IL-2 nor are they capable of responding to IL-2 when it is added exogenously. It appears that signals emanating from the T-cell Ag receptor complex coordinate the transcriptional activation of both the IL-2 genes and the genes encoding for IL-2 receptor. IL-2 receptors are absent on resting T cells and are solely expressed by Ag-activated T cells; they appear within hours of activation. The membrane half-life of unoccupied high-affinity receptors is 150 minutes, whereas subsequent to IL-2 binding these receptors disappear 10 times more rapidly (half-life is 15 minutes). IL-2 receptors are found on immature thymocytes, suggesting the role of IL-2 in maturation as well as proliferation of T cells.

Three variables determine the onset of cell cycle progression: IL-2 concentration, IL-2 receptor density, and the duration of IL-2 receptor interaction. An initial threshold of triggered IL-2 receptors must accumulate before a move is made to replicate DNA. Consequently, at the level of the individual cell, progression to DNA replication and mitosis is a quantal all-or-none decision that is determined precisely by a finite number of IL-2 receptor interactions.

Antitumor Effect of IL-2

LAK cells are derived from a population of peripheral blood lymphocytes exposed to IL-2. They possess the ability to lyse a broad spectrum of fresh tumor cells that are resistant to lysis by NK cells. Lymphocytes and other cells derived from normal tissues are resistant to LAK cytolysis [13].

In therapy with LAK cells, lymphocytes are removed from the patient, activated by IL-2 in culture, and then readministered to the patient. The adoptively transferred LAK cells divide in vivo when IL-2 is administered concomitantly. Allogeneic LAK cells are almost as effective as syngeneic LAK cells in therapy. Thus, the mechanism of antigen recognition by LAK cells is MHC-independent. Although high doses of recombinant IL-2 alone can mediate the therapeutic effect in part, the magnitude of the reduction of metastatic disease in animal models is much greater when LAK cells are also administered [14].

Thus, the antitumor effect of high-dose IL-2 may reflect (1) direct tumor cytolysis mediated by LAK cells induced in vivo; (2) induction of other lymphokines; or (3) stimulation of proliferation and cytotoxic function of cytotoxic T lymphocytes, NK cells, and macrophages.

Pharmacokinetics

The half-life of IL-2 is 1 to 2 hours. IL-2 is cleared primarily through the kidneys, although it is not excreted in its active form. The dose, route, and schedule of IL-2 administration are critical. With higher doses of IL-2, LAK cells appear in the circulation and the NK cytotoxicity is augmented. More side effects are observed with high doses. When intravenous administration of IL-2 over 2 hours was compared to subcutaneous injection or continuous infusion of the same dose over 24 hours, it was found that the 2-hour infusion resulted in the highest peak level of IL-2, with a half-life of approximately 30 minutes, whereas the subcutaneous injection and the 24-

hour infusion resulted in lower but more prolonged serum levels. The 24-hour continuous infusion was also associated with more toxicity and immunomodulation: A dramatic increase in the percentage and absolute number of cells expressing IL-2 receptor was reported with continuous intravenous IL-2. When the daily dose of IL-2 was divided into 15-minute infusions every 8 hours, the toxicity was reduced further [15].

Clinical Activity

Melanoma and renal cell carcinoma are the solid tumors most sensitive to IL-2 treatment. Reports from the National Cancer Institute indicate that the response to IL-2 plus LAK cells is significantly superior to IL-2 alone ($p < 0.02$). IL-2 and LAK cell therapy also seems to be effective in non-Hodgkin's lymphoma [16]. In its present form, however, this therapy is expensive and associated with side effects.

Reports of combined IL-2 and LAK cell therapy in colorectal cancer are disappointing.

In vitro brain tumors are sensitive to IL-2 and LAK cell therapy. In animal models with brain tumors, this therapy also yielded positive results [17]. Ongoing studies in humans seem to show some effectiveness of IL-2 and LAK cells in brain tumors [18].

Future Perspective

Although LAK cells improve the therapeutic benefit associated with IL-2 administration, these promiscuous killer cells have relatively weak antitumor activity, and so attempts have been made to find improved LAK cells with more specific cytolytic activity [19].

IL-4 is capable of synergizing with IL-2 to produce improved LAK cells compared with those induced by either agent alone. In vivo trials with these "super LAK cells" are under way in murine models.

Tumor-infiltrating lymphocytes (TILs) are lymphoid cells that infiltrate tumors and can be isolated and expanded in vitro. They are 50 to 100 times more effective than LAK cells in mediating tumor regression when transferred into tumor-bearing mice. TILs from some patients with melanoma are uniquely reactive against the tumor from which they are derived and do not lyse normal cells or other cancers with similar histologic features. Clinical trials of TILs in humans have begun. The adoptively transferred cells are effective in the absence of administered IL-2, although low doses of IL-2 may enhance their therapeutic efficacy. Successful therapy with TILs depends on immunosuppression of the host, with either high-dose cyclophosphamide or total body irradiation, at the time of treatment. This is in contradistinction to LAK cell therapy, in which cyclophosphamide does not increase efficacy. The other advantage of TILs therapy is that the lower dosage requirement for IL-2 administration might reduce the side effects of therapy.

Toxicity

The toxicity and immunomodulation of IL-2 are dose-dependent and are maximum with continuous infusion compared to 2-hour infusion or divided doses given every 8 hours. Toxicity is common at doses of 10,000 U/kg given every 8 hours for 5 days, but some patients could tolerate 30,000 U/kg every 8 hours for 5 days, and current trials incorporating IL-2 and LAK cells are utilizing 100,000 U/kg every 8 hours for 5 days [15]. Toxicity is usually short-lived and reversible over 1 to 2 weeks. Hypotension is the predominant consideration for withholding therapy.

Flulike Symptoms

Fever, chills, myalgias, rigors, malaise, and anorexia are the most common side effects associated with IL-2 therapy. Their severity increases with increasing dosage. Fever usually develops 2 to 4 hours after beginning IL-2 infusion and resolves within 6 hours of terminating the infusion.

Capillary Leak Syndrome

Increased capillary permeability leading to massive edema and intravascular volume depletion characterize the capillary leak syndrome, which may be associated with hypotension and renal failure. This syndrome is also seen more with continuous infusion of IL-2. During treatment, patients must be monitored in an intensive care unit, with judicious administration of colloid or crystalloid solutions when the central venous pressure (CVP) falls below 3 to 4 cm H_2O. When the CVP increases to 6 cm H_2O, dopamine (1–5 μg/kg/minute) is added. If the blood pressure cannot be maintained on dopamine alone or if supraventricular tachycardia occurs, phenylephrine hydrochloride (1–5 μg/kg/minute) is indicated. Excessive fluid replacement might result in increased pulmonary edema, and furosemide or other diuretics should be administered if the CVP is 8 to 12 cm H_2O and blood pressure is adequate to maintain adequate urine output. If grade IV life-threatening toxicity occurs, dexamethasone may be given.

Cardiovascular Effects

Hypotension is a common side effect of IL-2 therapy, especially with higher doses. It is usually the predominant consideration in withholding therapy. Myocardial infarction, angina, and arrhythmias have also been reported with IL-2 treatment.

Renal Toxicity

Azotemia is not an uncommon side effect of IL-2 therapy. Cessation of IL-2 is usually followed by spontaneous diuresis and normalization of serum creatinine over 3 to 5 days. If spontaneous diuresis does not occur, the use of diuretics is effective. An elevation of creatinine to 2.0 to 3.5 mg/dl is common and reversible on discontinuation of therapy.

Bone Marrow Changes

Lymphocytes decrease during IL-2 infusion. Rebound lymphocytosis is observed thereafter, and the lymphocyte counts return to normal before the next infusion. Rebound lymphocytosis is greater after higher rather than lower doses and is greater also after the 24-hour infusion than after the 2-hour or 15-minute infusion, implying that in vivo activity of IL-2 is enhanced by the continuous maintenance of elevated serum IL-2 levels. Near-maximum rebound lymphocytosis was observed 1 day after discontinuation of IL-2 infusion.

Eosinophilia, anemia, and thrombocytopenia are also observed with IL-2 administration (especially with the continuous infusion).

Gastrointestinal Disturbances
Nausea, vomiting, glossitis, and diarrhea are reported in patients on IL-2 therapy. There may be a transient and moderate elevation in serum bilirubin (usually < 5 mg/dl).

Other Side Effects
Transient confusion, dyspnea, erythematous rash, pruritis, and nasal congestion have been observed with IL-2 therapy. Potential side effects after intrathecal administration of IL-2 and LAK cells are headache, fever, nausea, vomiting, meningitis, and hydrocephalus.

HEMATOPOIETIC GROWTH FACTORS

Perspective
With the development of semisolid culture systems supporting the growth of hematopoietic colonies, it was recognized that hematopoietic precursor cells are unable to survive and proliferate in vitro unless specifically stimulated [20]. This led to the discovery of a group of specific regulatory glycoproteins that stimulate cell proliferation and at least some aspects of the functional activities of these various hematopoietic subpopulations [1]. Those regulatory glycoproteins are often called *colony-stimulating factors* (CSFs) because of their ability to induce the formation of colonies when bone marrow is suspended in vitro.

Production and Biological Activity
Hematopoietic CSFs are produced by many tissues in the body (fibroblasts, endothelial cells, monocytes, and lymphocytes) after stimulation with bacterial endotoxin, monokines, or lectins (see Table 15-1). They are essential to survival, proliferation, and differentiation of hematopoietic progenitor cells in vitro. The biological activity of these regulatory factors is measured by their ability to stimulate the development of colonies of differentiated cells from progenitor cells in soft agar culture system. They are classified based on the type of cells found in these colonies (Fig. 15-2).

Classification of CSFs
G-CSF is the granulocyte CSF, which stimulates neutrophils, increases neutrophil phagocytic activity, and enhances superoxide production. *M-CSF (CSF₁)* is the macrophage CSF, which stimulates monocytes and increases monocyte antibody-dependent cytotoxicity and monocyte tumoricidal activity. *GM-CSF* (granulocyte-macrophage CSF) stimulates neutrophils, eosinophils, and monocytes. It also enhances a variety of functions of mature granulocytes, including increased phagocytic activity and increased superoxide production, and it increases monocyte antibody-dependent cytotoxicity and tumoricidal activity. It also induces α-IF and IL-1. *IL-3* or *multi-CSF* supports multilineage colonies and stimulates neutrophils, eosinophils, monocytes, megakaryocytes, mast cells, and erythroid colony formation by bone marrow cells. It also enhances monocyte tumoricidal activity.

Action of Individual CSFs
G-CSF and M-CSF are postulated to support the growth and proliferation of only relatively late progenitor cells that are already com-

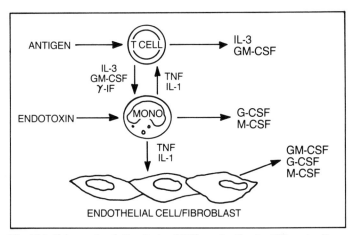

Fig. 15-2. Colony-stimulating factor (CSF) production by different cell types. Monocytes (MONO) and T cells are activated by endotoxin and antigen, respectively, to produce granulocyte (G) and macrophage (M) CSF directly or to induce CSF production in other cells. (IL-1 = interleukin-1; IL-3 = interleukin-3; γ-IF = gamma-interferon; TNF = tumor necrosis factor.) (Modified from J. D. Griffin, Clinical applications of colony stimulating factors. *Oncology* 2:16, 1988.)

mitted to their respective lineage (Fig. 15-3). GM-CSF, in contrast, is presumed to interact additionally with somewhat earlier progenitor cells that are still capable of differentiating into neutrophils, eosinophils, or monocytes. The multiplicity of activities attributable to IL-3 is believed to be a consequence of its ability to support the growth of cells from relatively early pluripotent progenitors to mature cells of multiple lineage.

The cross-induction of CSF makes it difficult to attribute an activity to a particular CSF in a mixed culture system. Also, synergistic interaction between IL-1 and CSF in hematopoiesis has been observed. IL-1 acts on highly purified stem cells to synergize with GM-CSF or M-CSF in stimulating colony formation. IL-1 alone has no colony-forming ability.

The cDNA and genes encoding for G-CSF, M-CSF, GM-CSF, and IL-3 have been molecularly cloned. These cDNA clones are valuable for studying the molecular biology of CSFs as well as for large-scale production of recombinant growth factor proteins.

Granulocyte-Macrophage Colony-Stimulating Factor

As stated previously, GM-CSF is a potent inducer of neutrophil, eosinophil, and monocyte proliferation, and its functions include the induction of aggregation, enhancement of antibody-dependent cytotoxicity, enhancement of direct tumor cytotoxicity, and enhancement of phagocytic activity. In the presence of erythropoietin, the cloned factor has some ability to support the proliferation of erythroid and megakaryocytic progenitor cells, as well as progenitor cells that give rise to mixed colonies having all myeloid elements.

In cultures containing GM-CSF, the final size achieved by colonies and the number of colonies developing can be modified by a variety

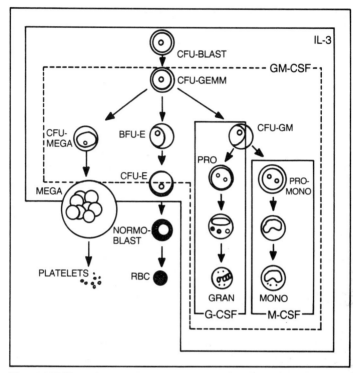

Fig. 15-3. Differentiation of hematopoietic progenitor cells in response to colony-stimulating factor (CSF). Cell compartments responsive to growth factors are enclosed by boxes. (CFU = colony-forming unit; CFU-BLAST = blast CFU; CFU-GEMM = CFU for granulocytes, erythrocytes, megakaryocytes, and monocytes; CFU-E = erythroid CFU; CFU-GM = granulocyte-monocyte CFU; BFU-E = burst-forming unit–erythroid; MEGA = megakaryocyte; GM-CSF = granulocyte-macrophage CSF; IL-3 = interleukin-3, also known as multi-CSF; PRO = promyelocyte; PROMONO = promonocyte; GRAN, G = granulocyte; MONO = monocyte; M = macrophage; RBC = red blood cell.) (Modified from J. D. Griffin. Clinical applications of colony-stimulating factors. *Oncology* 2:18, 1988.)

of accessory factors. Prostaglandin E (PGE) appears to inhibit macrophage colony-forming cells selectively. Macrophages have been shown to produce PGE in response to CSF stimulation in vitro. In serum-free cultures, GM-CSF exhibits little capacity to stimulate granulocyte colony formation, but such stimulation is enhanced by the addition of hydrocortisone.

Pharmacokinetics

GM-CSF has a biphasic serum clearance with an initial half-life of 7 minutes and a second half-life of approximately 2 hours. The use of ^{125}I-labeled GM-CSF revealed the presence of receptors on granulocytes, monocytes, and eosinophils [20]. The number decreases with increasing maturation. Mature eosinophils exhibit half the receptor number of neutrophils. There are no GM-CSF receptors on lymphoid or erythroid cells.

Clinical Activity

Phase 1 and 2 trials of GM-CSF have shown that GM-CSF caused a dose-dependent and dramatic rise in peripheral white blood cell (WBC) counts in various normal or diseased individuals when administered over periods of days to months. GM-CSF generated increased numbers of neutrophils at relatively low doses but also increased eosinophil and monocyte counts at higher doses and, occasionally, induced an increase in platelets, lymphocytes, and erythroids [21].

In patients with myelodysplastic syndrome who were treated with GM-CSF, a dose-dependent increase in the WBC count was observed. During the rest period between GM-CSF cycles, the WBC count declined but was often higher than before therapy. Some patients showed an increase in platelet count and a decrease in red blood cell transfusion requirements [22].

In other groups with bone marrow failure, a dramatic increase in WBC count was also achieved on GM-CSF therapy. It mainly consisted of increases in granulocytes, bands, eosinophils, and monocytes. Furthermore, in some patients, responses were observed in multiple cell lineages. The basis of this multilineage stimulation is not well understood: These responses may be due to a direct effect of GM-CSF on the progenitor cells or they may be mediated by the release of mediators such as IL-1 [23].

In neutropenic patients with AIDS, a dose-dependent increase in the WBC count was obtained with GM-CSF. With higher doses of GM-CSF, the neutropenia was corrected and leukocytosis achieved. Although increases in eosinophils, monocytes, and lymphocytes were observed with high-dose GM-CSF, the inversion of the T helper/suppressor ratio was unchanged in these patients [21].

In patients undergoing bone marrow transplantation, GM-CSF markedly accelerated the rate of recovery of circulating granulocytes and shortened the period of aplasia. It was also used to shorten the period of neutropenia in patients receiving ablative chemotherapy [24].

In summary, beneficial effects on bone marrow function associated with decreased incidence of infection were reported with GM-CSF therapy in patients with myelodysplastic syndrome, aplastic anemia, and AIDS. In cancer patients who were receiving ablative chemotherapy or bone marrow transplantation, GM-CSF had the potential for allowing the use of higher doses of cytotoxic drugs and irradiation. GM-CSF attracts neutrophils and inhibits their migration. Its role in treating local infections is being investigated.

Toxicity

Phase 1 and 2 trials indicate that GM-CSF is relatively nontoxic compared with the earlier biological response modifiers [24]. The most common side effects are not life-threatening and reverse promptly on discontinuation of the drug. They include the following. *Fever* usually is responsive to antipyretics but occasionally requires alteration of therapy. Sepsis should always be considered and ruled out in neutropenic patients, even when drug fever is highly suspected. *Phlebitis* may occur when GM-CSF is administered by peripheral veins. It is recommended that GM-CSF always be given through a central line, since no phlebitis or clotting problems have been reported with this mode of administration. The patient may experience *bone pains,* the severity of which seems to be related to WBC and granulocyte counts rather than directly to the GM-CSF dose. Bone pain is usually transient and responds to analgesics. Radiologic studies obtained in these patients were all within normal limits. The mechanism of bone pain is not well understood, but it could be related to the release of mediators from neutrophils. *Other side effects* include myalgias, flushing, malaise, decreased appetite, headache, diarrhea, and vomiting.

Patient Selection

GM-CSF was shown to stimulate both the proliferation and the differentiation of a human myeloid leukemia cell line [25]. The ultimate in vivo effect of this hormone in leukemia is not well known. In the M. D. Anderson Cancer Center experience with patients with myelodysplastic syndrome with increased blast cells, no leukemic transformation was reported [22]. On the contrary, GM-CSF treatment caused a decrease in both the percentage and the absolute numbers of blast cells in the bone marrow of those patients. Initially, all patients had a blast cell count of less than 20 percent. In a separate group of myelodysplastic syndrome patients whose bone marrow consisted of more than 20 percent blast cells before therapy, incrased blast cells were noted after GM-CSF was administered. These results suggest that care must be taken in selecting patients for GM-CSF treatment.

REFERENCES

1. Clark, S. C., and Kamen, R. The human hematopoietic colony stimulating factors. *Science* 236:1229, 1987.
2. Dinarello, C. A., and Mier, J. W. Lymphokines. *N. Engl. J. Med.* 317:940, 1987.
3. Isaacs, A., and Lindenman, J. Virus interference. 1. The interferons. *Proc. R. Soc. Lond. [Biol.]* 147:258, 1957.
4. Quesada, J. R., et al. Alpha interferon for induction of remission in hairy-cell leukemia. *N. Engl. J. Med.* 310:15, 1984.
5. Talpaz, M., et al. Therapy of chronic myelogenous leukemia. *Cancer* 59:664, 1987.
6. Roth, M. S., and Foon, K. A. Current status of interferon therapy in oncology. *Prog. Hematol.* 15:19, 1987.
7. Merigan, T. C. Human interferon as a therapeutic agent. *N. Engl. J. Med.* 318:1458, 1988.
8. Strander, H. Interferon treatment of human neoplasia. *Adv. Cancer Res.* 46:1, 1986.
9. Torti, T. M., et al. α-Interferon in superficial bladder cancer: A Northern California Oncology Group study. *J. Clin. Oncol.* 6:476, 1988.
10. Spiegel, R. J. The alpha interferons: Clinical overview. *Semin. Oncol.* 14(Suppl. 2):1, 1987.
11. Morgan, D. A., et al. Selective in vitro growth of T lymphocytes from normal human bone marrows. *Science* 193:1007, 1976.
12. Rosenberg, S. A., et al. Biological activity of recombinant human interleukin-2 produced in *Escherichia coli. Science* 223:1412, 1984.
13. Rosenstein, M., et al. Lymphokine-activated killer cells: Lysis of fresh syngeneic natural killer-resistant murine tumor cells by lymphocytes cultured in interleukin 2. *Cancer Res.* 44:1946, 1984.
14. Mulé, J. J., et al. The antitumor efficacy of lymphokine-activated

killer cells and recombinant interleukin 2 in vivo. *J. Immunol.* 135:646, 1985.

15. Thompson, J. A., et al. Influence of dose and duration of infusion of interleukin 2 on toxicity and immunomodulation. *J. Clin. Oncol.* 6:669, 1988.

16. Rosenberg, S. A., et al. Observations on the systemic administration of autologous lymphokine-activated killer cells and recombinant interleukin-2 to patients with metastatic cancer. *N. Engl. J. Med.* 313:1485, 1985.

17. Jacobs, S. K., et al. In vitro killing of human glioblastoma by interleukin-activated autologous lymphocytes. *J. Neurosurg.* 64:114, 1986.

18. Schimizu, K., et al. Phase I study of adoptive immunotherapy of human brain tumors with lymphokine-activated killer (LAK) cells and recombinant interleukin-2 (rIL-2) (abstract). Presented at International Meeting on Brain Oncology, Rennes, France, 1986.

19. Rosenberg, S. A., et al. A new approach to the adoptive immunotherapy of cancer with tumor infiltrating lymphocytes. *Science* 233:1318, 1986.

20. Metcalf, D. The molecular biology and functions of the granulocyte-macrophage colony-stimulating factors. *Blood* 67:257, 1986.

21. Groopman, J. E., et al. Effect of recombinant human granulocyte-macrophage colony-stimulating factor on myelopoiesis in the acquired immunodeficiency syndrome. *N. Engl. J. Med.* 317:593, 1987.

22. Vadhan-Raj, S., et al. Effects of recombinant human granulocyte-macrophage colony-stimulating factor in patients with myelodysplastic syndromes. *N. Engl. J. Med.* 317:1545, 1987.

23. Vadhan-Raj, S., et al. Stimulation of hematopoiesis in patients with bone marrow failure and in patients with malignancy by recombinant human granulocyte-macrophage colony-stimulating factor. *Blood* 72:134, 1988.

24. Brandt, S. J. Effect of recombinant human granulocyte-macrophage colony-stimulating factor on hematopoietic reconstitution after high-dose chemotherapy and autologous bone marrow transplantation. *N. Engl. J. Med.* 318:869, 1988.

25. Harris, P. E., et al. Distinct differentiation-inducing activities of gamma-interferon and cytokine factors acting on the human promyelocytic leukemia cell line HL-60. *Cancer Res.* 45:3090S, 1985.

SELECTED READINGS

Gastl, G., and Huber, C. The biology of interferon actions. *Blut* 56:193, 1988.

Griffin, J. D. Clinical applications of colony stimulating factors. *Oncology* 2:15, 1988.

Morris, A. G. Interferons. *Immunology* 1:43, 1988.

Sieff, C. A. Hematopoietic growth factors. *J. Clin. Invest.* 79:1549, 1987.

Smith, K. A. Interleukin 2: Inception, impact and applications. *Science* 240:1169, 1988.

IV

Complications of Cancer and Therapy

Acute Allergic Reactions: Anaphylaxis

Roberta A. Gottlieb

PERSPECTIVE

Anaphylaxis can occur with any substance. However, in chemotherapy it is most common with L-asparaginase, bleomycin, and etoposide (VP-16).

PRECAUTIONS

When L-asparaginase, white blood cell transfusions, or other products likely to cause anaphylaxis are being administered to a patient, a physician must be on the unit, and diphenhydramine (Benadryl), hydrocortisone, and epinephrine should be readily available.

TREATMENT

1. At the first sign of an allergic reaction (usually urticaria or nasal congestion), stop the infusion.
2. Administer diphenhydramine; 25 to 50 mg intramuscularly or intravenously may be sufficient.
3. In the presence of a more severe reaction such as generalized urticaria, swelling, hypotension, tachycardia, stridor, wheezing, or respiratory distress, proceed as follows:
   a. Delay absorption of antigen by placing a tourniquet proximally. This is not useful if the drug was administered intravenously.
   b. A 1 : 1000 solution of aqueous epinephrine 0.01 ml/kg, should be administered subcutaneously. If laryngeal edema is present, dilute the drug in 5 to 10 ml of normal saline and administer intravenously. This may be repeated 2 times at 20-minute intervals, the second and third doses being given subcutaneously. Have oxygen and intubation supplies ready.
   c. Monitor the blood pressure and central venous pressure. Restore blood pressure with albuminized saline (10 ml/kg of 5% albumin in normal saline).
   d. For bronchospasm, administer an aminophylline bolus (4 mg/kg) intravenously over 30 minutes. If bronchospasm is prolonged, continuous infusion of aminophylline and nebulized bronchodilators may be indicated.
   e. For severe or prolonged anaphylaxis (especially if the drug is cleared slowly from the system), give hydrocortisone, 10 mg/kg intravenously, followed by 16 mg/kg/day in divided doses every 4 to 6 hours.
4. Avoid subsequent exposure to the allergen. Patients who react to *E. coli* L-asparaginase should be switched to *Erwinia* L-asparaginase or PEG-asparaginase. Some protocols using VP-16 allow switching to VM-26. The reaction should be documented in the permanent medical record.

Cardiac Complications

Laura E. Ferguson and Roberta A. Gottlieb

CONGESTIVE HEART FAILURE

Perspective

Congestive heart failure arises when the heart is unable to meet a patient's circulatory needs. Two broad categories—high-output failure and low-output failure—should be considered.

High-Output Failure

In high-output failure (normal to elevated cardiac output), profound anemia leads to tissue hypoxia with a compensatory increase in cardiac output. Prolonged hypoxia, particularly of the cardiac muscle, leads to irreversible injury. Thyrotoxicosis or hyperpyrexia are conditions in which the basal metabolic rate and systemic circulatory needs are increased beyond the cardiac capacity. Arteriovenous malformations or fistulas lead to rapid shunting of blood through a low-resistance circuit. Treatment of high-output failure is directed toward identifying and correcting the causative factor(s).

Low-Output Failure

Low-output failure (low cardiac output) may be due to pericardial restriction caused by malignant effusion, radiation-induced fibrosis, or infection-related pericarditis. This possibility should be evaluated using echocardiography. Alternatively, arrhythmias induced by metabolic derangements and the toxic effects of drugs (anthracyclines, tricyclic antidepressants, and digoxin) should be ruled out by electrocardiography (ECG). Remember the antidote to digoxin overdose is phenytoin sodium (Dilantin). Myocardial dysfunction may be due to metabolic derangements (hypocalcemia, hypomagnesemia, and hypophosphatemia), nutritional deficits, radiation damage to the myocardium, myocarditis, and, most important, exposure to cardiotoxic drugs (anthracyclines, cyclophosphamide, and cytosine arabinoside in conjunction with cyclophosphamide). Valvular dysfunction caused by bacterial endocarditis should be considered particularly in the immunocompromised patient with a new murmur or an indwelling central venous catheter.

Fluid Overload

A third clinical category should be considered in the patient who presents with peripheral or pulmonary edema and normal cardiac function: Fluid overload is easily achieved in the patient with borderline or poor renal function who is receiving aggressive fluid therapy as is used with cisplatin infusions. Iatrogenic fluid overload can be avoided if daily fluid balance and weight are monitored.

Initial Stabilization of Patient

Initial stabilization of the patient with congestive heart failure should consist of the following:

1. Elevate the head of the bed 30 degrees.
2. Provide 30 to 50% oxygen (higher concentrations may decrease pulmonary vascular resistance and increase edema).
3. Administer a low maintenance dose of intravenous fluids (800–1200 liters/sq m/day of 5% dextrose in quarter-normal saline). Avoid sodium overload and add potassium only after adequate renal function is confirmed.
4. Sedation with morphine reduces anxiety and decreases cardiac preload but may cause hypotension and respiratory depression.
5. Diuresis is accomplished with furosemide, 0.1 to 0.5 mg/kg intravenously.
6. Low-dose dopamine, 2 to 5 μg/kg/min, will support renal and hepatic blood flow.
7. Monitor the patient's vital signs frequently, as well as his or her weight, intake, and output. ECG telemetry and pulse oximetry should be employed.

Laboratory Evaluation

Laboratory evaluation, which should immediately follow initial stabilization of the patient, includes:

Serum electrolytes, calcium, magnesium, phosphate, blood urea nitrogen, and creatinine levels
Complete blood cell counts
Urinalysis (to rule out nephrosis or nephritis)
Chest radiography
ECG
Echocardiography
Swan-Ganz monitoring, if clinically indicated

Treatment

Detailed recommendations for managing congestive heart failure are beyond the scope of this text. Basic principles are (1) to correct the underlying cause(s) where possible; (2) to consider cardiac inotropic agents, such as digoxin, and correct metabolic derangements; and (3) to obtain cardiologic consultation, especially when the cause is unclear (endocardial biopsy may be necessary) or management is difficult.

ANTHRACYCLINE CARDIOTOXICITY

Anthracycline (daunorubicin, doxorubicin) cardiomyopathy is characterized by degeneration of myocardial cells and myofibrillar lysis. Clinical features include arrhythmias and myocardial dysfunction to the point of congestive heart failure.

Contributing Factors

Contributing factors in anthracycline cardiotoxicity include the following.

Cumulative Dose

Although the relationship is nonlinear, cardiotoxicity is seen in 1 to 5 percent of patients who received a total dose of less than 550 mg/sq m of an anthracycline, compared with 30 percent in patients who received more than 600 mg/sq m [1, 2]. Many investigations limit the cumulative dose to 250 mg/sq m or less, based on a study that showed that 55% of children who received doxorubicin (median dose: 319 mg/sq m) had abnormal cardiac function by two-dimensional echocardiography, while no abnormalities of left ventricular function were seen in children who received less than 250 mg/sq m of doxorubicin [3].

Patient Age

Young children and infants are more likely to suffer cardiotoxicity from anthracyclines. Congestive heart failure has been seen in infants after a single dose of doxorubicin.

Associated Exposures

Exposure to chemotherapeutic agents, including cyclophosphamide, dactinomycin, and mithramycin, increases the risk and severity of cardiac injury induced by anthracyclines. Radiotherapy can contribute to cardiac injury by a separate mechanism and cause pericarditis or coronary artery disease.

Nutritional Status

Malnourished patients are more likely to sustain cardiotoxicity from anthracyclines.

Rate of Infusion

A lower *peak* blood level may be less deleterious to the heart (infuse over not less than 3–5 minutes). The merits of small frequent doses or continuous infusion versus bolus dosing are under investigation.

Type of Anthracycline

Doxorubicin is more cardiotoxic than daunorubicin.

Clinical and Subclinical Features

Arrhythmias and abnormalities of conduction may be detected in 11 percent of patients within a few days after anthracycline administration and may be transient. Abnormalities include supraventricular tachycardias, premature atrial contractions, and premature ventricular contractions. Left axis deviation, diminished R-wave voltages, and nonspecific ST- and T-wave changes may also be seen.

Patients with subclinical damage, which may not be detected by ECG or echocardiography, may decompensate because of fluid overload (secondary to poor renal function or overly aggressive hydration) or when an increased demand is placed on the heart, such as during pregnancy (even months to years after completing anthracycline therapy).

Treatment

Treatment of congestive heart failure caused by anthracycline toxicity is no different from that of other causes. However, because in many cases the damage is irreversible, the best treatment is prevention. The physician should be aware of risk factors and should carefully monitor cumulative dose and cardiac function. The latter is assessed by subjective history of the patient's exercise tolerance, weight gain, cardiovascular examination, ECG, and echocardiography.

There is some evidence that QT interval prolongation may predict subsequent fractional shortening measured by echocardiography. The corrected QT interval (QTc) is calculated according to the formula

Table 17-1. Antihypertensive medications

Drug	Dose	Route	Schedule	Comments
Hydrochlorothiazide (diuretic)	0.5–1.5 mg/kg	PO	1–2 times daily	Mild diuretic; increases serum glucose, calcium, uric acid, lipids; decreases potassium
Chlorothiazide (diuretic)	5–10 mg/kg	PO, IV	1–2 times daily	Same as for hydrochlorothiazide
Furosemide (Lasix) (diuretic)	1.0–5.0 mg/kg; max. 160 mg/dose	PO, IV	1–4 times daily	For use in patients with low glomerular filtration rate needing diuresis; metabolic alkalosis, hypokalemia may occur; ototoxic and nephrotoxic
Metolazone (Zaroxolyn) (diuretic)	2.5–10 mg/dose	PO	1–2 times daily	Use with furosemide in patients with low glomerular filtration rate
Spironolactone (diuretic)	0.5–2.0 mg/kg; max. 200 mg/day	PO	3–4 times daily	Potassium-sparing
Propranolol (beta-blocker)	1.0–4.0 mg/kg 0.025–1.0 mg/kg	PO IV	2–3 times daily 2 times daily	Avoid in asthma, congestive heart failure, heart block, diabetes; has central nervous system side effects
Hydralazine (Apresoline)	0.25–1.5 mg/kg; max. 4.5 mg/kg/day 0.4–0.8 mg/kg	PO IV	2–4 times daily Every 4–6 hours	Good for acute hypertensive crisis

Table 17-1. (continued)

Drug	Dose	Route	Schedule	Comments
Diazoxide (Hyperstat)	2.0–5.0 mg/kg; max. 5.0 mg/kg/dose; if first dose ineffective, repeat in 30 minutes	IV	Every 4–24 hours	Rapid-acting; use in hypertensive encephalopathy; may require concomitant furosemide; hyperglycemia may occur
Sodium nitroprusside	0.5–10 μg/kg/min	IV drip (cover in foil)		Monitor patient in intensive care unit; drug has very short half-life
Captopril (inhibitor of angiotensin I–converting enzyme)	0.3–2.0 mg/kg; max. 6 mg/kg/day	PO	3 times daily	More effect in 3 days; reversible neutropenia and nephrotoxicity may occur
Nifedipine (calcium channel blocker)	10 mg/dose; max. 20 mg/dose	PO, SL	3–4 times daily	Sublingually for rapid effect
Clonidine (Catapres) (Catapres-TTS)	0.1–0.3 mg TTS-1–0.1 mg/day	PO Patch	2–3 times daily Every week	Rebound hypertension may occur
Minoxidil	0.1–1.0 mg/kg; max. 100 mg/day	PO	2 times daily	Needs to be used with beta-blocker and diuretic

Key: PO = orally; IV = intravenously; SL = sublingually TTS = transdermal therapeutic system; max. = maximum dose.

$$QTc = \frac{\text{measured QT}}{\sqrt{R - R \text{ interval}}}$$

The QTc should not exceed 0.46; a prolonged QTc correlates with increased risk of cardiotoxicity with subsequent anthracycline exposure [4]. Some centers rely on endomyocardial biopsy to monitor children [5].

HYPERTENSION

Hypertension may occur in pediatric oncology patients, and its cause should be sought by the usual approaches. Antihypertensive medications are listed in Table 17-1.

REFERENCES

1. Von Hoff, D. D., et al. Risk factors for doxorubicin-induced congestive heart failure. *Ann. Int. Med.* 91:710, 1979.
2. Von Hoff, D. D., et al. Daunomycin-induced cardiotoxicity in children and adults. *Am. J. Med.* 62:200, 1977.
3. Lipshultz, S. E., et al. Abstract No. 790. *Blood* 70(Suppl. 1):234, 1987.
4. Bender, K. S., et al. QT interval prolongation associated with anthracycline cardiotoxicity. J. Pediatr. 105:442, 1984.
5. Pegelow, C. H., et al. Endomyocardial biopsy to monitor anthracycline therapy in children. *J. Clin. Oncol.* 2:443, 1984.

18

Pulmonary Complications

Respiratory Distress
Roberta A. Gottlieb

PERSPECTIVE
Multiple etiologies may give rise to respiratory distress. The clinician should work through the differential diagnosis carefully but only after instituting the basic measures of ensuring a good airway, adequate oxygenation, and, if necessary, ventilation. The following are indications for intubation:

Airway protection
Pulmonary toilet
Airway obstruction (present or impending)
Ventilation

DIFFERENTIAL DIAGNOSIS
As respiratory distress may be incited by many conditions, considerations in the differential diagnosis are extensive.

Airway Disorders
Typified by stridor, hoarseness, retractions, or wheezing, the possibilities include anaphylaxis (with laryngeal edema and bronchospasm), vocal cord paralysis (due to tumor invasion, surgical complication, or, rarely, vincristine toxicity), tracheal compression by mass (see section on Superior Vena Cava Syndrome), or foreign body (a possibility in any young child).

Pulmonic Processes
Pulmonic processes are characterized by an abnormal chest radiograph and include a large number of possibilities. Tumor infiltration can give rise to a local infiltrate or opacity on radiograph and may be accompanied by pleural effusion. Atelectasis, often seen postoperatively, is characterized by volume loss of the affected lobe. Pulmonary infiltrate may also represent pneumonitis due to bacteria, fungus, mycobacteria, protozoa (particularly Pneumocystis), and viruses. Pneumonitis can also be seen with leukostasis due to an elevated white blood cell count (particularly AML) or following a leukocyte transfusion. Eosinophilic pneumonitis is occasionally seen in children receiving GM-CSF. Fibrosis is associated with radiation to the lung fields and with certain chemotherapeutic agents including bleomycin, methotrexate, and busulfan. Also implicated are cyclophosphamide, cytosine arabinoside, procarbazine, and carmustine [1, 2]. Acute pulmonary edema may be seen with anaphylaxis, idiosyncratic reactions to drugs (including cytosine arabinoside), and congestive heart failure and fluid overload. A pneumothorax may also give rise to respiratory distress and should be considered in patients who have undergone central line placement or thoracentesis, or who have a thoracic malignancy.

Cardiac Disorders

Congestive heart failure and high-output failure are associated with tachypnea and ultimately with pulmonary congestion and respiratory distress. Pericardial tamponade may present similarly.

Central Nervous System Disorders

Aspiration may result from loss of gag and cough reflexes due to a brainstem tumor or seizure activity. The use of oral lidocaine for mucositis can also suppress the gag reflex. Hypoventilation and apnea may result from seizures, high-level spinal cord or brainstem compression, or drug administration (particularly anticonvulsants and narcotics). Hyperventilation may be seen with increased intracranial pressure (seek other signs) or anxiety (a diagnosis of exclusion).

Other Potential Causes

In evaluating the patient with respiratory distress, one should also consider the possibility of sepsis, metabolic acidosis, severe anemia, and shock.

EVALUATION

Physical Examination

Physical examination should focus on vital signs, mental state, gag reflex, air exchange, stridor, retractions, nasal flaring, careful auscultation, and percussion (although it is less useful in infants). A cardiac examination also should be performed. Abdominal examination is done to assess hyperinflation, use of abdominal muscles, splinting caused by pain, or a mass. Use of abdominal muscles in paradoxical fashion precedes apnea in infants. Look for cyanosis and capillary refill. *Remember* that anemic patients may not show cyanosis even with significant hypoxemia. Tachypnea and cyanosis without major distress suggests interstitial disease or cardiac disease.

Laboratory Studies

Laboratory studies should include arterial blood gases, pulse oximetry if available, and chest roentgenography (which may be unrevealing in neutropenic patients. Other studies are selected according to the suspected cause of distress. There is no reason to withhold oxygen while waiting for blood gas results. *Remember* that respiratory acidosis is treated with effective ventilation; administering sodium bicarbonate treats neither the problem nor the symptom.

TREATMENT

Basic supportive measures for management of respiratory distress include airway maintenance, oxygenation, and ventilation if necessary, as well as frequent or continuous monitoring. Specific management is dictated by the specific clinical entity. Determining the etiology of a pulmonary parenchymal process may require open lung biopsy. Such aggressive investigation is warranted so that appropriate therapy can be instituted promptly.

Superior Vena Cava Syndrome

Roberta A. Gottlieb and Joshua Halpern

CLINICAL FEATURES

Superior vena cava (SVC) syndrome is an uncommon but life-threatening condition that represents tracheal and vascular compression caused by an anterosuperior mediastinal mass (lymphoma, germ-cell tumors, neuroblastoma) or SVC obstruction (especially seen with thrombosed indwelling central venous catheters). Lymphomatous tracheal compression is a related entity. Presenting features are distention of the neck veins, edema above the clavicles or brawny facial plethora, symptoms of increased intracranial pressure, and respiratory distress with retractions, stridor, wheezing, cyanosis, nasal flaring, and occasional pleural effusion. Progressive vascular compression may result in thromboembolic phenomena and fatally increased intracranial pressure.

IMMEDIATE CARE

Rapid intervention is required. In the case of SVC syndrome caused by a clot, surgical correction of the obstruction is necessary. In the case of compression caused by a cancer, emergency radiotherapy or steroids (usually high-dose dexamethasone) are therapeutic. For lymphomas and seminomas, chemotherapy is as efficient as radiotherapy, with less long-term morbidity. Tracheal compression may be progressive and may not be fully relieved by intubation. A mixture of helium and oxygen (70 : 30) will decrease viscosity and turbulence in the severely obstructed airway and may buy time until definitive therapy is under way.

Irradiation will usually be started at high doses per fraction (3–4 Gy for three to four fractions per day), then continued at 2 to 3 Gy per fraction, to achieve a total of 30 to 40 Gy. The outcome depends on the histologic features of the primary tumor and the stage of the disease. Therapeutic intervention before histologic evaluation may affect the accuracy of diagnosis.

REFERENCES

1. Sostman, H.D., Matthay, R. A., and Putman, C. E. Cytotoxic drug-induced lung disease. *Am. J. Med.* 62:608, 1977.
2. Patel, A. R., et al. Cyclophosphamide therapy and interstitial pulmonary fibrosis. *Cancer* 38:1542, 1976.

SELECTED READING

Allegretta, G. J., Weisman, S. J., and Altman, A. J. Oncologic emergencies I: Metabolic and space-occupying consequences of cancer and cancer treatment. *Pediatr. Clin. North Am.* 32:601, 1985.

19

Renal Complications

Renal Failure
Roberta A. Gottlieb

Acute renal failure in the patient with cancer is frequently caused by tumor lysis or nephrotoxic drugs. However, one must rule out prerenal and obstructive causes, since these are easily reversed with appropriate therapy. The goal is to maintain homeostasis: fluid balance, metabolic parameters, and nutrition. Azotemia predisposes to infection, gastrointestinal bleeding, and delayed wound healing.

Use of a flow sheet is essential to good management. Parameters to follow are patient weights every 12 hours, strict intake and output, urine specific gravity or spot urine sodium and chloride and osmolarity (to monitor fractional excretion of sodium, FE_{Na}), serum electrolytes, blood urea nitrogen, creatinine, calcium, magnesium, phosphate, and uric acid levels, osmolarity, and pH.

$$FE_{Na} = \frac{urine_{Na} \times plasma_{Cr}}{plasma_{Na} \times urine_{Cr}} \times 100\%$$

Additional studies might include a complete blood cell count, chemistry panel (especially liver enzymes), and coagulation profile. Consider chest roentgenography in fluid-overloaded patients, electrocardiography (ECG) if hyperkalemia is present, and renal ultrasonography if obstruction is a possibility. A radionuclide glomerular filtration rate (GFR) scan provides information about the function of each kidney.

Monitor drug levels (especially aminoglycosides and vancomycin) and anticipate the need to adjust the dosage and schedule of renally excreted drugs.

FLUID MANAGEMENT
Fluid balance should be monitored. Short-term weight changes represent fluid. Use of central venous pressure or Swan-Ganz catheter monitoring may be necessary. If the FE_{Na} is low ($< 1\%$) and there is evidence of inadequate renal perfusion, correct with appropriate fluids.

If the FE_{Na} is elevated and renal perfusion is adequate, then replace insensible water loss. In infants, provide 10% dextrose in water and appropriate electrolytes at a dosage of 45 ml/kg/day. In children, the dosage is 300 to 400 ml/sq m/day or 30 to 40 ml per 100 calories expended.

Replace urinary losses (and excessive other losses, such as gastrointestinal losses) appropriately. Measure electrolyte contents to ensure correct replacement therapy.

In the patient whose kidneys can respond, furosemide with or without metolazone or chlorothiazide can aid fluid removal.

Low-dose dopamine (2–5 μg/kg/min) may enhance renal blood flow.

HYPONATREMIA

Possible Causes

Consider the possible origins of the hyponatremia. Pseudohyponatremia may be caused by hyperglycemia, hyperlipidemia, or hyperproteinemia. (Allow a drop of 1.6 mEq Na for each 100-mg/dl rise in glucose in excess of 100 mg/dl.)

Decreased Na and body water may be caused by renal disease or may be drug-induced ($FE_{Na} > 3\%$). If the FE_{Na} is less than 1 percent, extrarenal losses are likely.

Decreased Na with a normal or slightly increased body water level is an indication to restrict fluids. The syndrome of inappropriate antidiuretic hormone secretion (SIADH) may be caused by cyclophosphamide and vincristine and signaled by a urinary Na level in excess of 20 mmol/liter or FE_{Na} greater than 2 percent. Steroid use, hypothyroidism, and other causes also may result in a urinary Na level that exceeds 20 mmol/liter. In the case of decreased Na and edema, restrict fluids and treat the cause. In nephrotic syndrome, cirrhosis, or congestive heart failure, urinary sodium will be less than 10 or the FE_{Na} will be less than 1 percent. If there is renal failure, urinary Na will exceed 20 mmol/liter or the FE_{Na} will exceed 3 percent.

Fluid Restriction

When fluid restriction is necessary, initially replace insensible losses (plus excess gastrointestinal losses, if indicated). When absolutely necessary, complete deprivation of fluid will remove 300 to 400 ml/sq m/day of free water.

Immediate Care

Rapid correction of severe hyponatremia (for the symptomatic patient with seizures or coma) is essential; 12 ml/kg of 3% saline will raise the sodium level by 10 mEq/liter. Further correction can be more gradual. Infuse the saline solution over 30 minutes to 3 hours depending on the acuteness of the situation. Allow several hours for equilibration. Risks of such therapy include worsening fluid and sodium overload, worsening hypertension; and sudden shifts in osmolarity. Hyponatremia may also be ameliorated with furosemide (1 mg/kg), with milliliter-for-milliliter urine replacement using normal saline (urine losses will be approximately half-normal saline).

HYPERKALEMIA

Hyperkalemia is exacerbated by transfusions, hemolysis, tumor lysis, acidosis, administration of potassium-containing intravenous fluids, and renal failure. In mild hyperkalemia, there are no ECG changes and the potassium level is less than 6.0 mEq/liter. Potassium in intravenous fluids and oral sources should be stopped. Glucose should be given intravenously or orally, and the acid-base balance should be corrected.

If a high potassium level (manifest by K > 6.0 or peaked T wave in lead II on ECG) persists or continues to rise, sodium polystyrene sulfonate, (Kayexalate), 1 gm/kg/dose, can be given every 6 hours with 70% sorbitol orally (3–4 ml/gm resin) or a 20% sorbitol enema can be given as often as every hour; clear the colon after 30 minutes with 10% dextrose in water. One gram per kilogram should lower the potassium level 1 mEq/liter. Watch for hypernatremia and fluid overload. Remove necrotic tissue, debride wounds, and evacuate enclosed collections of blood. Also, avoid transfusions.

When hyperkalemia is severe, the potassium level is greater than 6.5 mEq/liter or ECG changes are seen. Peaked T waves, a broad QRS complex, and a prolonged P-R interval may or may not precede the loss of P waves, ventricular arrhythmias, or fibrillation. Management involves the following:

1. Administer 10% calcium gluconate, 0.5 ml/kg intravenously over 5 to 10 minutes and monitor the patient.
2. Give glucose (50% dextrose in water), 1 ml/kg, and follow it with a continuous infusion of 20% dextrose in water.
3. If hyperkalemia persists, administer insulin, 0.5 U/kg intravenously. The dose may be repeated in 20 to 30 minutes after glucose loading.
4. Give sodium bicarbonate, up to 1 ml/kg, to correct the acidosis or to drive potassium into cells transiently.
5. Continue Kayexalate enemas. Dialysis is needed if the potassium level exceeds 7.5 mEq/liter or if other treatment approaches are inadequate. Remember that hemodialysis is faster than continuous arteriovenous hemofiltration, which is faster than Kayexalate, which is faster than peritoneal dialysis to remove potassium.

METABOLIC ACIDOSIS

For metabolic acidosis, provide adequate calories (300 kcal/sq m/day) in the form of carbohydrates and fats to reduce acid production from gluconeogenesis (PO_4^{-3}, SO_4^{-2}, amino acids). As renal function improves, introduce high-utilization proteins or specialized total parenteral nutrition.

Sodium bicarbonate can be used to correct metabolic acidosis only if the patient's respiratory function is adequate. Most patients need 1 to 2 mEq/kg/day of bicarbonate, which may be increased by 1 mEq/kg as needed. Correcting the bicarbonate level beyond 15 mmol/liter without concomitant correction of hypocalcemia and hyperphosphatemia (which are common in tumor lysis) will exacerbate those metabolic derangements. Start phosphate binders early and do not administer intravenous calcium unless the patient is symptomatic (tetany or seizures).

INFECTIONS IN RENAL FAILURE

Risk factors for infection during renal failure are indwelling catheters and an immunosuppressed host. Signs of infection may be unreliable: Fever may be absent or minimal, and leukocytosis may be caused by azotemia or infection, as may altered mental status. Persistent hyperkalemia or acidosis may suggest infection.

Antibiotic prophylaxis is not indicated. Instead, the clinician should consider surveillance cultures. Suspected sepsis is treated with broad-spectrum antibiotics, pending culture and sensitivities. Monitor the levels of drugs, and adjust the doses and intervals of all drugs that are cleared renally.

INDICATIONS FOR DIALYSIS

A number of conditions are cause for performing dialysis, including the following:

1. A rapid rise in the blood urea nitrogen and creatinine levels or uremia severe enough to cause gastrointestinal, central nervous system, or hemorrhagic disorders, or pericarditis

2. Hyperkalemia in which the potassium level exceeds 7.5 or that is uncontrolled by other measures, especially in the case of ongoing production of potassium (as in tumor lysis, hemolysis, or hypercatabolic states)
3. Severe metabolic acidosis uncorrected by bicarbonate or for which bicarbonate therapy would cause hypernatremia or circulatory overload
4. Hypertension caused by fluid overload and unresponsive to medical therapy
5. Fluid overload leading to congestive heart failure or pulmonary edema
6. Patients with tumor lysis who have any of the following:
   Serum potassium in excess of 6 mEq/liter (nonhemolyzed sample)
   Serum uric acid in excess of 15 mg/dl
   Serum creatinine in excess of 10 mg/dl or rising rapidly
   Serum phosphorus in excess of 10 mg/dl or rising rapidly
   Symptomatic hypocalcemia
   Volume overload

Prepare for dialysis in any patient with rapidly progressing renal failure. Consult a nephrologist early.

These criteria for dialysis are conservative; in many cases it is appropriate to initiate dialysis much earlier, particularly in the case of acute tumor lysis.

Tumor Lysis Syndrome
Cynthia J. Tifft

A syndrome consisting of hyperuricemia, hyperkalemia, and hyperphosphatemia with hypocalcemia occurs following neoplastic cell lysis, particularly in lymphoma and leukemia. Metabolic abnormalities are particularly severe in patients with B cell lymphoma/leukemia, as a result of rapid tumor cell lysis and extreme sensitivity to chemotherapeutic agents. Lysis following chemotherapy can lead to renal failure and sudden death from hyperkalemia or hypocalcemia.

Clearance of the products of tumor lysis depends on renal excretion, hepatic metabolism, and phagocytosis by the reticuloendothelial system. Renal clearance is the primary mechanism for excretion of uric acid, potassium, and phosphate. Patients with already compromised renal function are therefore at higher risk for acute tumor lysis. Optimum management of patients at risk depends on evaluation of renal function prior to starting chemotherapy, adequate hydration, drug therapy, and close monitoring in the first week after initiation of chemotherapy.

TREATMENT
When possible, a 24-hour creatinine clearance should be obtained or estimated by patient length prior to initiating chemotherapy:

$$CrCl = \frac{0.55 \; L(cm)}{P \; Cr \; (mg/dl)}$$

(not accurate in patients older than 6 months of age or in cachexia) [1]. Hydration at 3 liters/sq m/day should begin 24 hours before chemotherapy if the patient can tolerate it. Allopurinol, 500 mg/sq m/day (or 100 mg three times/day) orally, will reduce hyperuricemia and uricosuria during tumor lysis. However, it results in significant xanthinuria, which may cause nephropathy [2]. Alkalinization of urine will increase the solubility of urate in renal tubules. To achieve this, begin with sodium bicarbonate, 40 mEq/liter, added to regular intravenous fluids, and titrate to keep the urine pH above 6. Do not include potassium chloride in intravenous fluids. Once chemotherapy is initiated, monitor frequently the potassium, calcium, and phosphate levels, as well as renal function.

COMPLICATIONS

The most serious complication of tumor lysis syndrome is the onset of renal failure with azotemia, oliguria, hyperuricemia, hyperkalemia, and hypocalcemia. Hyperkalemia can be treated acutely if the potassium level exceeds 6 mEq/liter or if there are ECG changes (monitor T wave, lead II) (see sections on Renal Failure and Hyperkalemia). While administering Kayexalate and in the face of marked hyperkalemia, begin dialysis preparations (a consultation with a renal specialist should already have been conducted).

Hypocalcemia can be treated by lowering serum phosphate with oral phosphate binders (aluminum hydroxide [Amphojel, ALterna-GEL]), and providing oral calcium supplementation. If the patient is highly symptomatic, hypocalcemia can be corrected with intravenous calcium. Calcium gluconate, 100 mg/kg/dose, is given by *slow* intravenous push while on cardiac monitor. Monitor for bradycardia. Calcium gluconate (10%) has 0.45 mEq of calcium per milliliter and is hypertonic, so dilute 1 : 1 with sterile water or 5% dextrose in water.

Patients who are worsening rapidly may require hemodialysis according to the following criteria:

Serum potassium in excess of 6 mEq/liter
Serum uric acid in excess of 10 mg/dl
Serum creatinine in excess of 10 mg/dl
Serum phosphorus in excess of 10 mg/dl
Symptomatic hypocalcemia
Volume overload with oliguria that is unresponsive to diuretics

In the case of acute tumor lysis, dialysis should be initiated early, as chemotherapy is likely to exacerbate the metabolic derangements. Patients who have decreased urine output during initial hydration therapy are likely to require dialysis [3].

Metabolic Disturbances
Roberta A. Gottlieb

Metabolic disturbances are a common occurrence in the child with cancer. The more common electrolyte disturbances, their causes and consequences, and appropriate treatment modes are presented in Table 19-1.

Table 19-1. Characterization of electrolyte disturbances common in the pediatric oncology patient

Disturbance	Causes	Consequences	Management
Elevated potassium level	Tumor lysis, acidosis, renal failure, hemolysis	Arrhythmias, peaked T waves on electrocardiogram	Correct the acidosis; give furosemide (Lasix), 1 mg/kg, and Kayexalate, 1 gm/kg per rectum; if severe, give glucose, insulin, and calcium, and perform dialysis
Diminished calcium level	Tumor lysis, hyperphosphatemia, T-cell acute lymphoid leukemia, rhabdomyolysis (early), renal failure	Seizures, altered mental status, carpopedal spasm, tetany, weakness, hyporeflexia, bradycardia	Stop alkalinization; give calcium, 0.5–1 gm orally 2–4 times daily; administer calcium gluconate, 100 mg/kg, intravenously; monitor the patient as therapy may worsen hypocalcemia if patient is hyperphosphatemic
Elevated phosphate level	Tumor lysis, renal failure, rhabdomyolysis (early)	Hypocalcemia, calcium phosphate nephropathy, weakness, coma	Oral phosphate binders (aluminum hydroxide [Dialume, antacids]); hydration and dialysis
Elevated uric acid level	Tumor lysis, diuretics	Nephropathy, renal failure	Hydrate with 3 liters/sq m/day; alkalinize urine (pH 7.0); allopurinol, 100 mg orally 3 times daily
Elevated sodium level	Dehydration, renal failure, DI, brain tumor, leukemia	Seizures, irritability	Monitor urine sodium level, weight; replace insensible losses and urine if DI present; rehydrate if dehydration present; correct *slowly* over 48–72 hr

Diminished sodium level	Overhydration, dehydration, SIADH (often caused by vincristine therapy), brain tumor, leukemia, chemotherapy	Seizures, irritability	Rehydrate if dehydrated; restrict fluids in presence of SIADH or CHF; replace volume losses if volume status normal or decreased—restrict fluids, give Lasix with saline replacement of urine output; if symptomatic, use 3% saline (12 ml/kg) to raise serum sodium level 10 mEq/liter
Diminished potassium level	Diuretics, corrected acidosis, amphotericin therapy	Weakness, ileus, QT prolongation	2–5 mEq/kg/day orally or 0.5 mEq/100 calories intravenously; phlebitis may occur if the potassium level exceeds 40 mEq/liter in intravenous fluid
Elevated calcium level	Malignancy affecting bone, hyperparathyroidism, sarcoid, rhabdomyolysis (late)	Abdominal pain, CNS symptoms, weakness	Hydrate with normal saline and administer furosemide (1 mg/kg); steroids are useful in paraneoplastic syndromes; rarely, calcitonin (4 IU/kg given every 12 hrs SQ or IM), mithramycin (15–25 µg/kg IV push), or dialysis may be necessary. *Never give phosphate.*
Diminished phosphate level	Malnutrition, new TPN, renal tubular dysfunction, rhabdomyolysis (late)	Hemolysis, cardiac dysfunction, glucose intolerance	Oral phosphate, 1–2 gm/day in four divided doses, or phosphate, 0.5–1.5 mmol/kg intravenously over 6 hr, if serum phosphate level is less than 1.0 mg/dl.
Diminished magnesium level	Cisplatin therapy, diuretics, gastrointestinal losses	Seizures, altered mental status, tetany	Magnesium gluconate, 500 mg orally 3 times daily or 5–30 mEq/liter intravenously over 12–24 hr

Key: DI = diabetes insipidus; SIADH = syndrome of inappropriate antidiuretic hormone secretion; CHF = congestive heart failure; CNS = central nervous system; TPN = total parenteral nutrition.

REFERENCES

1. Schwarz, G. J., et al. A simple estimate of glomerular filtration rate in children derived from body length and plasma creatinine. *Pediatrics* 58:259, 1976.
2. Band, P. R., et al. Xanthine nephropathy in a patient with lymphosarcoma treated with allopurinol. *N. Engl. J. Med.* 7:354, 1970.
3. Stapleton, F. B., et al. Acute renal failure at onset of therapy for advanced stage Burkitt lymphoma and B cell acute lymphoblastic lymphoma. *Pediatrics* 82:863, 1988.

20

Gastrointestinal Complications

Nausea and Vomiting
Melissa M. Hudson

Many chemotherapeutic agents cause nausea and vomiting. Chief among these are cisplatin, cytosine arabinoside, cyclophosphamide, doxorubicin, dactinomycin, dacarbazine, etoposide, lomustine, procarbazine, 5-azacytidine, methotrexate, and 6-mercaptopurine. A variety of agents available to control or preferably prevent these side effects are listed in Table 20-1. Regimens associated with predictable nausea and vomiting should be accompanied by scheduled, not PRN, antiemetics. Relaxation techniques are helpful in patients who experience anticipatory nausea and vomiting (see Chap. 27).

Diarrhea
Roberta A. Gottlieb

Diarrhea is a frequently encountered problem in the pediatric patient, and the possible causes are more numerous in the immunosuppressed host.

EVALUATION

General Principles
The patient history should include date and type of last chemotherapy, expected and experienced reactions, antibiotic use, exposures to illnesses, level of activity, intake, urine output, frequency and character of stools, and the presence of fever and vomiting. The patient's underlying disease and degree of immunosuppression should be taken into consideration.

Physical examination should address vital signs, hydration status, mucosal integrity (mouth and anus), abdominal examination, and associated findings. Typhlitis or appendicitis may present with diarrhea and abdominal pain. *Remember* that peritoneal signs are minimal in the neutropenic patient.

Laboratory Studies
Obtain a complete blood cell count, electrolyte, blood urea nitrogen, and creatinine levels, urinalysis, stool guaiac and fecal leukocyte determinations (Wright's stain is preferable), *Clostridium difficile* toxin detection, examination for ova and parasites (including *Cryptosporidium*), and blood, urine, and stool cultures. Abdominal flat plate and upright radiographs (portable studies are nondiagnostic) are indicated if the examination suggests ileus, obstruction, or perforation. Endoscopy may be diagnostic in *C. difficile* colitis, graft-versus-host disease, cytomegalovirus enterocolitis, and parasitic infection.

DIFFERENTIAL DIAGNOSIS
See Table 20-2.

Table 20-1. Agents useful in controlling nausea and vomiting

Drug	Dose	Route	Schedule	Comments
Phenothiazines (antiemetics)				
Prochlorperazine (Compazine)	0.1 mg/kg/dose 0.05 mg/kg/dose	PO, PR IM	q6–8h q6–8h	Do not use IV route in children; do not use in children younger than 2 years or who weigh < 10 kg
Promethazine (Phenergan)	0.25–0.5 mg/kg/dose	PO, PR, IM, IV	q4–6h	Sedation, EPS are side effects
Chlorpromazine (Thorazine)	0.5 mg/kg/dose 0.5 mg/kg/dose 0.5 mg/kg/dose max. in children <5 years is 75 mg/day	PO PR IM, IV	q4–6h q6–8h q6–8h	Sedation, EPS are side effects
Butyrophenones (block dopamine receptors in chemoreceptor trigger zone)				
Haloperidol (Haldol)	Adults: 2 mg/dose	PO, IM	q4–6h	Sedation, EPS are side effects
Droperidol (Inapsine)	0.1 mg/kg Adults: 2–5 mg/dose	IM, IV	q4–6h	Premedicate with diazepam. Hypotension, sedation, hallucinations, EPS may occur
Metoclopramide (Reglan)	Preschoolers 0.1 mg/kg/dose 2 mg/kg/dose 1–2 mg/kg/dose	PO PO Slow IV drip	q2–6h q2–6h q2–6h	Drowsiness, EPS, diarrhea may occur

Benzodiazepines (useful because of antianxiety and amnesic effects)				
Lorazepam (Ativan)	0.03–0.05 mg/kg/dose; max. 4 mg/dose; Adults: 2–6 mg	IV PO	q6h q8–12h	Respiratory depression, drowsiness are side effects
Diazepam (Valium)	0.04–0.2 mg/kg/dose; max. 0.6 mg/kg/8h; 0.03–0.4 mg/kg/dose; adults: 2–10 mg/dose	IV, IM PO	q2–4h q6–8h	Respiratory depression, drowsiness, hypotension are side effects
Antihistamines (anticholinergic and central nervous system actions)				
Diphenhydramine (Benadryl)	1–2 mg/kg/dose Adults: 10–50 mg/dose (max. 300 mg/day)	IV PO	q6–8h	Drowsiness, dizziness, disturbed coordination are side effects
Miscellaneous				
Dexamethasone (Decadron)	4–8 mg/sq m loading dose, followed by 2–4 mg/sq m/dose	IV	q6h	Adjunct to other antiemetic therapy
Scopolamine	0.5 mg transdermal	Patch	Worn behind ear, change every 3 days	Ipsilateral pupillary dilatation may occur
Dronabinol (delta-9-tetrahydrocannabinol, [THC, Marinol])	Adults: 5–20 mg	PO	q2–4h	Drowsiness, dizziness, dysphonia, tachycardia are side effects

Key: PO = orally; PR = per rectum; IM = intramuscularly; IV = intravenously; max. = maximum dose; EPS = extrapyramidal symptoms.

Table 20-2. Possible causes of diarrhea in the pediatric cancer patient

Possible cause	Laboratory study
Infectious causes	
Shigella	Routine stool culture
Salmonella	Routine stool culture
Campylobacter	Special culture media needed
Yersinia	Special culture media needed
Traveler's diarrhea (*Escherichia coli* strains)	Special techniques required
Clostridium difficile	Antigen detection and special culture needed
Rotavirus and related viruses	Viral culture
Cytomegalovirus	Viral culture, intestinal biopsy
Giardia lamblia	Microscopic examination, electron microscopy for ova and parasites; duodenal aspirate
Entamoeba histolytica	Microscopic examination for ova and parasites
Cryptosporidium	Microscopic examination
Microsporidia	Microscopic examination
Yeast	Frequently isolated but rarely causative
Treatment-induced causes	
Cytosine arabinoside, 5-fluorouracil, methotrexate, mercaptopurine, alkylating agents, anthracyclines	Diagnosis by history, exclude other causes
Antibiotics (direct effect or by alteration of gut flora)	Stool culture, *C. difficile* toxin detection and culture
Radiation (cytotoxic effect causes loss of mucosa)	Diagnosis by history, endoscopy, biopsy features
Graft-versus-host disease	Diagnosis by endoscopy, biopsy features, clinical setting
Other causes	
Hypoproteinemia (bowel wall edema)	Serum albumin, protein
Lactose intolerance (common among Hispanics)	Stool-reducing substances, pH, D-xylose excretion, breath hydrogen test
Malabsorption syndromes (usually not watery stools)	Stool fat quantitation and specific other tests

TREATMENT

Isolate the patient until a contagious cause is ruled out. Rehydrate orally with Pedialyte RS or similar oral rehydration solution if possible or intravenously if necessary. Nutritional support is important in protracted diarrhea. Management is directed toward the specific etiologic agent; thus, diagnosis should be pursued vigorously.

Constipation
Roberta A. Gottlieb

Certain drugs cause severe constipation, especially vinca alkaloids (vincristine, vinblastine) and narcotics (morphine, codeine, and meperidine). Prevention is the key: Stool softeners and lubricants (mineral oil, 15 ml orally) should be employed as needed. Children in the process of toilet learning are at special risk if they are also receiving one or more of the agents listed earlier. Stool softeners include docusate sodium (Colace), 5 mg/kg/day; malt soup extract (Maltsupex), senna concentrate (Senokot), and lactulose (Cephulac). The dosage is age-related:

Age	Maltsupex or Senokot	Lactulose
1 month–1 year	½ tsp twice daily	¼–½ tsp 2–4 times daily
1–5 years	1 tsp twice daily	2–4 tsp 3–4 times daily
5–15 years	2 tsp twice daily	2–3 tbsp 3–4 times daily

Additional therapy may include magnesium sulfate or sodium sulfate by mouth. Rectal manipulation in the form of suppositories or enemas is contraindicated in the immunocompromised patient.

Parents of pediatric cancer patients should be aware of the risk of constipation and should be sure the patient's diet includes natural lubricants (prune juice, tomatoes, olive oil) and fiber (green vegetables, fruits, bran, and whole grain products).

Ileus and Intestinal Obstruction
Roberta A. Gottlieb

PERSPECTIVE

Ileus often follows vincristine therapy. Obstruction may be related to primary tumor, surgical complications, radiation injury, or abscess formation. Inflammation and perforation of the cecum (typhlitis) are seen in patients with leukemia.

EVALUATION

1. Obtain a careful history with attention to the patient's primary disease and recent therapy, previous operations, and duration and severity of symptoms.

2. Perform a physical examination with attention to fever, presence or absence of bowel sounds, distention, tenderness, masses, and fecal impaction. Rectal examination is contraindicated in the neutropenic patient. Remember that the immunosuppressed patient may not show typical features of peritonitis.
3. Perform a diagnostic radiographic evaluation with flat plate and upright or decubitus films. Portable films are of poor quality and may be misleading.
4. Additional studies based on the clinical impression may include ultrasonography or computed tomography with contrast enhancement, upper and lower gastrointestinal series, and occasionally endoscopy.

TREATMENT

Surgical consultation should be initiated if obstruction or typhlitis is suspected. (Also see the section on Surgical Complications in Chap. 14.) Allow bowel rest with suction decompression (Cantor tube or tungsten-weighted nasoduodenal tube) and intravenous fluids. Intubation may be contraindicated in the neutropenic or thrombocytopenic patient or in the case of mucositis. Gastrointestinal losses should be replaced with an appropriate electrolyte solution. Narcotics will further decrease bowel motility and so should be avoided. In the neutropenic patient, empiric antibiotic therapy should be instituted and should cover intestinal flora including clostridia. Therapy may be instituted while evaluation is still under way.

SELECTED READING

Craig, J.B., and Powell, B.L., Review: The management of nausea and vomiting in clinical oncology. *Am. J. Med. Sci.* 293:34, 1987.
Morrow, G. R. Management of Nausea in the Cancer Patient. In S. Rosenthal, J. R. Carignan, and B. D. Smith (eds.), *Medical Care of the Cancer Patient.* Philadelphia: Saunders, 1987. Pp. 38–388.

21

Hematologic Complications

Nancy Collins O'Brien

DISSEMINATED INTRAVASCULAR COAGULATION

Disseminated intravascular coagulation (DIC) is an acquired, unregulated activation of coagulation and fibrinolysis characterized by multiple hemostatic abnormalities. It is a symptom, not a disease, and is always associated with an underlying disease state.

Clinical Features

Acute DIC typically occurs in very ill patients (e.g., purpura fulminans); the exception is the patient with acute promyeloid leukemia (APL) beginning on cytoreductive therapy. Hallmarks include (1) moderate to severe purpura, (2) oozing at surface injuries, (3) variable degrees of circulatory failure and shock, and (4) variable degrees of hemorrhage.

Chronic DIC results from low-grade activation of coagulation or partial compensation (e.g., the Kasabach-Merritt syndrome). Among its features are (1) an asymptomatic or mildly symptomatic patient (who may progress to serious hemorrhage or acute DIC), (2) thrombocytopenia, (3) variable purpura, and (4) variable venous thrombosis.

Associated Conditions

Bacterial cell walls can activate the clotting cascade. Acute DIC is associated with gram-negative sepsis, meningococcemia, and beta-hemolytic streptococcus. Varicella may occasionally cause DIC. Promyelocytic leukemic blast cells release large amounts of a procoagulant, which is best controlled by scheduled fresh-frozen plasma (FFP) and platelets. In some cases, heparin may be necessary. Transfusion reactions, drug reactions, and hemorrhage (especially into a closed space such as a necrotic tumor or as a postoperative complication) can also lead to DIC. Neuroblastoma may also precipitate a consumptive coagulopathy, especially when treatment is initiated. L-Asparaginase, owing to its effects on hepatic synthesis of clotting factors and inhibitors, can precipitate a coagulopathy.

Giant hemangioma or lymphangioma (Kasabach-Merritt syndrome) or intravenous catheters can lead to low-grade consumption of platelets and fibrin deposition, with subsequent localized and low-grade chronic intravascular coagulation. The coagulation profile may be only slightly abnormal.

Laboratory Evaluation

Approach to Workup

Initial tests include the following:

Platelet count, blood smear examination, prothrombin time (PT) and partial thromboplastin time (PTT)
Thrombin clotting time (TCT) if PT and PTT are prolonged
Ivy bleeding time if bleeding tendency is not clinically apparent. (This is to be avoided in patients in whom DIC is obvious.)

Confirmatory tests include the following:

Fibrinogen and degradation products titer
Factors II, V, and VIII levels
Antithrombin-III level

Other tests aimed at identifying the underlying cause of DIC if it is
not apparent

Laboratory Abnormalities

All of the following abnormalities may accompany DIC, but items 1
through 6 *must* be present to substantiate a diagnosis of DIC:

1. Thrombocytopenia ($< 150 \times 10^9$/liter or steadily falling)
2. Prolonged PT, PTT, and TCT. PTT may be short and PT normal in
   patients with APL
3. Decrease in plasma fibrinogen
4. Increase in fibrin and fibrinogen degradation products
5. Decrease in factors II, V, VIII, and antithrombin-III
6. Prolonged Ivy bleeding time
7. Fragmentation of red blood cells on smear

Differential Diagnosis

Conditions to consider in the differential diagnosis include the following:

Parenchymal liver disease (factor VIII level is usually normal, except in advanced cases)
Vitamin K deficiency (platelet count, TCT, factors V and VIII, and
fibrinogen degradation products normal)
Heparin effects (platelet count, factors II and VIII, and fibrinogen
degradation products normal; PT less affected than PTT)
Microangiopathic disease (only platelet count and bleeding time are
abnormal)

Treatment

The underlying disease should be treated aggressively, including
chemotherapy and surgery, if indicated. Supportive care consists of
supplying red blood cells for anemia or FFP and red blood cells for
hypovolemia or shock; assessing and managing specific organ failure, especially renal failure; and supplying FFP (10–15 ml/kg) and
platelets (5 U/sq m) for acute bleeding.

Intravenous heparin should be used only if the preceding measures fail. *Remember* that heparin activity is dependent on an adequate antithrombin-III level! The dosage is a 50-U/kg bolus followed
by 20 to 50 U/kg/hour by continuous infusion (preferred) or 50 to 100
U/kg every 4 hours. Use PT to follow progress and to distinguish
between continuing DIC and heparin effects. In the case of APL, 5 to
10 U/kg/hour is often sufficient to achieve the goal of normalizing
(not prolonging) the PTT. If DIC responds to heparin treatment,
continue it until *all* plasma factors and platelet counts have stabilized at normal levels.

Prognosis

The prognosis depends on the degree of severity of DIC and the
prognosis of the underlying disease.

TRANSFUSION THERAPY

Transfusion of blood products is critical in the treatment of childhood cancer. Nevertheless, blood products should be used only when absolutely necessary.

Risks

The general risks of transfusions include the following:

Transmission of infectious diseases, such as human immunodeficiency virus, cytomegalovirus, Epstein-Barr virus, hepatitis B, non-A non-B hepatitis, human T-cell leukemia virus type I, malaria, and syphilis
Transfusion reactions
Volume overload
Graft-versus-host disease in immunocompromised recipients
Sensitization of patients to blood products

Also, the religious beliefs of some patients preclude blood component therapy, although court-ordered protection of children may supervene.

Red Blood Cell (RBC) Transfusions

The decision to transfuse RBCs should be based on the clinical assessment of the patient and not the hematocrit alone. Important factors to consider are (1) hemoglobin concentration; (2) rate of onset of decreased hemoglobin level; (3) host tolerance of decreased hemoglobin level (assess vital signs); (4) oxygen requirements and metabolic rate; (5) rate of ongoing blood loss (is there active bleeding or risk of bleeding due to coagulopathy, thrombocytopenia, or sites of potential hemorrhage?); (6) expectations of marrow output; (7) arterial oxygen saturation; (8) associated conditions such as pneumonia or sepsis; and (9) long-term transfusion needs. However, the *only* indication for RBC transfusion is to prevent or reverse tissue hypoxia.

Packed RBCs have a hematocrit of 60 to 90 percent and a shelf life of 21 to 35 days depending on the anticoagulant used. They may be washed or filtered to remove most leukocyte contamination (which reduces febrile or urticarial reactions) or irradiated (20 Gy will inactivate lymphocytes) to reduce the risk of graft-versus-host disease in the immunocompromised patient.

Calculation of Rate

A RBC transfusion rate of 10 ml/kg over 2 hours is acceptable in uncompromised patients, whereas patients with heart failure should generally receive no more than 2 ml/kg/hour. Diuretics may be useful in patients with compromised cardiac, pulmonary, or renal function. If a transfusion will take longer than 4 hours, split the blood into multiple smaller transfusions.

Calculation of Volume

The volume and rate of the transfusion depend on the patient's cardiac and pulmonary status. In general, the volume of packed RBCs needed may be calculated in deciliters as follows:

$$\text{Volume (dl)} = \frac{(\text{PBV})\,(\text{Hbd}) - (\text{PBV})\,(\text{Hba})}{23\,(\text{gm/dl})}$$

where PBV =   patient blood volume (dl) (Note: A normal adult blood
               volume of 70–75 ml/kg is reached by 3 months of age.
               From birth to 3 months, the approximate blood volume
               is 80–85 ml/kg, whereas that of a premature infant is
               100–105 ml/kg.)

   Hbd =   desired hemoglobin concentration (gm/dl)
   Hba =   actual hemoglobin concentration (gm/dl)

Platelet Transfusions

Thrombocytopenia is common in childhood cancer and may be a
result of direct marrow infiltration with tumor or of myelosuppression from chemotherapy or radiotherapy. Other causes include
drugs, increased consumption, or trapping in splenomegaly. The
need to transfuse platelets should not be based on the platelet count
alone. Various factors, such as drugs (aspirin and other nonsteroidal
anti-inflammatory agents, and certain antibiotics), fever, sepsis, uremia and other toxins, and age of the platelets, adversely affect platelet function. Remember that when platelet function is inhibited by
circulating platelet toxins (such as drugs), transfused platelets will
also be affected.

Thrombocytopenia Associated with Bone Marrow Failure

In thrombocytopenic patients with bone marrow failure, bleeding is
rare when the platelet count is higher than $30,000/\mu l$. When the
count is lower than $20,000/\mu l$, the risk of spontaneous bleeding increases markedly, especially in leukemic patients. In many centers,
such patients are transfused prophylactically to raise their platelet
count to 40,000 to $50,000/\mu l$. It is important to know that such
prophylaxis is costly, entails the same risks as any transfusion, and
may sensitize the patient, thus rendering subsequent transfusion
useless.

   Patients who are bleeding require more aggressive transfusion,
with attention to clinical cessation of bleeding, *not* a certain platelet
count. Continued bleeding despite a platelet count of $100,000/\mu l$ or
higher is not attributable to thrombocytopenia, and one must search
for other causes.

   Prophylactic platelet transfusion may be indicated for invasive
procedures when the platelet count is fewer than $50,000/\mu l$ (in the
case of lumbar puncture or bone marrow aspiration) or fewer than
$100,000/\mu l$ (in the case of central line placement or surgery).

Dosage

A unit of transfused platelets initially contains at least 5.5×10^{10}
platelets, with 50 to 70 percent going into the circulating blood
volume and the remainder being trapped by the spleen. A transfusion of 4 U/sq m is usually a good starting point. Desired platelet
increment (PI) can be calculated more precisely as follows:

$$PI\ (/\mu l) = \frac{(5.5 \times 10^{10}) \times (\text{no. of units given}) \times 0.5}{(\text{patient blood volume in ml}) \times 10^3}$$

Platelets should be administered through a standard $170\text{-}\mu$ blood
filter. In children it is important to specify the volume in which the
platelets are to be infused.

Granulocyte Transfusion

Overwhelming infection in the face of immunosuppression is a common cause of death in children with cancer and, consequently, the idea of white blood cell transfusions has great theoretical benefit. Its clinical usage is a subject of great controversy [1, 2]. However, it is generally agreed that such transfusions are of use only in severely neutropenic patients with sepsis. Granulocyte transfusion is generally considered warranted if all the following conditions exist in a given patient:

1. The granulocyte count in peripheral blood is 200/μl or less.
2. There is documented or highly suspicious infection or sepsis.
3. The patient has failed to respond to 24 to 48 hours of appropriate antibiotic therapy.
4. The expected duration of neutropenia is less than 7 days.
5. Bone marrow recovery is expected if infection is controlled.
6. There is an available donor who will continue to be available for the expected duration of neutropenia.

IDIOPATHIC THROMBOCYTOPENIC PURPURA OF CHILDHOOD

Perspective

Idiopathic thrombocytopenic purpura of childhood (ITP) is characterized by acute peripheral thrombocytopenia (< 100,000 platelets/μl) occurring in association with increased bone marrow platelet production and a decreased platelet life span. It is usually acute and self-limited but can be recurrent or chronic.

The onset of ITP is variable, with a peak noted at age 2 to 5 years. The annual incidence in the United States is at least 4 per 100,000. There is no sex predilection or seasonal peak [3].

Etiology

The term *idiopathic* is a misnomer as ITP is now known to be caused by increased reticuloendothelial destruction of platelets to which immunoglobulin G (IgG) is bound. It is unclear whether this IgG is a specific antiplatelet autoantibody or an IgG–viral antigen complex. Because ITP is a heterogeneous disease, there may be more than one mechanism at work.

Evaluation

Clinical Features

The hallmark of ITP is purpura (often petechial) with an otherwise normal physical examination. Affected children appear well except for their bruising, and so the presence of other abnormalities suggests another disease. Onset may be associated with a viral illness, thrombocytopenia often beginning 1 to 3 weeks after the illness resolves. Epistaxis is a common bleeding complication, but oral and gastrointestinal bleeding, hematuria, and intracranial hemorrhage are rare.

Laboratory Studies

Besides thrombocytopenia of varying degree, blood cell counts should reveal no other abnormalities. The blood smear will show reduced numbers of platelets that typically are larger than normal. The platelet count is less than $40,000/\mu l$ in 80 percent of children, and the mean platelet volume *may* be elevated. Coagulation tests are rarely indicated and are generally normal, except for the bleeding time, which is prolonged and should not be performed. Testing for platelet-associated IgG, if available, is positive in 85 percent of cases but is *not* specific for ITP. Other laboratory tests may be performed to rule out other disorders, including direct and indirect Coombs' testing, and tests for antinuclear antibody, other tissue autoantibodies, and quantitative immunoglobulins.

Bone marrow aspiration is helpful in the diagnosis of ITP, showing normal or increased megakaryocytes and no abnormalities in other cell lines. The majority of pediatric hematologists perform bone marrow aspiration on ITP patients to allay fears and anxieties regarding more sinister disorders and because marrow examination has been recommended before corticosteroid therapy is initiated, since the use of steroids could mask an undiagnosed acute lymphoid leukemia. It is noteworthy that isolated thrombocytopenia in an otherwise well patient is an unusual presentation of childhood acute lymphoid leukemia.

Complications

Although it occurs rarely (in fewer than 1% of patients), intracranial hemorrhage is a devastating complication of childhood ITP. Risk factors include a platelet count of fewer than $20,000/\mu l$, hypertension (a well-known side effect of steroid therapy), and head trauma.

Treatment

There are two components of the management of childhood ITP: general supportive care and specific pharmacologic therapy.

Supportive Care

Supportive care is most easily understood in terms of the benign natural history of ITP. The physical activity of new-onset ITP patients should be restricted, and contact sports and playground activity must be curtailed. Most children are no safer in a hospital than at home. Parents should be given a list of antiplatelet drugs to avoid, including aspirin, phenothiazines, antihistamines, glyceryl guaiacolate, and certain antibiotics. Immunizations and intramuscular injections should be avoided while thrombocytopenia is present.

Specific Pharmacologic Therapy

The issue of whether and when to use specific drug therapy for ITP is a hotly debated one among pediatric hematologists. There is no doubt that treatment with either corticosteroids or intravenous IgG results in earlier return to safe platelet counts. The assumption is made that safe platelet counts correlate with decreased bleeding complications. Much less clear is whether one therapeutic modality is better than the other. Intravenous IgG is much more expensive than oral corticosteroids but has fewer side effects, and studies suggest that certain patients respond more rapidly to intravenous IgG than to steroids [4]. Unfortunately, it carries with it the risk of infection or allergic reaction. Steroids have the advantage of low price and are used for relatively short periods of time, making side effects less important in the choice of therapeutic approach.

The decision regarding whether to treat ITP and by what method must be reached for each individual patient. The severity of symptoms, young age, and other factors may shift the balance toward treatment. Dosages are as follows:

Prednisone: 2 mg/kg/day orally for 2 weeks;
                    taper over third week
Intravenous IgG: 0.4 to 0.5 gm/kg/day intrave-
                    nously for 5 days; subsequent
                    dose recommendations vary
                    widely

The routine use of platelet transfusions is not indicated in ITP because the antibody will also shorten the life span of transfused platelets. However, bolus infusions may be helpful in controlling life-threatening bleeding.

Prognosis

Ninety percent of children with ITP recover uneventfully in weeks to months. The diagnosis of chronic ITP is made when a platelet count of fewer than $100,000/\mu l$ persists for 6 months. Recurrent ITP occurs in 1 to 4 percent of patients and may be associated with viral illness and vaccinations [5].

REFERENCES

1. Higby, D. J., and Burnett, D. Granulocyte transfusions: Current status. *Blood* 55:2, 1980.
2. Laurenti, F., et al. Polymorphonuclear leukocyte transfusion for the treatment of sepsis in the newborn infant. *J. Pediatr.* 98:18, 1981.
3. Miller, C. R., Baehner, R. L., and McMillan, C. N. *Blood Diseases of Infancy and Childhood.* St. Louis: Mosby, 1984.
4. Imbach, P., et al. Intravenous Immunoglobulin Therapy in Immune Thrombocytopenic Purpura (ITP) and Other Immune Related Hemorrhagic Disorders in Childhood. In A. Morrell and U. E. Nydegger (eds.), *Clinical Use of Intravenous Immunoglobulins.* London: Academic Press, 1986. P. 178.
5. Nathan, D. G., and Oski, F. A. *Hematology of Infancy and Childhood* (3rd ed.). Philadelphia: Saunders, 1987.

22

Infectious Complications

Preventive Measures in the Immunocompromised Patient
Nancy Collins O'Brien

AVOID EPITHELIAL PENETRATION

Many episodes of illness in the susceptible host can be prevented by adhering to basic guidelines. The most important host defense is the epithelium: skin, respiratory and gastrointestinal epithelium, mucous membranes, and urinary epithelium. The first principle of prevention, therefore, is to avoid penetration of the epithelium. To this end, the following measures should be instituted:

Strict hand washing
No rectal examinations or thermometers
Stool softeners to prevent anal fissures
No bladder catheterization
Cleansing with povidone-iodine (Betadine) preparation before all skin punctures
Minimum blood workup; blood obtained via fingerprick rather than venipuncture whenever possible
Intravenous sites changed every 3 days; IV boards and dressings should be changed daily.
Diligent care of central lines; avoid opening a line more than once daily; continuous infusion with piggyback medications preferable to opening the port multiple times
Mask and gloves worn during lumbar punctures and bone marrow aspirations; gloves changed between procedures

PREVENT NOSOCOMIAL INFECTION

The second principle is to prevent nosocomial infection. The following measures should be instituted:

Strict hand-washing before and after contact with each patient
Gown and gloves worn when handling wounds or infected sites; wounds examined last or gown and gloves changed before touching "clean" areas, intravenous sites, and so on.
Patients with fever of unknown cause, diarrhea, or other infections (especially varicella) isolated

PREVENT SPECIFIC INFECTIONS

The third principle is to prevent specific infections. The following measures should be instituted:

Routine well-child immunizations continued, with the exception of oral polio and measles (live-virus) vaccine
Haemophilus influenzae b (Hib) vaccine given to patients and siblings younger than 4 years
Influenza vaccine administered each year in November; children younger than 12 should receive split virus vaccine rather than whole virus vaccine

Pneumocystis carinii pneumonia prevented by the administration of combined trimethoprim and sulfamethoxazole (5 mg/kg/dose of trimethoprim) 3 times weekly

Tuberculin skin testing of patient and family from areas where tuberculosis is endemic

Passive immunization for exposure to specific viral infections (varicella zoster virus, hepatitis, measles) (see section on Microorganisms Associated with Cancer Patients)

Infections in the Immunocompromised Patient

Robert W. Frenck, Jr.

Infection remains the leading cause of death in patients with cancer, primarily because of alterations in the host's defense mechanisms caused by the underlying disease, effects of therapy, or a combination of these.

GRANULOCYTOPENIA WITH FEVER

An inadequate number of granulocytes is the most important deficiency in the host's defense mechanisms in patients with neoplastic disorders. The risk of infection begins to increase when the absolute neutrophil count (ANC), which is calculated by multiplying the white blood cell count by the number of polymorphonuclear leukocytes plus bands, falls below $500/\mu l$. The risk is considered high (up to 70%) when associated with body temperatures ($> 38.3°C$) if the ANC is less than 100. Therefore, the febrile, granulocytopenic patient requires careful evaluation and treatment.

Evaluation

Patient History

The respiratory tract, skin (especially perirectal area), and mucosal surfaces are the most common sites of infection. Detailed questioning regarding cough, tachypnea, dyspnea, chest pain, skin sores, pain with defecation, pain with swallowing, and sore throat is required. Exposure to infectious diseases, a past history of infections, time of the last chemotherapy, and expected length of time until a normal granulocyte count returns is also important information to collect.

Physical Examination

Although a complete physical examination is required, special attention should be focused on the most frequent sites of infection. Detailed examination of the oropharynx, lungs, and perirectal area is critical. Also, evaluation of the skin—particularly the groin, axillae, and sites of skin disruption (intravenous catheters, bone marrow aspiration, fingerstick, and venipuncture sites)—needs to be performed. Lack of granulocytes frequently alters the inflammatory response of erythema and causes increased warmth, and pain; therefore, the practitioner must be attentive to subtle signs of inflammation. Repeated physical examinations may also be needed if the source of infection was not detected initially.

Laboratory Studies

Because the history and physical examination are often unremarkable, the laboratory evaluation must be broad in scope. Baseline blood tests should include a complete blood cell count, with differential and platelet counts, and determination of blood urea nitrogen, creatinine, serum glutamic oxaloacetic and pyruvic transaminase, and bilirubin levels. A urinalysis and urine culture are also required. (Note that granulocytopenic patients may have a urinary tract infection without white blood cells in the urine.) Aerobic and anaerobic blood cultures from two peripheral sites, or from one peripheral site and from one indwelling venous catheter, are needed.

Radiographic evaluation includes posterior and lateral chest radiographs, even if pneumonia is not suspected, and possibly sinus radiographs. Central nervous system (CNS) infections are uncommon, and so a lumbar puncture is required only if the patient has signs and symptoms suggestive of meningitis. An exception is the patient younger than 18 months old, in whom physical examination is less reliable so that lumbar puncture may be needed to rule out meningitis. Samples from skin lesions should be stained with Gram's stain and Tzanck stain and cultured, or a biopsy should be performed as needed. In addition, possible sites of infection elicited from the history and physical examination (e.g., sore throat, diarrhea, ear pain) should be cultured. Infections in neutropenic patients may be manifest by bleeding instead of pus formation, e.g., hemorrhagic tympanic membrane in otitis media.

Etiologies

There are five primary etiologies of fever in the granulocytopenic patient, and all occur with approximately equal frequency. The five etiologies are (1) bacteremia, (2) microbiologically defined infection without bacteremia, (3) a site of infection without microbiological confirmation, (4) a possible infectious cause (other infectious agents such as fungi, viruses, and parasites should be pursued), and (5) a noninfectious (chemotherapy and the like) or unexplained cause. Approximately 50 percent of bacteremias are caused by gram-negative rods (primarily *Escherichia coli,* and *Klebsiella* and *Pseudomonas* species), the other half being primarily attributable to gram-positive cocci. Knowledge of the common isolates from a practitioner's own institution is important because isolates can vary greatly between institutions.

Treatment

Empiric Therapy

It is well recognized that broad-spectrum antibiotic coverage should be instituted in the febrile, granulocytopenic patient immediately after an initial evaluation is completed, even if a site of infection has not been discovered. Therapy should be directed toward the common isolates from the institution and be synergistic; it should also be minimally toxic.

Multiple drug regimens have been proposed, but none have shown any definite superiority over others [1]. We use a two-drug combination of an aminoglycoside plus a semisynthetic penicillin (e.g., tobramycin plus ticarcillin). In patients receiving nephrotoxic chemotherapy, a third-generation cephalosporin with antipseudomonal activity (ceftazidime or cefoperazone) may be substituted for the aminoglycoside whenever possible [2].

Empiric therapy should be tailored to treat those organisms isolated from cultures of the patient. However, broad-spectrum coverage must be continued until there is resolution of the fever and granulocytopenia, to ensure optimum chances of recovery.

Length of Treatment

Resolution of granulocytopenia and fever is the most common outcome. Ten to fourteen days of antibiotic therapy is usually adequate treatment regardless of the original organism. Sometimes fever resolves but granulocytopenia persists. Continuing therapy for 5 to 7 afebrile days may be sufficient, though some advocate continuing antibiotic coverage until granulocytopenia resolves. If antibiotics are discontinued, the patient must be monitored closely and antimicrobial therapy must be reinstated if fever recurs.

Occasionally, patients remain febrile and granulocytopenic despite broad-spectrum antibiotic therapy. Adding better gram-positive coverage (vancomycin) after 5 days of fever has been recommended in patients at high risk for these infections (e.g., those with indwelling devices) [3]. Also, empiric antifungal therapy should be considered after 7 days of persistent fever since fungal infections are common in this situation and are difficult to diagnose before death.

RESPIRATORY INFECTIONS

Infections of the respiratory tract are the most common infections in the cancer patient. Using results of the chest roentgenogram and peripheral white blood cell count, a logical approach to evaluation and treatment of these patients can be constructed.

Etiologies

The causes of patchy infiltrate in the nongranulocytopenic patient are similar to those in the general population. Viral infections (respiratory syncytial virus and adenovirus) and routine bacterial pathogens (*H. influenzae* and *Streptococcus pneumoniae*) are the most common isolates. Standard antimicrobial therapy for pneumonia (e.g., cefuroxime or ampicillin and chloramphenicol) should be initiated.

In the case of granulocytopenia and a patchy infiltrate, gram-negative rods need to be considered in addition to the above-mentioned organisms. Initial therapy should include an aminoglycoside plus semisynthetic penicillin plus standard therapy. If the patient continues to worsen or is not improving by 72 hours after initiation of therapy, further evaluation (bronchopulmonary lavage, open lung biopsy) is necessary to check for resistant bacteria, fungal infections, or tuberculosis.

Interstitial infiltrate in the nongranulocytopenic patient is most commonly of viral etiology, but *P. carinii* should be considered. Patients with this illness typically have a dry cough, fever, and tachypnea, which later progresses to cyanosis, hypoxia, and respiratory alkalosis. Empiric therapy consists of trimethoprim and sulfamethoxazole. Again, more aggressive evaluation of the patient, including open lung biopsy, is needed if the patient is not responding to treatment by 72 hours or earlier in some patients.

In the granulocytopenic patient, interstitial pneumonia may be caused by gram-positive or gram-negative bacteria, viruses (including cytomegalovirus [CMV]), or *P. carinii*. Therefore, therapy needs to include broad-spectrum antibiotics plus trimethoprim and sulfa-methoxazole. Aggressive, early evaluation is warranted to provide optimum treatment.

Evaluation

Initial evaluation requires obtaining sputum for Gram's staining, acid-fast staining, and culture for bacteria, mycobacteria, *Mycoplasma,* respiratory viruses, *Legionella pneumophila, Chlamydia,* and fungus. Blood cultures and a tuberculin skin test should also be done.

Bronchopulmonary lavage may be performed. Although the yield is only 70 to 75 percent, lavage is a relatively easy and noninvasive procedure. In addition to testing as for sputum, the lavage sample should be submitted for methenamine silver staining, potassium hydroxide preparation, and cytologic evaluation for CMV. Lung aspirate may be of use.

Open lung biopsy is the most invasive and yet most sensitive test. It is warranted for a patient who is deteriorating or not improving by 72 hours after therapy is begun and whose disease cannot be diagnosed by lavage.

CENTRAL VENOUS CATHETER INFECTIONS

Central venous catheter infections have become a common problem because of the frequent use of such devices. Diagnosis is made on the basis of (1) a positive blood culture from the catheter but a negative peripheral culture, (2) a positive culture from both sites and a heavier growth of bacteria from the central line culture, or (3) possibly a positive peripheral blood culture without another source of infection. *Staphylococcus epidermidis* is the most common isolate, requiring treatment with vancomycin.

In a patient who appears to have sepsis or a patient with an infection along the track of the catheter (manifested by purulence from the catheter site or redness along the track), immediate removal of the catheter is recommended. Otherwise, an attempt may be made to treat the infection with the catheter in place. Inability to eradicate the infection, persistent fever after 2 days of appropriate therapy, or clinical worsening of the patient again mandates removal of the catheter. Using these criteria, approximately 70 percent of infections can be treated without removing the catheter.

ESOPHAGITIS

Dysphagia, odynophagia, and retrosternal pain are the classic complaints from patients with esophagitis. *Candida* species and herpes simplex virus (HSV) are the most common infectious agents associated with esophagitis in the immunocompromised host, but occasionally, bacteria (usually gram-positive organisms) have been found to be the cause of infection.

Obtaining a barium esophagogram has been advocated for initial evaluation of the problem. However, a high false-positive rate and an inability to differentiate reliably among infectious etiologies have diminished the usefulness of this test [4]. Flexible endoscopy with esophageal brushings is a procedure with low morbidity and a much higher specificity than barium esophagography. Brushings should be sent for potassium hydroxide wet smear, Papanicolaou's staining, and Gram's staining, plus cultures for fungus, herpesvirus, and bacteria. Empiric therapy can be guided by visual assessment during endoscopy but needs to be adjusted depending on the results of the brushings.

INTESTINAL INFECTIONS

Diarrhea is a common complication of cancer patients and is usually a side effect of chemotherapy. When diarrhea is caused by an infectious agent, the pathogens responsible are typically the same as in the general population. However, immunosuppression and granulocytopenia predispose cancer patients to certain enteric illnesses.

In one study, *Clostridium difficile* was found in the stool of 12 percent of cancer patients, most likely because of repeated antibiotic therapy. Symptomatic diarrhea developed in a majority of these patients within a week. Abdominal pain, fever, and diarrhea, are the classic symptoms, and there is usually a history of antibiotic administration. Diagnosis is confirmed by culturing the organism from the stool and identifying *C. difficile* toxin. The infection typically responds quickly to vancomycin therapy.

Salmonella (especially *S. typhimurium* in patients with the acquired immunodeficiency syndrome [AIDS]) and *Aeromonas* species are other bacteria commonly associated with diarrhea in cancer patients. Three parasites—*Giardia lamblia, Cryptosporidium,* and *Strongyloides stercoralis*—have also been found to be more frequent pathogens in immunocompromised hosts. (For discussion of these organisms, see the section on Microorganisms Associated with Cancer Patients.

Typhlitis is an uncommon illness almost exclusively limited to children with acute lymphoid leukemia and granulocytopenia; it is characterized by a patchy inflammation of the bowel and is usually restricted to the cecum. Fever, abdominal pain, and watery diarrhea are frequently the presenting symptoms. Physical signs of abdominal distention and pain (often the right lower quadrant) and decreased bowel sounds mimic appendicitis. Septicemia, most commonly caused by gram-negative bacteria, occurs in up to 70 percent of the patients. If diagnosis is made early and broad-spectrum antibiotic therapy instituted promptly, surgical removal of the necrotic cecum may be avoided. The granulocytopenic patient tolerates surgery poorly and will have poor wound healing. Antibiotic coverage for *Clostridium septicum* is mandatory [5]. (see Chap. 14).

Microorganisms Associated with Cancer Patients
Robert W. Frenck, Jr.

BACTERIA

Gram-negative enteric bacilli (especially *E. coli, Klebsiella* species, and *Pseudomonas aeruginosa*) continue to represent a large proportion of the pathogens in cancer patients. However, over the past 10 years, in many institutions gram-positive organisms (principally coagulase-negative staphylococci) have become the most common of the bacterial pathogens isolated.

Gram-Negative Bacteria

The common clinical manifestations of gram-negative infections are pneumonia, urinary tract infections, septicemia, perirectal cellulitis, and skin infections, including ecthyma gangrenosum, a necrotizing lesion often associated with *P. aeruginosa*. The combination of an aminoglycoside and semisynthetic penicillin is usually effective against these organisms.

Gram-Positive Bacteria

Cellulitis, osteomyelitis, abscess, and septicemia are common presentations of gram-positive organisms. *Staphylococcus aureus* is a frequent isolate, generally gaining entrance through the skin or an indwelling catheter. Coagulase-negative staphylococci have become pathogens of major importance, usually associated with an existing vascular or CNS catheter. Routine empiric therapy against coagulase-negative staphylococcus does not appear warranted, since delaying initiation of antibiotics until after the organism has been isolated has not caused increased morbidity and the treatment (vancomycin) is extremely costly.

Pneumococcal and group A streptococcal infections are uncommon, but they deserve special attention in the splenectomized patient.

Nocardia Species

The incidence of infection with *Nocardia asteroides* and *Nocardia brasiliensis* is increased in the immunocompromised patient. Although the respiratory tract is the major portal of entry, the organisms may also gain entry through the mouth or skin. Pneumonia is a common presentation, often progressing to consolidation or abscess formation. Hematogenous spread to the brain occurs in approximately 30 percent of patients [6]. The combination of pneumonia and neurologic symptoms should suggest the diagnosis of a *Nocardia* infection.

Mycobacteria

Children with cancer do not seem to be at an increased risk for infection with *Mycobacterium tuberculosis,* although the overall incidence is rising. However, patients with AIDS have been found to be at a significantly increased risk for *M. avium-intracellularis.* Infections may be manifest as generalized lymphadenopathy, pneumonia, diarrhea, and septicemia. Although therapy for this infection includes ansamycin, clofazimine, isoniazid, and ethambutol, the efficacy is questionable.

VIRUS

Children with cancer tolerate many common viral infections with few or no sequelae. Most serious viral infections in the immunocompromised host are caused by the herpesvirus group; HSV, varicella zoster virus (VZV), CMV, and Epstein-Barr virus (EBV).

Herpesviruses

Herpes Simplex Virus

In the normal host, HSV infections are usually mild and self-limited and characterized by vesicular and ulcerative lesions. However, in the immunocompromised host, HSV can cause substantial morbidity and mortality. Lesions resemble those in normal hosts except there are increased numbers and the course is prolonged. Major sites of infection are the oral mucosa, esophagus, skin (localized or generalized as in eczema herpeticum), and eye. Disseminated infections most commonly involve the lung, liver, and CNS [7]. A study of mouth ulcers in cancer patients revealed that 50 percent of these ulcers were caused by HSV, especially if the ulcers occurred on the lip or palate [8]. Diagnosis is often made based on the clinical findings, and it may be confirmed by demonstrating intranuclear inclusions or by growing the virus in culture. The base of vesicles should be scraped to obtain best results for Tzanck staining and culture. Topical acyclovir may be used to treat mild to moderate HSV lesions. Intravenous acyclovir (15–30 mg/kg/day in divided doses every 8 hours) should be used for serious infections. The main complication of acyclovir therapy is precipitation of crystals in the kidney. This can be prevented by good hydration and administration of the drug over a period of at least 1 hour.

Varicella Zoster Virus

Primary exposure to VZV results in chickenpox, usually a self-limited disease that can cause fulminant disease in an immuno-compromised host. Visceral dissemination occurs in up to 32 percent of patients, with a 7 percent mortality [9]. The lung is the most commonly involved organ, and symptoms of lung involvement are fever, dyspnea, and nonproductive cough. Dissemination to the CNS, liver, gastrointestinal tract, and lymph nodes also occurs, especially if the absolute lymphocyte count falls below 500/μl. Diagnosis is based on clinical findings and rarely requires laboratory confirmation.

Herpes zoster represents a reactivation of a prior VZV infection. Patients with altered cellular immunity, primarily Hodgkin's disease, run a much greater risk of developing herpes zoster. The disease is mainly self-limited even in the immunocompromised host, but dissemination occurs in up to 25 percent of these patients [9].

Following exposure to VZV, individuals at risk should receive varicella zoster immune globulin (VZIG) within 96 hours. The dose of VZIG is 12.5 U/kg, with a maximum of 625 U. Also, chemotherapy should be withheld during the incubation period of 21 days. If lesions develop, therapy with intravenous acyclovir should be initiated immediately (30 mg/kg/day in divided doses every 8 hours) and continued for 7 to 10 days [10]. Intravenous acyclovir has also been found to slow the progression, speed healing, and prevent dissemination of zoster lesions. Oral acyclovir (50 mg/kg/day in divided doses 5 times daily) is probably sufficient for mild infections.

Cytomegalovirus

CMV is ubiquitous and can be found in the urine of up to 20 percent of asymptomatic children [6]. Common symptoms include fever, rash, hepatitis, retinitis, esophagitis, colitis, pneumonitis, and CNS abnormalities. A fourfold rise of antibody titer or presence of immunoglobulin M (IgM) against CMV may be diagnostic. Finding cytomegalic cells with large intranuclear inclusions, the classic cellular change of CMV-infected cells on cytologic evaluation, is also indicative of an acute infection. It is possible to culture the virus, but growth may take 3 to 4 weeks. Until recently, treatment of CMV was unsuccessful. However, a new drug, gancyclovir, shows promise for treating CMV retinitis, esophagitis, and colitis [11].

Epstein-Barr Virus

The incidence of EBV infections in patients with lymphoproliferative diseases is approximately double the rate in the general population [12]. Infections are usually mild, manifested by characteristic symptoms of infectious mononucleosis, possibly with increased viral shedding. Specific EBV serology, IgM to EBV capsid antigen (IgM-VCA), IgG-VCA, and antibody to the EBV nuclear antigen may be helpful in determining the presence of an acute EBV infection. To date, no effective therapy is available.

Respiratory Viruses

Respiratory viral infections, including respiratory syncytial virus (RSV), influenza A and B viruses, parainfluenza, and adenovirus, are typically well tolerated by the immunocompromised host. However, viral shedding is prolonged, and cases of severe infections have been reported [13, 14]. Infection with these viruses should be considered in any febrile patient with associated lower respiratory tract symptoms and chest radiographic abnormalities, especially during the winter months. Isolation of these viruses from the pharynx or throat strongly supports an acute infection, often allowing discontinuation of multiple antibiotics. Rapid diagnosis of RSV infections can be made using an indirect fluorescent antibody test.

Treatment of respiratory viral infections had previously been only supportive, but recently, specific therapy has been developed. Amantadine is effective for the prophylaxis and treatment of influenza A virus. To prevent disease, the drug is given every 12 hours (5–8 mg/kg/day, maximum 200 mg/day) during an outbreak. Initiation of amantadine therapy within 48 hours of onset of symptoms will shorten the length and severity of illness. The main toxicity is CNS-related, with symptoms of insomnia, decreased concentration, and fatigue in up to 25 percent of patients. Ribavirin is a broad-spectrum virustatic agent with activity against RSV, influenza A and B, parainfluenza, and adenovirus, but to date it is licensed only for use in RSV pneumonia. Treatment with this medicine should be initiated in patients at high risk (immunodeficient patients or those with underlying heart and lung disease or if a severe infection (hypoxia or cyanosis) develops. Administration of ribavirin is by nebulizer (20 mg of ribavirin per milliliter of water delivered for 12–18 hours/day) to nonintubated patients. Use in intubated patients should be attempted only by experienced personnel because of the possibility of drug precipitation in ventilator tubing. Toxicity appears to be minimal.

Measles (Rubeola)

Rubeola infections are rarely encountered in the United States owing to the high rate of immunization. However, infections in the immunocompromised host can be severe, with up to 30 percent mortality. The two major complications common in an immunocompromised host are giant-cell pneumonia and an atypical encephalitis. If exposed to measles, immunocompromised, seronegative patients should receive IgG (0.5 ml/kg, maximum 15 ml) immediately. Live vaccine should not be given as this may result in severe complications. Treatment of established infections is supportive.

Hepatitis

Hepatitis can occur in cancer patients as a primary infection resulting from hepatitis A, hepatitis B, or non-A, non-B hepatitis virus, or as a secondary infection caused by EBV, CMV, HSV, or toxoplasmosis. The term *viral hepatitis* is commonly used to refer to infections caused by the first three agents.

Hepatitis A is caused by a 27-nm RNA virus with an average incubation period of 30 days, ranging from 15 to 50 days. The period of greatest infectivity is during the 2 weeks before jaundice occurs. Transmission is through the fecal-oral route. Viremia is of short duration, and so transmission by blood is rare. The clinical illness has an abrupt onset of fever, malaise, anorexia, nausea, and abdominal discomfort. In children, most infections are asymptomatic and not accompanied by jaundice. Diagnosis is made by the finding of antihepatitis A IgM in the patient's serum. Immune globulin given within 2 weeks of exposure is protective against developing infection.

Hepatitis B is caused by a 42-nm DNA virus with an average incubation period of 60 to 90 days, ranging from 45 to 160 days after exposure. The disease is transmitted by contact with contaminated blood products or by absorption through mucosal surfaces of infected secretions, such as saliva or semen. The onset of disease is insidious and may include anorexia, malaise, nausea, vomiting, abdominal pain, arthralgia, and jaundice. Diagnosis of an acute or chronic infection is made through serologic measurement of hepatitis B surface antigen (HB_sAg), "e" antigen (HB_eAg), and their antibodies. Patients should be considered infectious as long as HB_sAg is present. Treatment consists of hepatitis B immune globulin (HBIG), which should be administered immediately if the patient has had percutaneous or mucosal exposure to bodily fluids of persons known to have hepatitis B. If the HB_sAg status is unknown, the exposed person should receive immune globulin pending results of the HB_sAg test. If a donor is found to be HB_sAg-positive, then the patient receiving the donor's blood products should receive HBIG. In the patient at risk for repetitive exposure to hepatitis B, hepatitis B vaccine series should be initiated along with administration of HBIG (0.06 ml/kg intramuscularly, repeated in 1 month; minimum dose is 0.5 ml).

Non-A, non-B hepatitis is probably caused by at least two different agents. No laboratory tests are available to confirm the diagnosis, so this illness becomes a diagnosis of exclusion in patients receiving blood products. No specific recommendations have been made with regard to prophylaxis, but it is reasonable to apply the recommendations for prophylaxis against hepatitis A.

FUNGI

Invasive fungal infections are a cause of morbidity and mortality in increasing numbers of immunocompromised patients. Most fungal infections occur in patients with hematologic malignancies, especially acute leukemia. Granulocytopenia, glucocorticoid administration, broad-spectrum antibiotic therapy, and indwelling vascular catheters are also predisposing factors for fungal infections. Hyperglycemia and preexisting tissue damage have also been associated with an increased incidence of *Aspergillus* infections. *Candida* and *Aspergillus* species are the cause of most fungal infections in cancer patients, but *Cryptococcus* infection is prevalent among patients with altered cellular immunity, such as Hodgkin's disease.

Specific Fungi

Candida *Species*

The gastrointestinal tract and bloodstream are the major sites of primary infection by *Candida* organisms. Once disseminated, *Candida* can infect any organ, but the liver, lungs, meninges, eyes, heart, and kidneys are the most commonly involved [15]. Diagnosis is difficult because of nonspecific signs and symptoms and a low percentage of positive blood cultures (30–50 percent), even in autopsy-proved cases of disseminated disease [16]. Infection should be considered if *Candida* is cultured from a closed body space or multiple body sites of individuals at high risk.

The significance of *Candida* isolated from indwelling vascular catheters is controversial [16]. Many advocate that removal of the catheter is sufficient treatment, whereas others recommend catheter removal plus a 2-week course of therapy with amphotericin B in an attempt to prevent dissemination. Another issue regards isolation of *Candida* from the urine. When associated with an indwelling urinary catheter, this finding usually represents local disease and can be treated with catheter removal and a short course of amphotericin B. However, if there is no history of a urinary catheter being used, a positive urine culture may represent disseminated disease.

Aspergillus *Species*

Aspergillus are ubiquitous organisms that primarily cause respiratory illness; infections disseminate in approximately 30 percent of immunocompromised hosts [6]. The organisms have a propensity for invading blood vessels, causing thrombosis and infarction. Thus, in patients at risk for fungal infections who develop multiple thrombi or evidence of pulmonary embolism, the diagnosis of *Aspergillus* needs to be considered. *Aspergillus* may also cause hemorrhagic bronchopneumonia, pulmonary cavitation with fungal balls and, occasionally, a rhinocerebral infection with involvement of the sinuses progressing into the nose, palate, and base of the skull. Again, diagnosis is difficult since *Aspergillus* is infrequently cultured from the sputum or is a common sputum contaminant in the normal host. However, if the organism is cultured from an immunocompromised host, it should be considered evidence of infection and therapy should be initiated.

Cryptococcus *Species*

The lungs are the site of primary infection by *Cryptococcus* organisms and, in normal hosts, the infection may resolve without therapy. Patients with altered cell-mediated immunity often have dissemination, with the CNS being the most frequent site of distal infection. Patients complain of headache, vertigo, nausea, and vomiting. Physical findings consist of fever, nuchal rigidity, stupor, focal neurologic abnormalities, and evidence of increased intracranial pressure. Cerebrospinal fluid examination will show an elevated white blood cell count (lymphocyte predominance), elevated protein level, and low glucose level. The India ink test is positive in 60 percent of patients [17]. Cryptococcal antigen assay is a very sensitive test that can aid in diagnosing this infection.

Therapy

Multiple drugs are available for treating fungal infections. However, amphotericin B is the most effective drug for susceptible organisms, although it is associated with multiple side effects. Most patients experience transient chills, rigors, and fever during amphotericin B administration. These symptoms can often be prevented by pretreating with diphenhydramine and acetaminophen and adding 25 to 50 mg of hydrocortisone to the infusion mixture. The kidneys are the main target of injury. Azotemia and hypokalemia are common findings. Elevation of the serum creatinine often occurs with prolonged amphotericin B administration and may necessitate dose reduction. Anemia may also develop when the drug is used for more than 30 days.

A test dose of 0.1 mg/kg (maximum 1.0 mg) should be administered and the patient closely monitored for anaphylaxis or other adverse reactions. If no major problems develop, the patient should be given 0.5 mg/kg/day of amphotericin B. Although this dose is usually sufficient for the treatment of most *Candida* infections, *Aspergillus* infections require a higher dose, up to 1.0 mg/kg/day. The total dose of amphotericin B varies depending on the infection, but a range of 20 to 30 mg/kg appears to be sufficient in most instances [6]. *Aspergillus* infections also often require surgical intervention with resection of large fungal balls and debridement of necrotic tissue.

Resolution of granulocytopenia and the underlying immunocompromised state seems to be the most important factor for eradicating fungal diseases.

PARASITES

Pneumocystis carinii

P. carinii is a protozoan parasite of global distribution. Antibody to *P. carinii* is present in nearly 100 percent of normal children, which indicates that most infections in cancer patients are a reactivation of latent organisms. Although children with leukemia are at greatest risk, it may also be seen in those with solid tumors or after bone marrow transplantation. An interstitial pneumonia is the most common infection. Patients typically present with fever, cough, retractions, and tachypnea. The chest radiograph generally has diffuse hazy infiltrates but may be atypical, with lobar consolidation.

Trimethoprim and sulfamethoxazole in combination is the primary antibiotic treatment (20 mg/kg/day of TMP). However, if patients with documented *P. carinii* infection are not responding after 48 to 72 hours, they may benefit from pentamidine therapy instead (see the section on respiratory infection).

Toxoplasmosis

Toxoplasma gondii is an intracellular parasite acquired by ingesting cyst-containing meat or oocysts in cat excreta. As with *P. carinii*, most infections are reactivations of a previous illness. The CNS is the principal organ affected by toxoplasmosis, with necrotizing encephalitis of the gray matter being the most common finding. The disease is particularly prevalent in AIDS patients and is a major cause of encephalitis in this population. Signs and symptoms reflect the CNS involvement. The diagnosis depends on histologic confirmation or serologic findings. The Sabin-Feldman dye test is the standard serologic test, although measuring IgM against *Toxoplasma* has begun to replace it. Therapy consists of pyrimethamine plus sulfadiazene. The optimum duration of therapy has not been determined but many patients receive treatment for 1 year or longer.

Strongyloides Species

Strongyloides stercoralis is an intestinal nematode that infects a large portion of the world's population, expecially in Asia. Infections are usually asymptomatic and may persist for decades. However, in an immunocompromised host, particularly one who is receiving corticosteroids, the hyperinfection syndrome may develop [18], in which the noninvasive rhabdoid larvae transform to filiform larvae and then burrow through the intestinal wall into the bloodsteam and migrate to the lungs. Patients often complain of abdominal distention, fever, and diarrhea, along with cough, wheezes, and hemoptysis. Additionally, the syndrome is frequently associated with gram-negative bacteremia, presumably from bacteria leaking through the defect in the intestine. Immunosuppressed patients from an endemic area who exhibit such symptoms plus persistent bacteremia should be evaluated for strongyloidiasis. Diagnosis is made by isolating larvae from the stool or duodenum. Treatment consists of administering thiobendazole for 5 to 7 days, although longer courses of therapy may be required.

Cryptosporidia

Cryptosporidia are protozoan parasites that infect the gastrointestinal tract of many species of mammals. Normal hosts can be infected from close contact with animals and develop a self-limited diarrheal illness. Immunocompromised patients usually have a more severe course, with diarrhea persisting for months to years and resulting in malnutrition. Diagnosis is based on demonstration of cryptosporidial cysts in the stool. No specific therapy is available, and termination of the infection is most likely dependent on resolution of the immunosuppression.

REFERENCES

1. Wade, J. C., Johnson, D. E., and Bustamonte, C. I. Monotherapy for empiric treatment of fever in granulocytopenic cancer patients. *Am. J. Med.* 80(Suppl. 5C):85, 1986.
2. Pizzo, P. A., et al. A randomized trial comparing ceftazidime alone with combination antibiotic therapy in cancer patients with fever and neutropenia. *N. Engl. J. Med.* 315:552, 1986.
3. Rubin, M., et al. Gram-positive infections and the use of vancomycin in 550 episodes of fever and neutropenia. *Ann. Intern. Med.* 108:30, 1988.
4. Wheeler, R. R., et al. Esophagitis in the immunocompromised host: Role of esophagoscopy in diagnosis. *Rev. Infect. Dis.* 9:88, 1987.
5. Alpern, R. J., and Dowell, V. R., Jr. *Clostridium septicum* infections and malignancy. *J.A.M.A.* 209:385, 1969.
6. Pizzo, P. A. Infectious complications in the child with cancer. *J. Pediatr.* 98:341, 1981.
7. Wong, K. K., and Hirsch, M.S. Herpesvirus infections in patients with neoplastic disorders. *Am. J. Med.* 76:464, 1984.
8. Greenberg, M. S., et al. Oral herpes simplex infections in patients with leukemia. *J.A.M.A.* 114:483, 1987.

9. Feldman, S., Hughes, W. T., and Daniel, C. B. Varicella in children with cancer: Seventy-five cases. *Pediatrics* 56:388, 1975.

10. Whitley, R. J., et al. Vidarabine therapy of varicella in immunocompromised patients. *J. Pediatr.* 101:125, 1982.

11. Jacobson, M. A., and Mills, J. Serious cytomegalovirus disease in the acquired immunedeficiency syndrome (AIDS). *Ann. Intern. Med.* 108:585, 1988.

12. Sumaya, C. V. Epstein-Barr virus infection: The expanded spectrum. *Adv. Pediatr. Infect. Dis.* 1:75, 1986.

13. Rivkin, M. J., and Aronoff, S. C. Pulmonary infections in the immunocompromised child. *Adv. Pediatr. Infect. Dis.* 2:161, 1987.

14. Rosenow, E. C., Wilson, W. L., and Cockerill, F. R. Pulmonary diseases in the immunocompromised host. *Mayo Clin. Proc.* 76:473, 1984.

15. Gold, J. W. Opportunistic fungal infections in patients with neoplastic disease. *Am. J. Med.* 76:458, 1984.

16. Hawkins, C., and Armstrong, D. Fungal infections in the immunocompromised host. *Clin. Haematol.* 13:599, 1984.

17. Musial, C. E., Cockerill, F. R., and Roberts, G. D. Fungal infections of the immunocompromised host: Clinical and laboratory aspects. *Clin. Microbiol. Rev.* 1:349, 1988.

18. Wong, B. Parasitic diseases in immunocompromosed hosts. *Am. J. Med.* 76:479, 1984.

SELECTED READINGS

Basson, W. J., and Brady, M. T. Management of infections in children with cancer. *Hematol. Oncol. Clin. North Am.* 1:801, 1987.

Culbert, S. J., and Pickering, L. K. Principles of Total Care—Physiologic Support. In W. W. Sutow, D. J. Fernbach, and T. J. Vietti (eds.), *Clinical Pediatric Oncology* (3rd ed.). St. Louis: Mosby, 1984. P. 267.

23

Endocrine System Complications

Robert N. Marshall

Most endocrine problems that arise in children as a consequence of a malignant disease and its treatment will be basically similar to the same conditions in otherwise healthy children. There are some differences, however, that may influence the choice of diagnostic studies and the type of treatment selected. In this chapter, the endocrine disorders most likely to be encountered are discussed, with suggestions concerning their management.

HYPERGLYCEMIA

Elevated blood glucose levels may occur under a variety of circumstances. Important considerations are detection, etiology, and treatment options.

Detection

Abnormal carbohydrate metabolism can be identified easily, using one or more of the following tests.

Urine Dipsticks

Glycosuria usually indicates that the blood glucose level has risen above the renal threshold for reabsorption (160–180 mg/dl for most children with normal renal function) for some period of time since the last voiding. Clinically evident polyuria is not usually present until blood glucose values in excess of 300 mg/dl have been present long enough to create an osmotic diuresis. The presence of urine ketones with glycosuria indicates a more severe degree of impaired glucose utilization than glycosuria alone. Isolated ketonuria is most often associated with inadequate carbohydrate intake or some other catabolic state.

Blood Glucose

Since normal glucose levels are variable, it is important to note the time at and conditions under which the specimen was obtained. Specimens taken during fasting (normal < 120 mg/dl) and 2 hours after a meal (normal < 140 mg/dl) are helpful reference points to identify the degree of hyperglycemia if it is present. Whole blood glucose values are approximately 15 percent lower than serum or plasma levels on the same specimen. If capillary blood is tested with disposable test strips, meticulous attention must be paid to technique details. Oral and intravenous glucose tolerance tests are rarely needed, except under special circumstances to identify subtle degrees of altered glucose metabolism.

Glycohemoglobin

The glycohemoglobin test is an excellent one for determining whether clinically significant hyperglycemia has been occurring regularly during the preceding weeks or months. Results will be altered by conditions that affect red blood cell turnover, such as hemorrhage, transfusions, and hemolysis. Some methods may be affected by hemoglobinopathies.

Etiology and Management

Most hyperglycemic states encountered in pediatric oncology patients are the result of insulin insensitivity rather than diminished insulin secretion. Pharmacologic doses of glucocorticoids are the most frequently encountered cause of glucose intolerance. (A primary adrenal or pituitary tumor causing Cushing's syndrome will rarely induce similar hyperglycemia.) In most patients, it will be mild and transient, requiring no specific treatment except temporary diet modification. It can be severe, however, and persist after the steroids have been discontinued. This is more likely if there is a strong family history of diabetes. There is usually sufficient residual insulin activity to prevent ketonuria, and laboratory documentation of the resistance by an elevated insulin level is helpful to distinguish this type of glucose intolerance from insulinopenic diabetes. Treatment with exogenous insulin is indicated if fasting blood glucose values exceed 150 mg/dl, postprandial values are in excess of 200 mg/dl, or if the treatment associated with the high glucose values will continue for more than a few weeks. However, some patients are very difficult to manage if tight glucose control is attempted. In this case it may be appropriate to restrict glucose and decrease the prednisone dose, and reserve insulin use for patients with ketosis or a glucose in excess of 500 mg/dl. Because of the insensitivity to insulin, relatively high doses of insulin may be necessary to restore normal glucose levels. A test dose of 0.25 U/kg of regular insulin, given subcutaneously before a meal, can be used to estimate insulin sensitivity. If there is minimal or no change in the glucose level within 4 to 6 hours, the total daily dose needed is probably greater than 1.0 U/kg/day. Treatment can usually be managed with NPH or Lente insulin alone, without regular insulin. However, regular insulin is appropriate in patients whose insulin needs are changing rapidly. If there is minimal fasting hyperglycemia, a single morning dose often is sufficient. Oral hypoglycemic agents have not been shown to be effective.

L-Asparaginase affects both pancreas and liver and can cause hyperglycemia. This effect is exacerbated by the concomitant use of steroids for remission induction in leukemia and may be more difficult to manage.

Transient hyperglycemia can occur after severe physiologic stress or during rapid hydration with glucose-containing intravenous fluids. Temporary glucose intolerance may also be seen while refeeding patients who have been in negative caloric balance for several days or weeks. An insulin-deficient diabetic state is sometimes encountered in patients who develop pancreatic toxicity from L-asparaginase therapy. Management of these patients is similar to that of children with type I diabetes.

HYPOGLYCEMIA

Detection

Hypoglycemia should be suspected in certain clinical situations, particlarly if suggestive symptoms occur. Most episodes consist of signs of the catecholamine response: pallor, sweating, tachycardia, tremor, dilated pupils, and so on. Altered behavior and consciousness occur as the blood glucose level drops lower, depriving the brain of adequate substrate. Convulsions are a late manifestation and are of particular concern because they may create additional demands for glucose and oxygen that are already limited.

Etiology

A drop in blood glucose level should be anticipated whenever intravenous glucose is abruptly discontinued, particularly the higher concentrations used in parenteral nutrition formulas. Malnourished patients and those with massive tumors are at risk. Insulin-secreting tumors are rarely encountered in children beyond the neonatal period. Patients with adrenal insufficiency and those with pituitary deficits (especially growth hormone and adrenocorticotropic hormone [ACTH] deficiency) are prone to hypoglycemia caused by postprandial decreased glucose production. Occasionally, severe liver disease, such as a fulminant hepatitis, may induce hypoglycemia. Among the list of drugs that may cause a low blood glucose level, salicylates are the most likely to be involved in this age group. Factitious hypoglycemia can be caused by extreme leukocytosis if the cells are not promptly separated from the serum or plasma.

Treatment

Treatment consists of oral or intravenous glucose support until the etiology can be identified and corrected. In a conscious patient who can eat or drink, in most cases a small amount of milk or juice will relieve symptoms within 5 to 10 minutes. Intravenous glucose at a rate of 3 to 7 mg/kg/minute is sufficient to maintain normal glucose levels except in situations such as hyperinsulinism in which there is increased utilization of glucose. In an emergency, glucose gel applied to the oral mucous membranes will correct most hypoglycemic episodes in an unconscious patient if venous access is compromised. Bedside glucose monitoring is particularly helpful to follow these patients since information on a single drop of capillary blood can be obtained immediately.

SYNDROME OF INAPPROPRIATE ANTIDIURETIC HORMONE SECRETION

Etiology

The syndrome of inappropriate antidiuretic hormone secretion (SIADH) is a condition in which antidiuretic hormone (ADH) secretion persists despite hypotonic plasma. Antineoplastic drugs, such as vincristine and cyclophosphamide, are a recognized cause of SIADH. It may also occur following cerebral injury caused by infection, abscess, or hemorrhage. SIADH commonly follows surgical intervention for craniopharyngiomas or midbrain tumors. Diabetes insipidus is often present for the first 3 to 5 postoperative days, but SIADH can abruptly supervene as ADH begins to leak from damaged cells. Other causes of this syndrome include pulmonary disease, anesthesia, and some pain relief medications.

Detection

Clinical symptoms are related to fluid retention and eventual water intoxication. Early symptoms, such as headache, irritability, muscle weakness, and loss of appetite, are nonspecific and frequently difficult to distinguish in the presence of the precipitating condition. As the process becomes more severe, patients become nauseated and confused and begin to have seizures. If not recognized and managed appropriately, SIADH can be fatal. Anticipation and prevention are particularly desirable to avoid the complications of this disorder.

The characteristic findings in SIADH include the following:

1. Hyponatremia and hypoosmolarity
2. Absence of volume depletion
3. Concentrated urine relative to plasma
4. Continued urinary excretion of sodium (urine sodium > 30 mEq/ liter)
5. Normal renal and adrenal function
6. Absence of edema, weight loss, hypotension, dehydration, or hypokalemia
7. Improvement of hyponatremia and urine sodium loss by fluid restriction

Low levels of blood urea nitrogen and uric acid are common findings that are not characteristic of other causes of hyponatremia. This syndrome must be distinguished from other common causes of hyponatremia, such as adrenal insufficiency, salt depletion caused by diarrhea and vomiting, hypercalcemia, and osmotic losses from tumor lysis.

Treatment

Treatment consists of restriction of fluid and elimination of the underlying disorder where possible. In extreme, life-threatening cases, infusion of 5 to 10 ml/kg of 3% saline and administration of furosemide has been recommended to promote a rise in the serum sodium concentration and a water diuresis. In the absence of severe neurologic symptoms, a more gradual correction is preferred.

HYPOTHALAMIC-PITUITARY DEFICIENCIES

The pituitary gland is vulnerable to damage by certain tumors, irradiation, and surgical trauma. The hypothalamus is necessary for normal pituitary function, and a variety of clinical disorders can arise from injury to one or both of these important structures. Growth hormone (GH) secretion appears to be the most sensitive to these insults, followed by gonadotropin regulation and secretion; ACTH and thyroid-stimulating hormone (TSH) are relatively more resistant to damage. Surgical trauma is more likely to affect ADH secretion by the posterior pituitary gland than a primary hypothalamic-pituitary tumor or irradiation. Prolactin is different from the other pituitary hormones in that the hypothalamus has an inhibitory effect on its secretion rather than a stimulatory one. For this reason, elevated prolactin levels can be a useful marker of hypothalamic disorders that leave the pituitary intact.

The type and extent of radiation damage on the secretion of pituitary hormones depends on the total dose received by the hypothalamic and pituitary areas and the duration of the course of treatments. A series of treatments spread over 6 weeks will be less likely to affect pituitary function than a similar radiation dose given to the same areas during a shorter period of time. As a general guide, pituitary deficiencies are a common occurrence when cranial radiation doses of 25 Gy (1 gray = 100 rad) or more are administered, and deficits become probable at levels greater than 40 Gy. High-dose, more intense regimens of radiotherapy may cause immediate pituitary deficits, but the more commonly used dosage schedules may inflict damage that may not affect hormone secretion for several years. Because of this relatively long latency period, the history and clinical examination are the best guides to the need for laboratory testing to detect pituitary problems.

Growth Hormone Disorders

Since GH is most commonly affected, growth rates should be calculated from careful measurements of the child's height at each visit and compared with standard growth velocity charts. Serial plots of heights are also important, but this is a less sensitive way to detect early growth failure. Spinal irradiation may have an effect on growth independent of pituitary GH secretion. Similarly, the more temporary and reversible effects of chemotherapy and glucocorticoids on growth need to be considered before assuming that pituitary problems are responsible. In children who are well nourished and older than 4 years, somatomedin C (insulinlike growth factor I) levels are a useful screening tool. It is also helpful to obtain a radiograph of the left hand and wrist for bone age analysis to determine whether the characteristic delay in skeletal maturity is present and to estimate remaining height potential. Hypothyroidism needs to be ruled out or treated before reliable testing of GH secretion can be done. A single random level of serum GH is useless. Confirmation of suspected GH deficiency requires at least two separate stimulation tests of GH secretion. Even standard testing may fail to detect subtle hypothalamic defects in GH regulation (neurosecretory GH deficiency), and a therapeutic trial of treatment with biosynthetic GH may be necessary to establish this diagnosis when it is strongly suspected.

Other Types of Hypothalmic-Pituitary Dysfunction

Other types of hypothalamic-pituitary dysfunction can also be inferred from clincial symptoms. Central nervous system lesions and their treatment are associated with both precocious puberty and delayed or absent puberty. Early breast development in girls (before age 8) or testicular enlargement in boys (before age 9) may be amenable to suppression with analogs of the gonadotropin-releasing hormone. Inhibition of early puberty often is necessary to prevent early epiphyseal closure and secondary short stature. This is particularly important if GH or TSH deficiency is also present and contributing to growth failure. On the other hand, gonadotropin deficiency can cause absent, delayed, or incomplete pubertal development, depending on the area and degree of damage. This needs to be considered whenever pubertal development has not started by age 13 years in girls or 14 years in boys. Stimulation testing with gonadotropin-releasing hormone is more helpful than single, randomly drawn levels of luteinizing hormone (LH) and follicle-stimulating hormone (FSH). It is sometimes difficult to distinguish between gonadotropin deficiency and constitutional delay as the cause of delayed puberty in adolescents, particularly in males, in whom the latter is relatively common. In boys with constitutional delay, normal pubertal progression is often "triggered" by a short, 3-month course of testosterone injections. Treatment of gonadotropin deficiency consists of gradually increasing doses of androgens or estrogens over a period of 2 to 3 years to achieve full secondary sexual development. (Even after many years of such treatment, it is often possible to achieve normal testicular and ovarian activity with fertility by switching to more complex regimens of gonadotropin-releasing hormone infusion or frequent injections of gonadotropins.) Bone age radiographs should be obtained at intervals to ensure that skeletal maturation does not exceed gains in height age, so that nearly full growth potential is achieved. CNS leukemia can result in hyperpituitarism responsive to intrathecal chemotherapy or radiotherapy. Precocious puberty is occasionally seen in acute lymphoid leukemia.

ACTH Deficiency

ACTH deficiency is characterized by complaints of weakness, fatigue, arthralgia, anorexia, abdominal pain, and vomiting. Symptoms are most likely to be present at times of stress, such as in infectious illness or trauma. If the deficiency is severe and uncorrected, hypotension and shock can occur. A morning cortisol level (preferably obtained by 8:00 A.M.) or a cortisol value obtained during acute stress that is less than 15 μg/dl is suggestive of adrenal insufficiency. An ACTH stimulation test may be needed to determine whether the defect is adrenal or at the pituitary level. The ACTH deficiency may be iatrogenic, following long periods of suppression by high doses of glucocorticoid treatment. This is an uncommon problem in children who have been treated for 6 weeks or less. Nonetheless, it is wise to give children who have been on suppressive doses of glucocorticoids for a month or more supplements of glucocorticoids before operations, before stressful procedures, and during severe illnesses until steroid treatment has been discontinued for 1 year. Physiologic oral replacement doses of hydrocortisone are 8 to 12 mg/sq m/day, divided into two or more doses. A larger morning dose is usually given to simulate the normal diurnal rhythm of secretion. A twofold or threefold increase is sufficient to cover stressful situations. When vomiting prevents oral steroid treatment or when an adrenal crisis is suspected, rapid correction is needed with at least 10 mg/kg/day of hydrocortisone sodium succinate (Solu-Cortef) given intravenously or intramuscularly.

Hypothyroidism

Excessive sleep requirements, weight gain despite lack of appetite, cold intolerance, and constipation are some of the common symptoms among children with hypothyroidism. Secondary (pituitary) and tertiary (hypothalamic) hypothyroidism are indicated when both thyroxine (T_4) and TSH levels are low. If a triiodothyronine (T_3) resin uptake level is not also low or at the low end of normal, hypoproteinemia or a low thyroid-binding globulin level should be suspected rather than TSH deficiency. Secondary hypothyroidism can be distinguished from tertiary by an absent TSH response to thyrotropin-releasing hormone. The prolactin response to thyrotropin-releasing hormone can also be measured to gain additional information about hypothalamic or pituitary damage. A single daily dose of 1.5 to 2.0 μg/kg of synthetic L-thyroxine (e.g., Synthroid, Levothroid) is usually sufficient replacement for hypothyroidism. Slightly higher doses are needed in infants and very young children.

Diabetes Insipidus

Diabetes insipidus usually presents with obvious symptoms of excessive thirst and urination with nocturia or enuresis. The urine remains clear in color throughout the day. Tumors of the hypothalamus, surgical trauma, histiocytosis, and CNS leukemia are the usual causes among pediatric oncology patients. If a central nervous system lesion also affects the centers for thirst regulation, severe hypernatremic dehydration can occur, and treatment may be very difficult to regulate. Unless the patient is severely dehydrated, urine specific gravity usually remains lower than 1.010 (< 300 mOsm/liter). Serum osmolarity is slightly increased in most cases, and the plasma ADH level will be inappropriately low for the osmolarity. In partial diabetes insipidus, a water deprivation test may be needed to establish diagnostic criteria and to rule out other causes of polyuria. The drug of choice for hormone replacement is 1-desamino-8-D-arginine vasopressin or DDAVP, which can be given by nasal insufflation in one or two daily doses. To avoid water intoxication, successive doses should not be given until a brief diuresis has occurred. By giving a dose at bedtime, sleep disturbance by nocturia can be avoided. The usual dose of 1.25 to 5.0 μg will usually achieve rapid urinary concentration which lasts approximately 8 to 24 hours in most patients. In patients with partial diabetes insipidus, chlorpropamide may be used to enhance the effect of the limited ADH that remains, and it may also improve the sense of thirst in some patients with hypodipsia.

OVARIAN AND TESTICULAR DYSFUNCTION

The gonads are susceptible to damage by both chemotherapy and irradiation. The prepubertal gonad is much more resistant to these insults than pubertal ovaries and testicles. Cyclophosphamide, chlorambucil, and busulfan are some of the drugs that commonly affect gonadal function. Recovery is sometimes seen after several years of hypofunction. Mature testicles may be damaged with as little as 5 to 10 Gy of irradiation, but ovaries appear to be less sensitive, with dysfunction becoming evident at two to three times this dose. The seminiferous tubules and fertility are usually lost before Leydig cell destruction occurs or testosterone production ceases. A decrease in testicular volume is usually evident. The testicles are a common site of relapse in leukemia, and the radiation doses used to treat this complication cause almost total destruction of the testicle, even in prepubertal boys. Because of their location, the ovaries are more likely to be included in the irradiation field for common abdominal tumors. A variety of clinical consequences may follow, from minor menstrual irregularities to primary amenorrhea, depending on the radiation dosage and activity of the glands. By age 10 to 12 years, LH and FSH values become elevated if extensive gonadal damage has been sustained. In younger children, and in lesser degrees of gonadal injury, a gonadotropin-releasing hormone stimulation test may be needed to show abnormally elevated gonadotropins. As with gonadotropin deficiency, these patients are given androgens or estrogens at the appropriate age to create a normal time sequence of pubertal progression.

HYPOTHYROIDISM

It is sometimes necessary to remove nearly all or part of the thyroid gland to remove various types of thyroid tumors. A single lobe is often sufficient to maintain normal thyroid function. Large doses of radiation to the neck can also reduce the amount of functioning tissue. The normal thyroid gland is relatively radioresistant, but iodides and some types of iodide-containing contrast agents may increase the thyroid gland's susceptibility to radiation damage.

Normal T_4 levels may be maintained by an increase in TSH secretion. In such cases of compensated hypothyroidism, chronic hyperstimulation of the remaining gland may predispose it to adenoma formation. Although such patients may be clinically euthyroid, thyroid replacement is advisable in these patients with sustained elevations of TSH. The goals of treatment are to suppress the TSH level to the normal range of 1 to 5 μU/ml and to keep the patient free of hypothyroid or thyrotoxic symptoms. The target range of serum T_4 for most patients who have average levels of thyroid-binding proteins is usually 8 to 12 μg/dl. If more than 3.0 μg/kg/day of L-thyroxine is needed to achieve TSH suppression in school-age children, noncompliance with treatment should be suspected. If overtreatment is suspected, highly sensitive assays of TSH are available on special request in most laboratories; these assays will detect TSH values of less than 0.5 μU/ml, which indicate excessive dosage if normal pituitary function is present.

24

Neurologic Complications

Seizures

Roberta A. Gottlieb

MANAGEMENT

Management of generalized status epilepticus involves the following immediate steps:

1. Clear the airway and suction, supply oxygen, and provide glucose. Start an intravenous line, and draw blood to check the metabolic parameters, especially glucose.

2. Lorazepam (0.05–0.15 mg/kg intravenously) or diazepam (0.1–0.3 mg/kg IV) should be infused at a rate no faster than 1 mg/minute. The maximum diazepam dose is 10 mg intravenously for children older than 5 years. Lorazepam is longer-acting and causes more sedation, whereas diazepam is short-acting and causes respiratory depression.

   Be prepared to intubate the patient. Lorazepam and diazepam should be used with great caution or avoided in children already on other anticonvulsants such as phenobarbital. These drugs cannot be given through a central venous catheter. If there is no intravenous access, administer diazepam rectally (cut the needle off a butterfly infusion set); absorption occurs within 5 minutes.

3. Phenytoin sodium (Dilantin) is provided in a loading dose of 10 to 15 mg/kg intravenously at a rate slower than 1 mg/kg/minute. Infusion over more than 30 minutes is preferable if lorazepam or diazepam have controlled the seizure. Dilute the Dilantin in normal saline, *not* dextrose (in which it will precipitate). This drug cannot be given through a central venous catheter. Hypotension and cardiac arrhythmias may occur; so the patient must be monitored during infusion. Absorption by the intramuscular route is slow and erratic.

   The goal is to achieve a trough blood level of 10 to 25 μg/ml. The maintenance dose is 4 to 7 mg/kg/day intravenously or orally once or twice daily. Dosage increases of 1 mg/kg/day should increase the trough blood level approximately 3 μg/ml. One may start with a small oral or intravenous bolus each time the dose is increased.

   Nystagmus on primary gaze may occur if the blood level exceeds 20 μg/ml; ataxia is sometimes seen at levels exceeding 30 μg/ml; and dysarthria and lethargy are seen at levels greater than 40 μg/ml. Blood level rises are nonlinear.

4. A loading dose of phenobarbital (15 mg/kg) is given at a rate of 100 mg/minute. In most cases, the patient can be given one ampule (135 mg) and observed; if the seizure persists, this approach may be repeated. Phenobarbital may be given intravenously or intramuscularly. It causes respiratory depression and sedation, especially if it is administered by intravenous push or with diazepam.

   The goal is a blood level of 20 to 45 μg/ml. The maintenance dose is 5 mg/kg/day intravenously or orally once or twice daily. Dosage increases of 1 mg/kg/day should increase the blood level by 5 μg/ml. One may start with a small bolus each time the dose is increased.

Excessive somnolence or coma may be seen at a blood level in excess of 50 μg/ml.

ETIOLOGY

Determination of the etiology of seizures should be pursued vigorously while therapy is under way.

1. Test glucose, electrolyte, calcium, and magnesium levels and correct any abnormalities. Hyponatremia due to SIADH can be caused by vincristine.
2. Obtain a baseline blood cell count, blood urea nitrogen, and creatinine level for each patient. Blood cultures, too, should be drawn, and antibiotic therapy instituted in patients at risk. Remember that a coagulopathy resulting in intracranial hemorrhage or infarct may be caused by L-asparaginase treatment.
3. In the case of a patient who is already on chronic anticonvulsants who presents with seizures, assume the anticonvulsant levels are in a moderate range.
4. Consider drug-induced seizures, particularly in patients receiving high-dose methotrexate.
5. Evaluate the patient for possible increased intracranial pressure.

FAILED MANAGEMENT

Failure to control seizures with these measures should prompt early consultation with a neurologist. Continue the supportive measures of oxygen and glucose supply and intubate the patient if necessary.

Other miscellaneous agents used to treat seizures are as follows:

Paraldehyde, 0.15 to 0.3 ml/kg intramuscularly, with the dose split between two sites; alternate routes are intravenously or per rectum. Paraldehyde dissolves plastic tubing, so it should be mixed in a glass syringe with an equal volume of mineral oil to give per rectum. The dose may be repeated in 1 hour.

Valproic acid per rectum (not usually available).

Lidocaine by intravenous drip.

Increased Intracranial Pressure
Bernard L. Maria and Joshua Halpern

PERSPECTIVE

Within a fixed space (the cranial vault), an increase in the volume results in a rapid rise in pressure. Intracranial volume increases can occur in three groups: those affecting the brain parenchymal space, cerebrospinal fluid (CSF) space, and vascular space. Increased volume in the brain parenchymal space may result from tumor (primary or metastatic), hemorrhage, edema (cytotoxic or vasogenic), or abscess. In the CSF space, increased production of fluid (choroid plexus tumor), poor flow (e.g., stenosis of aqueduct of Sylvius, fourth ventricle outflow, shunt malfunction), or decreased absorption (infection or carcinomatous meningitis, subarachnoid hemorrhage) may be responsible for increased volume. Increased volume in the vascular space may be attributable to hyperemia, vascular malformation, or sinus thrombosis.

DIAGNOSIS

Signs and symptoms of increased intracranial pressure are as follows:

1. Headache, change in behavior, nausea, vomiting, lethargy
2. Changes in pupillary reaction to light and impaired upward gaze
3. False localized signs (e.g., sixth nerve palsy)
4. Seizures of new onset or increased frequency
5. Abnormalities of station, gait, or coordination (hydrocephalus can produce a picture of paraparesis)
6. Papilledema (may take a week to develop). Remember that papillitis, due to leukemia or infection, may appear similar but is associated with early loss of visual acuity.
7. Findings on computed tomography (CT) scans of brain

MANAGEMENT

Dexamethasone (0.5–1.5 mg/kg in an intravenous loading dose, followed by 0.25–0.5 mg/kg/day intravenously in divided doses every 6 hours) reduces peritumoral edema and may effectively reduce intracranial pressure. If signs of herniation are present, institute immediate hyperventilation (lower the carbon dioxide tension to 20–30 mm Hg to induce cerebral vasoconstriction). Mechanically ventilated patients may require sedation (morphine). Many patients may also require paralysis with pancuronium. In extreme cases, hypothermia, ventriculostomy, or induction of barbiturate coma may be necessary.

Surgical decompression and complete excision of tumor is ideal treatment whenever possible.

Several temporizing measures may be undertaken. The patient should be positioned so that the head is elevated to 30 degrees and positioned midline to prevent jugular compression. Fluids should be restricted to one-half to two-thirds the maintenance level. Mannitol (0.25–1 gm/kg intravenously) may be given as needed until the serum osmolarity reaches 320. Also furosemide (1–2 mg/kg intravenously) may be useful in conjunction with mannitol, but blood pressure, fluid balance (weight), and osmolarity must be monitored.

If increased intracranial pressure is due to a central nervous system tumor and surgical intervention is not possible, then radiotherapy is indicated immediately after initiating steroid therapy. The doses of radiation are similar to those for spinal cord compression (three to four large fractions of 3–4 Gy each, followed by 2–3 Gy per fraction to a total dose of 30–40 Gy), except where higher doses are indicated for definitive treatment (50–60 Gy/5–7 weeks).

Spinal Cord Compression
Roberta A. Gottlieb and Joshua Halpern

PERSPECTIVE

Spinal cord compression may be produced by intradural lesions (usually primary central nervous system tumors) or extradural pressure attributable to primary or secondary vertebral tumors. Spinal cord compression that lasts more than 24 hours may produce irreversible neurologic damage. Thus, therapy should commence on an emergency basis.

SIGNS AND SYMPTOMS

Pain, often characterized as a vague, deep ache, may be the earliest symptom. The patient may complain only of aching thighs. In some cases the pain is pinpoint in location and associated with tenderness to percussion. Nerve root involvement may cause beltlike distribution of the pain or radiating pain to the groin or leg. Recurrent, chronic backache may be the only clue to an epidural tumor.

The weakness that accompanies spinal cord compression is often subtle, with loss of endurance. Weakness is usually proximal; the patient may have difficulty arising from a chair. A baby may stop walking and demand to be carried. The upper extremities may be spared.

Sensory changes are usually vague (heavy feet, dysethesia). On examination, sensory changes may be limited to a discrete level and exhibit a dermatomal pattern, which may not correspond to the site of compression). A hyperesthetic band at or above the sensory level may be patchy, with areas of paresthesia or sparing.

The ataxia that can occur may be confusing: It can mimic cerebellar pathologic processes or there may be true Romberg's sign. The patient's gait is worse in the dark; there is an associated loss of sense of position.

Bowel and bladder involvements are generally late findings unless there is a primary intraspinal tumor. Constipation and urinary retention precede incontinence. Urgency, frequency, and accidents are major signs.

DIAGNOSIS

1. The patient history should identify symptoms, underlying disease, date and type of last therapy (especially intrathecal medications), radiation dose and fields, recent fever, any trauma, and medications taken (especially prednisone and methotrexate, which cause osteoporosis and therefore vertebral body collapse). Lymphoma, leukemia, abscess, and primary bone tumors are common causes of spinal cord compression. Primary spinal tumors or paravertebral dumbbell tumors such as neuroblastoma or rhabdomyosarcoma and subarachnoid metastases (especially from medulloblastoma, ependymoma, and malignant astrocytoma) are other causes of spinal cord compression. Intrathecal medications administered to thrombocytopenic patients may result in postlumbar puncture hematoma and acute paraplegia.
2. Careful physical examination should document *quantitative* motor strength and assess gait. Sensory examination should detect sensory levels; the spine must be inspected and percussed. Reflex testing should include deep tendon reflexes. The Babinski reflex and superficial reflexes (anal wink, cremasteric muscle, abdominal muscles) should also be tested, and attention should be paid to rectal tone. Also cranial nerve testing should not be omitted.
3. Immediate consultation with a neurologist is advised. In addition, a neurosurgeon and radiotherapist should be involved early.
4. Plain film roentgenography of the spine is useful for ruling out bony destruction and subluxation.

5. Myelography or CT-myelography or magnetic resonance imaging with gadolinium enhancement is employed.
6. Pulmonary function should be tested if the lesion is at a high level.

TREATMENT

In the treatment of spinal cord compression, lumbar puncture is absolutely contraindicated unless myelography is carefully performed by a radiologist. The patient should be immobilized (logrolling), relieved of pain and sedated. Bladder drainage and stool softeners are used if needed. Quantitation of strength should be performed daily; the patient must be monitored for deterioration. A 100-mg bolus of dexamethasone is infused intravenously and followed by rapid taper and institution of definitive therapy. Chemotherapy is beneficial in cases of Ewing's sarcoma, neuroblastoma, leukemia/lymphoma, and selected other malignancies. Surgical decompression should be considered for single-level lesions, lesions of unknown histology, and patients with an expected long survival.

Radiotherapy is the standard treatment for multiple-level lesions, for advanced metastatic disease, for bulky unresectable lesions, and in inoperable patients. Radiotherapy should be administered concomitantly with steroids. It is usually started with three to four large fractions (3–4 Gy each) and then continued with 2 to 3 Gy per fraction to a total cumulative dose of 30 to 40 Gy.

Meningeal Carcinomatosis

Joshua Halpern

Meningeal carcinomatosis (leptomeningeal metastasis) is uncommon in pediatric solid tumors (with the exception of parameningeal rhabdomyosarcoma). Childhood acute lymphoid leukemia and lymphomas may extend to the CSF and present a picture of meningeal carcinomatosis. Intrathecal chemotherapy is currently recommended and has been administered with varying degrees of success, depending on the nature of the primary tumor. Whenever a myelogram, CT scan, or magnetic resonance image shows a deposit of tumor in the craniospinal axis, radiotherapy to the area is recommended. Radiation is also delivered to clinically suspicious areas, based on the neurologic examination, even when the imaging procedures are negative in these areas. The dose delivered is usually 30 Gy in 10 daily fractions of 3 Gy each.

Pain Management

Roberta A. Gottlieb

Children with cancer experience pain related to their disease and sometimes related to its therapy. It is important to determine the etiology of pain and to correct its cause whenever possible. Where the pain is expected to diminish and resolve over a short period of time, medication should be administered as needed. However, in the

Table 24-1. Recommended dosages and available forms of pain medications

Drug	Recommended dosage	Available forms (other than IV)
Acetaminophen (Tylenol)	10–20 mg/kg PO q4–6h	Tablet: 325 mg Elixir: 160 mg/5 ml Drops: 100 mg/1 ml
Codeine[a]	0.5–1 mg/kg PO q4–6h 0.5–1 mg/kg IM q4h (max. 120 mg)	Tablet: 15 mg, 30 mg, 60 mg
Morphine	0.1–0.2 mg/kg IV q4h (max. 15 mg) 0.3–0.5 mg/kg PO q4–6h	Sol.: 10 mg/5 ml or 20 mg/5 ml Tablets: 15 mg, 30 mg
Methadone[b]	0.2–1.0 mg/kg q6h (may need decrease after 2–3 days)	Sol.: 5 mg/5 ml or 10 mg/5 ml Tablet: 5 mg, 10 mg
Hydromorphone[c] (Dilaudid)	0.05–0.1 mg/kg PO q4–6h 0.015–0.03 mg/kg IV q4h (max. 4 mg) Adult: 1 suppository PR q6–8h	Tablet: 1 mg, 2 mg, 3 mg, 4 mg No liquid form (except with guaifenesin) Suppository: 3 mg

Codeine combination forms:

	Acetaminophen (mg) +	Codeine (mg)
Tylenol #1	300	7.5
Tylenol #2	300	15
Tylenol #3	300	30
Tylenol #4	300	60
Elixir/5 ml	120	12

Table 24-1. (continued)

Drug	Recommended dosage	Available forms (other than IV)
Meperidine[c] (Demerol)	1–2 mg/kg IV q3–4h (max. 125 mg) 1–3 mg/kg PO q4h	Syrup: 50 mg/5 ml Tablets: 50 mg, 100 mg
Oxycodone[c]	0.5–1.5 mg/kg PO q4–6h	Sol.: 5 mg/5 ml Tablets: 5 mg

Oxycodone[c] + acetaminophen	Adult, moderate pain: 1 capsule or tablet PO q6h
	Adult, severe/tolerant: may exceed usual dosage
		Tylox capsules or Percocet scored tablets:
		    Oxycodone 5 mg
		    Acetaminophen 325 mg

Hydrocodone bitartrate + acetaminophen	Adult, moderate pain: 1 tablet PO q6h
	Adult, severe/tolerant: 1 tablet q4h or 2 q6h
		Vicodin scored tablets:
		    Hydrocodone 5 mg
		    Acetaminophen 500 mg

Naloxone (Narcan)	0.01 mg/kg IV or IM or SC to reverse narcotics; may repeat q2–3min	Adult ampule: 0.4 mg/ml Neonatal ampule: 0.02 mg/ml

[a]Dependence less than with morphine. May produce more constipation than other narcotics. Consider stool softeners or lactulose early in use.

[b]Long plasma half-life (17–24 h), but analgesic effect only 6 to 8 hours. Can accumulate, so dose should be decreased after 2 to 3 days or severe sedation and toxicity may ensue.

[c]Similar narcotics with no proved advantages. Plasma half-life of Demerol is only 3 to 4 hours.

Key: IV = intravenously; PO = orally; IM = intramuscularly; max. = maximum dose; PR = per rectum; SC = subcutaneously; sol. = solution.

Source: Adapted from G. K. McEvoy (ed.). *American Hospital Formulary Service Drug Information.* Bethesda, MD: American Society of Hospital Pharmacists, 1989; and P. G. Lacouture, P. Gaudreault, and F. H. Lovejoy. Chronic pain of childhood: A pharmacologic approach. *Pediatr. Clin. North Am.* 31:1133, 1984.

Table 24-2. Recommended dosages and route of administration of sedatives

Medication	Dosage and route	Comments
Chloral hydrate (Noctec)	25–100 mg/kg PO or PR	30–45 min before procedure; wide margin of safety; no analgesia
Diazepam (Valium)	0.1–0.3 mg/kg IV or IM	Amnesic effect; risk of respiratory depression
Midazolam (Versed)	0.05–0.10 mg/kg IV or IM	Titrate gradually (max. 5 mg)
Lorazepam (Ativan)	0.05–0.10 mg/kg IV or IM	Less respiratory depression than diazepam but more risk of emesis
Droperidol (Inapsine)	0.1–0.2 mg/kg IV	Premedicate with chloral hydrate; occasional hallucinations
Fentanyl (Sublimaze)	2–3 μg/kg IV	Respiratory depression up to 4 hours; reversible with naloxone; effect lasts 30–60 min
Pentobarbital (Nembutal)	2–4 mg/kg PO, PR, or IM	Respiratory depression; avoid extravasation; low doses increase pain sensitivity

case of a child with pain of a known cause not being remedied, analgesia should be provided on a routine schedule. Anxiolytics and psychotherapy are beneficial in some circumstances, while surgical or electrical nerve blockade may be useful in others. Nonsteroidal anti-inflammatory agents including aspirin are not listed here because of their effect on platelet function and gastric mucosa; these effects are troublesome in children with cancer although their antiprostaglandin properties are useful in controlling metastatic bone pain. Remember also that chemotherapy or radiotherapy may offer effective palliation of pain related to tumor.

Recommended dosages and available forms of pain medications are listed in Table 24-1. In addition to the agents listed in the table, one can convert from one analgesic to another. Equivalent doses (in mg) are shown in the table below:

Morphine	Codeine	Methadone	Dilaudid	Demerol	Oxycodone
IV 10	120	10	1.5	75	15
PO 60	200	20	7.5	300	30

Sedation
Roberta A. Gottlieb

Children with cancer undergo many procedures that require immobilization or that are painful. A play therapist may be helpful in preparing a child to tolerate these procedures, whether a CT scan, radiation treatment, or bone marrow aspiration. Hypnosis has been used successfully in selected children. General anesthesia should be considered when a procedure is prolonged and painful or where the procedure is associated with the risk of complications if the child struggles (e.g., percutaneous central venous catheter placement or liver biopsy). Sedation is not a substitute for general anesthesia in providing good analgesia, and severe anxiety can overcome much of the sedative effect. In addition, since intravenous contrast dye is associated with a lowered seizure threshold, this should be kept in mind when selecting a sedative for CT scans. Sedation for painful procedures should provide analgesia as well. Table 24-2 lists some commonly used sedation methods.

25

Complications of the Nose and Mouth

Epistaxis
Roberta A. Gottlieb

ANTERIOR BLEEDING

Anterior nosebleeding is usually septal. It is managed in the following manner:

1. Hold the length of the nose firmly for 5 minutes.
2. Correct coagulopathy and thrombocytopenia if present. Some patients benefit from systemic steroids.
3. Salted pork fat has been used with good results; it swells to fit the nare, has disinfectant properties, and can be removed without dislodging clots [1].

In patients who are not myelosuppressed, one may attempt to pack the nose as follows:

1. Constrict the nasal vessels with 4% cocaine (maximum dose in 1 hour is 2.5 mg/kg or 1 ml of spray per 15 kg), or 4% lidocaine and 1% phenylephrine.
2. Clear the nasal passages with gentle suction and attempt to visualize the bleeding vessel (an invisible source indicates a posterior nose bleed).
3. Cauterize the bleeding vessel with silver nitrate for 15 seconds. This may be repeated, unless bleeding worsens.
4. If necessary, pack the nose (ideally with Gelfoam or Avitene [microfibrillar collagen], which does not have to be removed).
   a. A nasal speculum is used to expand the external nare.
   b. Bayonet nasal forceps are used for packing.
   c. Begin packing in the superoposterior region of the nasal cavity, then fill in the posteroinferior area, and finally, fill the anteroinferior area. If packing gauze is used, be sure to leave both ends extending out front.

POSTERIOR BLEEDING OR UNCONTROLLABLE ANTERIOR BLEEDING

In cases of posterior nosebleeding or uncontrollable anterior bleeding, an ear, nose, and throat surgeon should be consulted to achieve vascular control. Be sure that any coagulopathy is corrected. Support with blood transfusions if necessary. An orogastric tube may be helpful.

Oral and Dental Care for the Child with Cancer
Béla B. Toth and A. Bruce Carter

PERSPECTIVE

The oral cavity is a common site for immediate and late complications of cancer therapy. Adverse effects on the oral cavity depend on the type of cancer, the treatment regimen, and the age of the child receiving therapy. Surgery, radiotherapy, and chemotherapy are known to induce immediate tissue reactions (pain, mucosal break-down, mucositis, bleeding, or infection), as well as long-term se-quelae (trismus, hypoplastic facial development, xerostomia, dental malformation, dental maldevelopment, and accelerated tooth de-cay). Late anatomic anomalies are observed as more patients sur-vive into adulthood [2,3].

Comprehensive workup and treatment of the oncology patient must include evaluation of the oral cavity and institution of preven-tive measures. Many complications associated with the oral cavity are precipitated by preexisting, correctable, or preventable condi-tions [4]. The primary issues of oral and dental management of children with cancer are prevention of oral and dental disorders, acute complications of therapy, and long-term consequences. Thus, the goals of oral and dental care for the pediatric oncology patient are: (1) to prevent infectious complications, (2) to lessen potential cancer treatment complications, and (3) to minimize oral and dental sequelae. In this section we outline a simple approach to prevention as well as to the recognition and management of oral complications associated with anticancer therapy.

PREVENTIVE MEASURES

Education

One of the most important benefits of the oncologic pretreatment oral and dental evaluation is the opportunity to educate patient and family about oral care and hygiene. Both nursing staff and physicians should emphasize oral hygiene with not only patients but the families as well. This can be accomplished by instructing the patient in the appropriate use of toothbrushing aids and mouth rinses. Recommended oral care is outlined in Table 25-1. The pa-tient and the patient's family should be educated regarding the possibility that chemotherapy will produce neutropenia, throm-bocytopenia, and associated oral complications of infection and bleeding, as well as mucositis. Patients can minimize the cyclic, therapy-induced oral complications by maintaining good oral care practices and by modifying dietary habits. Patient and family should also be informed of late effects, such as xerostomia and facial and dental maldevelopment.

Hygiene

To maintain excellent oral hygiene and prevent or reduce oral com-plications, it is of utmost importance that dental plaque be kept at a minimum. Dental plaque is a microcosm of oral flora, and any other opportunisitic organism that enters the oral cavity will also colonize plaque. Because of its location (at the tooth surface of the gumline), plaque can cause tissue irritation (gingivitis) or bacteremia. As gin-givitis intensifies and the plaque (bacterial mass) accumulates, bacteremia becomes more frequent and is cause for concern, espe-cially if granulocytopenia or an indwelling central venous catheter is present.

Swishing cannot remove dental plaque; only brushing will remove plaque. A special "chemobrush" (Periodontal Health Brush, Inc., Osseo, WI) is recommended for use during periods of granulocy-topenia and thrombocytopenia (platelets < 40,000/μl). If thrombocy-

Table 25-1. Oral care plan for pediatric oncology patients

I. Intact mucosa
   A. Mucosal care
      1. Hydrogen peroxide 0.5% (standard 3% solution is diluted 1:4 with water), rinse and gargle 2–3 times
      2. Salt and soda rinse (½ tsp. each of salt and baking soda added to 1 qt. water) to remove residual debris and hydrogen peroxide
   B. Regular plaque removal with chemobrush, which is rinsed with hydrogen peroxide and water after use
   C. Decay prevention with stannous fluoride gel application at bedtime
   D. Hematologic parameters monitored; oral mucosa inspected for signs of bleeding, infection, erythema, or ulceration
   E. No abrasive food or mouthwashes containing phenol or alcohol
II. Mucositis
   A. Mucosal care (see I.A); no hydrogen peroxide if its use is painful; cool rinses with salt and soda
   B. Use of chemobrush or, if not tolerated, a sponge toothbrush
   C. Regular oral care followed by topical medications, if indicated
III. Oral bleeding
   A. Mucosal care with gentle salt and soda rinses only
   B. No manipulation of mucosa
   C. Topical hemostatic medications, if indicated
   D. Soft foods only

topenia is present, the patient should be monitored for oral trauma and bleeding by either the patient or the parents of the patient. Trauma caused by abrasive or irritating foods may precipitate or intensify oral complications. For example, an oral complication will occur with the repeated use of mouth rinses containing irritating ingredients such as alcohol or phenol, which compromise the mucosal lining. Therefore, eating irritating foods and using irritating mouth rinses are highly discouraged during periods of myelosuppression.

Evaluation

During the initial oncologic evaluation, all patients should receive a comprehensive oral and dental evaluation to document existing pathologic processes. The oral examination should include visualization of the teeth and the oral soft tissues (lips, cheeks, tongue, hard and soft palates, floor of mouth, and gingiva). Panographic and bitewing radiographs are taken to detect more extensive decay, possible dental abscesses, stage of tooth development (exfoliation of deciduous teeth), and any osseous pathologic findings. This workup will identify dental problems requiring immediate corrective measures before radiotherapy or chemotherapy is instituted and will allow the clinician to anticipate subsequent complications or late effects. If the patient is too ill or myelosuppressed to undergo dental treatment, septic foci and potential oral complications should be documented and eliminated when conditions permit. The pediatrician should be informed of the findings.

Sedation

If oral or dental treatment is needed—be it biopsy, extraction, or dental restoration—all aspects of the child's current situation should be considered. The oncologic workup is typically a very stressful period for the child and parents. Many children will revert to a more infantile behavior during stressful procedures. Although patience, understanding, and behavior modification techniques are helpful in gaining a child's cooperation, sedation or general anesthesia is sometimes indicated. When necessary, the anxious pediatric dental patient can be managed by meperidine (2 mg/kg) and promethazine (1 mg/kg) administered orally. As with any sedation technique, precautions include appropriate patient selection with complete medical history and consultation, monitoring of the patient's vital signs, ability to manage any potential complications, and supervision by trained personnel (see Chap. 24).

Because many oncologic workups will require invasive procedures (e.g., biopsy or staging laparotomy) that may necessitate the use of general anesthsia, dental treatment may be performed concurrently. The institution of cancer therapy cannot be postponed for long, and so the time available for dental treatment may be limited; multiple appointments under local anesthesia may be impractical. If extensive dental treatment is necessary, consideration should be given to carrying out all dental procedures in a limited number of appointments with the aid of sedation or in one appointment under general anesthesia. Dental treatment should be restricted to correcting those problems that pose a high risk for complications during cancer treatment. Procedures should cause as little tissue trauma as possible so that the initiation of cancer treatment is not unduly delayed. Treatment of less urgent problems can be postponed.

Dental Intervention Before Chemotherapy

When indicated, biopsy of tumor-associated lesions, cultures of oral sites of infection, and treatment procedures should be performed. Areas that cause tissue irritation, such as dental calculus and gingival opercula associated with erupting teeth, should be corrected to help maintain the integrity of the mucosal lining. Thus, orthodontic bands should be removed, and faulty, chipped dental restorations or tooth cusps should be smoothed, rounded off, or replaced. A tooth mucosal guard can be fabricated to protect the tongue or buccal mucosa from biting trauma or friction. A deciduous tooth that is mobile, and therefore close to being shed, might cause bleeding or gingival infection if shed during a period of myelosuppression, and so it should be extracted. The pediatrician should monitor deciduous teeth for mobility, so that any mobile tooth can be extracted before a course of chemotherapy rather than allowing it to be shed during a period of myelosuppression. Teeth that are nonsalvageable or abscessed must be extracted. Any tooth with decay that extends into the pulp, with no evidence of infection at the root apex, can be saved with appropriate dental therapy. Because the soft-tissue wound from extraction of a deciduous tooth heals rapidly, there should be no inordinate delay in starting chemotherapy. However, if a permanent (adult) tooth is removed, a delay is necessary since the extent of tissue injury (soft and osseous) is much greater, thus requiring more time for healing. The delay in starting therapy depends on the difficulty of extraction and on the type of therapy (expected onset, severity, and duration of myelosuppression or mucositis).

Dental Intervention Before Radiotherapy

Because of the risks of oral complications associated with the head and neck irradiation, the patient and family must understand the importance of oral hygiene before, during, and after radiotherapy. Irradiation causes immediate and long-term damage to oral and dental tissues, and so certain dental treatments should be implemented before treatment is started [5]. First, radiation mucositis is an early complication associated with higher doses of radiation and restricted to the mucosal areas included in the treatment fields. Therefore, any causes of local tissue irritation should be eliminated. Second, because radiation may cause progressive fibrosis and avascularity with a marginal healing potential, oral surgical procedures should be accomplished before radiotherapy is undertaken. Nonsalvageable teeth should be removed. Third, if the patient is to receive mantle radiation, mandibular wisdom teeth should be removed because of their proximity to the radiation treatment field. If they are retained, complications such as gingival and periodontal pocket infections, dental decay, and pain may develop. If the patient is to have general anesthesia for a biopsy or laparotomy, removal of the wisdom teeth can be done concurrently.

At the time of the preradiation dental examination, removal of the permanent teeth that lie in the radiation treatment field should be considered if poor oral hygiene is found or if it is believed that the patient and family will be unable to comply with a mandatory oral care plan. Such recommended treatment may appear overly aggressive; however, poor hygiene will lead to accelerated dental decay with increased risk of dental abscesses and osteoradionecrosis. Dental repair during and after radiation treatment is difficult because of poor wound healing.

If the treatment fields are known at the time of the initial dental evaluation, an intraoral radiation stent can be fabricated to position maxilla or mandible away from the radiation fields. Patient compliance with a stent is important to minimize radiation damage to the mandible.

TREATMENT

Dental Interventions

Even with appropriate pretreatment interventions and adherence to the oral hygiene protocol, the patient may need dental intervention during chemotherapy. Each oral or dental manipulation should be considered in terms of tissue trauma that can lead to possible hemorrhage, local infection, or bacteremia. No oral or dental procedure should be undertaken without first determining where the patient is in the course of the chemotherapy (e.g., approaching a nadir of myelosuppression). Laboratory studies should include the granulocyte and platelet counts and coagulation profile. If these hematologic parameters are not respected, even simple manipulations (i.e., dental probing or cleaning) may precipitate a complication such as hemorrhage or infection. Dental procedures (cleaning, dental fillings, extractions, biopsy, and the like) may be performed in patients with absolute granulocyte counts greater than $1000/\mu l$ and with platelet counts greater than $50,000/\mu l$ if the coagulation profile is normal. Antibiotic coverage for gram-positive and anaerobic organisms is used when the procedure causes moderate tissue damage (such as a biopsy), when there is risk of bacteremia (extractions), or when the patient is granulocytopenic or has an indwelling central venous catheter.

Dental problems that develop during radiotherapy should be managed with some consideration given to the irradiated tissues' tolerance to manipulation. It is advisable to keep dental procedures as simple as possible so as not to damage an already compromised mucosa. Irradiation impairs bone healing and is a contraindication for dental extraction, periodontal surgery, and surgical endodontics [5]. (A more complete discussion follows in the section on long-term follow-up in this chapter.) Placement of a temporary filling into a defective tooth is advisable if the tooth is symptomatic and located in an area where there is mucositis. Permanent dental restorations (silver amalgam filling) can be done for symptomatic teeth out of the field of radiation. Routine dental treatment may be deferred until after radiation treatment or the resolution of mucositis.

Pericoronal gingival tissue tags associated with erupting teeth can be a source of inflammation, infection, and pain secondary to biting trauma. The area should be copiously irrigated several times daily with hydrogen peroxide solution followed by saline to remove any entrapped food debris and bacteria. When the irritation begins to resolve and when thrombocytopenia and granulocytopenia resolve, the gingival tag sould be removed.

Oral Complications

Pain

Pain from the oral structures is a common finding with the oral complications associated with cancer therapy (e.g., infection, mucositis, or hemorrhage). The etiology of persistent pain *must* be identified and treated. Do not mask the symptom with narcotic analgesics or topical anesthetic agents. Infection can arise from three possible sites: the tooth (abscess), the gums (gingivitis), and the oral mucosa (mucositis).

ABSCESSED TOOTH An abscessed tooth causing a toothache should be considered for immediate extraction with appropriate supportive measures, such as anitbiotics and correction of thrombocytopenia or coagulopathy. If the pain is from a fractured or lost filling, then appropriate dental therapy can be provided. Routine interventions should be delayed until just before the next course of chemotherapy, when the patient has the least myelosuppression. Pain from deep decay or pulp necrosis is poorly managed with analgesics and requires corrective dental treatment.

STOMATITIS Stomatitis (including abscesses or gingivitis) may be mistakenly treated as mucositis, which results in a marked delay of appropriate therapy. It is imperative that appropriate cultures be taken and that the microbiological results be correlated with the mucosal pathologic process.

MUCOSITIS Mucositis is an ulcerative response that develops when chemotherapy or radiation arrests the normally rapid cellular turnover of the mucosal lining. The oral surfaces included in the radiation treatment fields may develop mucositis. The initial tissue reaction is seen as an edematous and erythematous response, which progresses to small, scattered areas of ulceration. As therapy continues, the ulcerations enlarge to a point at which the entire mucosa is denuded. Such areas are highly vulnerable to superinfection (stomatitis) and are extremely painful. Mucositis will persist, even after radiotherapy has been completed, until there is cellular recovery and the superinfection is cleared.

The duration and severity of mucositis associated with chemotherapy is variable and depends on several factors: the drugs used, their dosage and schedule of administration, and local oral factors. Resolution of mucositis does not parallel hematologic recovery but depends on oral hygiene and the presence of irritating factors.

The mucosa must be kept moist and free of debris. If vomiting occurs, it is important to maintain mucosal integrity by rinsing out the corrosive gastric acid secretions. Plaque must be eliminated to reduce bacterial colonization and infection of the mucosal ulcers, by using a chemobrush or spongelike toothbrush. This should be followed with diluted hydrogen peroxide rinses and salt and soda rinses (see Table 25-1). If there is pain other than an immediate stinging sensation, the hydrogen peroxide should be eliminated and only the salt and soda solution should be used. With a clean oral cavity, the mucositis can be assessed for possible superinfection by bacteria, fungi, or viruses. Because mucositis is often associated with superinfection, microbiological studies should be considered (i.e., Gram's stain, Tzanck smear, and bacterial, fungal, and viral cultures). If topical therapy is indicated, a clean oral cavity makes the medication more effective. (For treatment of specific infections, see Chap. 22.)

If no superinfection is present, Sucralfate suspension (The University of Texas M.D. Anderson Cancer Center Pharmacy Formulation; patent pending) is gently swished around the oral cavity after cleansing. This suspension coats the eroded, raw areas and forms a film that can protect the tissues from invading bacteria, reduce irritation (pain reduction), and possibly promote healing. If this suspension is used in conjunction with other oral or topical agents, it should be used last because its coating action on the mucosal surfaces will interfere with the effectiveness of those other agents.

Topical anesthetizing agents cause undue irritation and numbness, resulting in greater trauma to the compromised mucosa. However, a diluted topical anesthetic is sometimes used; a 1:2 dilution of unflavored lidocaine hydrochloride (Xylocaine 2% viscous solution) can allow oral hygiene and enteral nutrition to be continued without further tissue trauma caused by chemical irritation.

If tissue breakdown tends to occur in one specific location (site-specific mucositis [i.e., cheeks or lateral edges of tongue]) a soft polypropylene mucosal tooth guard can be fabricated to create a smooth, frictionless surface between the oral tissues and the teeth.

Bleeding

Bleeding from the oral cavity need not occur when there is profound thrombocytopenia or a coagulopathy. All too often this preventable complication results from mucositis or infection, trauma from teeth and food substances, or poor oral hygiene practices [6]. Even with normal-appearing oral soft tissues, profound thrombocytopenia (platelet count $< 20,000/\mu l$) may result in bleeding and calls for frequent assessment. The mouth must be kept moist. The oral hygiene regimen (hyrdogen peroxide, salt and soda rinses, and plaque reduction with a chemobrush) should continue as long as there are no sites of active bleeding or blood clots.

For evaluation of oral bleeding, clotted blood and mucus should be gently rinsed from the mouth to permit visualization of the bleeding sites [3]. Moist gauze pressure packing should be applied to bleeding sites. Agents such as Gelfoam or topical thrombin may also be useful. Prolonged bleeding may occur because of the fibrinolytic nature of the saliva. In such situations, ε-aminocaproic acid (Amicar) can be used. Mucosal injury may occur as a result of self-induced trauma (i.e., toothpick, fingernails, dental floss, or even routine oral hygiene practices).

Manipulation of hemorrhagic sites or removal of the blood clots by mechanical cleansing (toothbrush, sponge brush, or oral swabs) or even the use of the mildest dilution of hydrogen peroxide solution can reinitiate or prolong bleeding. Under these circumstances, gentle rinsing with tepid saline, a salt and soda solution, or water is recommended. The diet should be restricted to soft, custardlike food or liquids; hard, coarse, or abrasive foods (i.e., popcorn, crackers, cereals, chips, or hard candy) should be avoided.

Xerostomia

Xerostomia is a progressive condition that results from radiation damage to the salivary glands. The degree of damage depends on the treatment fields (size of field and unilateral versus bilateral fields) and the dose of radiation received. It also depends on the degree of recovery of the irradiated glandular tissues, on the ability of nonirradiated salivary glands to compensate, and on which salivary glands are irradiated.

During radiotherapy, saliva will change from a normal watery consistency to a viscous, ropy, or foamy texture, which may progress to dryness. The recommended oral care plan is similar to the mucositis protocol (see Table 25-1): (1) Swish diluted hydrogen peroxide gently for 30 seconds, and (2) rinse with a salt and soda solution. This rinsing procedure is done at least twice, until the oral mucosa feels clean to the patient or until there is undue discomfort from the radiation-induced mucositis. Reduction of the thick mucous secretions and the accumulated oral microorganisms will decrease pain as well as minimize the risk of infection to areas of mucositis. Topical agents used for infection or pain are more effective once the saliva is thinned.

Bone Marrow Transplantation

Special mention should be made of bone marrow transplant patients. If total body irradiation is used for conditioning and cell reduction, then a greater degree of xerostomia is found. Another complication that must be kept in mind is graft-versus-host disease (GVHD) with oral mucosal involvement. Such mucosal involvement may mimic mucositis, interfere with nutrition, cause pain, and mask infectious processes. Vigilance for bacterial, fungal, and herpetic pathogens is necessary to distinguish infection from the onset of GVHD in the oral cavity. In addition to cultures, visual inspection by an experienced clinician may obviate the need for diagnostic biopsy.

Artificial Implants and Antibiotic Prophylaxis

Children with implants such as ventricular shunts, intramedullary rods placed for limb salvage, or central venous catheters are at risk for serious infection from the bacteremia associated with dental procedures. Specific guidelines for antibiotic prophylaxis have been developed to reduce the risk of infections in patients with these special prostheses, as follows [7,8,9]:

I. Patients requiring endocarditis prophylaxis (standard risk: procedures causing gingival bleeding; bronchoscopy; biopsy or surgery of respiratory tract; certain gastrointestinal or genitourinary procedures)
    A. Oral regimen
        1. Adults and children heavier than 27 kg: penicillin V, 2 gm, 1 hour preoperatively; then 1 gm 6 hours later
        2. Children lighter than 27 kg: penicillin V, 1 gm, 1 hour preoperatively; then 500 mg 6 hours later
        3. Penicillin-allergic patients: erythromycin, 20 mg/kg (maximum dose 1 gm) 1 hour preoperatively; then 10 mg/kg (maximum dose 500 mg) 6 hours later
    B. Parenteral regimen: penicillin G, 50,000 U/kg (maximum dose 2 million U) intramuscularly or intravenously, 30 to 60 minutes preoperatively; then 25,000 U/kg (maximum dose 1 million U) 6 hours later.
II. Patients with prosthetic heart valves, prosthetic hips, joints, or limb-salvage prostheses (high-risk)
    A. Ampicillin, 50 mg/kg (maximum dose 1–2 gm) intramuscularly or intravenously, plus gentamicin, 2 mg/kg (adults 1.5 mg/kg) intramuscularly or intravenously, followed by 1 gm penicillin V 6 hours later, *or* repeat ampicillin and gentamicin regimen 8 hours later
    B. For penicillin-allergic patients: vancomycin, 20 mg/kg (maximum dose 1 gm), by intravenous infusion over 1 hour, starting 1 hour before procedure; no repeat dose necessary.
III. Patients with central venous catheters or neutropenia, undergoing oral procedures: same as I.A, but loading dose only.

LONG-TERM FOLLOW-UP

Tooth Decay Prevention

The importance of oral care and hygiene, which includes flossing and brushing, are always stressed to cancer patients to keep tooth decay and periodontal disease at a minimum. Once the complications of acute treatment (i.e., surgery, radiotherapy, or induction chemotherapy) have subsided, a complete decay prevention program must be implemented [10]. This consists of brushing on a 0.4% stannous fluoride gel once daily after the regular oral care regimen has been completed. This fluoride exceeds what is provided in regular fluoride-containing toothpastes. It is best applied at bedtime, so that it can stay in contact with the tooth surfaces for an extended period of time. This decay prevention program of flossing, brushing, and fluoride gel application is strongly recommended during and even after completion of therapy.

Postsurgical Follow-Up

If a surgical appliance was not fabricated at the time of orofacial surgery, the pediatric patient should be referred to a maxillofacial prosthodontist to fabricate a prosthesis that will fill in any oral defect and enhance rehabilitation. If a prosthesis was made and inserted at the time of operation, then the patient must be followed for re-adaptation of the surgical prosthesis as the wound heals and the postsurgical scarring produces new tissue boundaries.

Postsurgical fibrosis (trismus) can produce a limited oral opening. Mouth-opening exercises should be instituted immediately postoperatively, even though compliance may be a problem this early in the postsurgical course. Tongue blades are placed between the occlusal surfaces of the teeth, parallel to the dental arch. The tongue blade is gently inserted into the middle, forcing open both jaws by one tongue blade thickness. An additional tongue blade is inserted only after the first blade is accommodated with ease. It is important to maintain and not lose any degree of oral opening; thus, measurements are taken regularly to permit accurate assessment. It should not be left to clinical impression. Electrophysiotherapy may be of added benefit [4].

Because of the surgical defect and a limited oral opening, the patient may need extra care, special oral care instruction, and hygiene aides for optimum maintenance of the teeth and oral tissues. The decay prevention program (see Table 25-1) is instituted for all patients who have undergone head and neck surgery.

Follow-Up After Radiotherapy

The pediatric patient who has received radiotherapy to the head and neck requires long-term follow-up. The age of the patient and the dose of radiation are major factors that determine abnormal dental formation. The long-term effects of radiotherapy on the oral cavity include xerostomia, trismus, abnormal development of teeth and bony structures, and the potential for osteoradionecrosis.

Xerostomia

Xerostomia that results from head and neck irradiation, is highly variable in pediatric oncology patients, since glandular tissue may regenerate or undergo functional compensation. Salivary substitutes have varying degrees of acceptance. Water is universally accepted, well tolerated, and least expensive.

Trismus

The severity of postradiation fibrosis (trismus) depends on the age of the patient, the dose and type of radiation, and the treatment fields. To prevent decreased oral opening caused by radiation fibrosis, the patient must start oral opening exercises as soon as possible after the completion of therapy. The same forms of exercises and therapy listed for postsurgical trismus (tongue blades and electrophysiotherapy) should be applied to this group of patients. Frequent measurements of the oral opening must be done to assess any progressive fibrosis.

Abnormal Development of Teeth and Bony Structures

Tooth malformation, malalignment, and facial asymmetry produced by soft-tissue fibrosis and bony hypoplasia may arise from head and neck irradiation. Very often, the parents of the child who is now cured express great interest in orthodontic treatment to correct the malpositioned teeth. However, the effect of radiation of the developing tooth structure and underlying bone gives rise to abnormally shaped roots and contraindicates orthodontic intervention. When the mandible or maxilla is not irradiated directly but is at the edge of the treatment fields, roots exposed to the peripheral scatter of the ionizing rays are abnormal. Orthodontic treatment is contraindicated because tooth movement and functional loads (once the tooth is in proper occlusion) would be excessive and could lead to exfoliation of the tooth due to the lack of root support.

Osteoradionecrosis

The decay prevention program utilizing fluoride is mandatory to prevent osteoradionecrosis (a form of chronic osteomyelitis) of the teeth. Xerostomia from the radiation effects on the salivary glands, along with the alteration in oral microflora, produces a situation in which there is potential for rampant decay [10]. *There must be strict compliance with fluoride use,* or the decay will progress rapidly. The decay is painless and progressive. By the time symptoms develop, large portions of the tooth surface have been destroyed, or the decay has extended into the pulp (nerve) with the production of a dental abscess. Soft-tissue and osseous necrosis ensues if there is damage to the mucoperiosteum covering the bones [11]. Osteoradiorecrosis may respond to antibiotic therapy and intensive wound care but might require hyperbaric oxygen therapy to promote angiogenesis and wound healing [12]. Every attempt is made to salvage any and all adult teeth by dental filling, crowns, and root canal therapy. The extent of restorative dentistry necessary may be so great as to represent a major clinical and financial burden; extractions of nonrestorable teeth, with the aid of hyperbaric oxygen therapy, may be the only alternative.

Routine dental prophylaxis (removal of calculus, polishing, and fluoride treatment), as well as dental filling, crowns, and root canal therapy are appropriate for a patient who has received radiotherapy to the mandible, maxilla, and associated soft tissues. However, because of the damaging effects of radiotherapy on bone and soft tissues (fibrosis and avascularity), there are certain dental procedures that are contraindicated: extraction, periodontal surgery, and surgical endodontics. In all of these situations there is marked disruption of the already compromised tissue and wound healing would be poor.

For the patient who has had radiation to fields including the jaw bones and salivary glands, preventive dentistry including fluoride use is the most important factor for controlling a very serious potential dental problem. Compliance is essential. Fluoride application takes minimal time and effort, yet the benefits are profound in reducing tooth decay and periodontal disease.

Follow-Up After Chemotherapy

If the pediatric oncology patient who is receiving chemotherapy has been seen and treated according to the established oral and dental care guidelines, then by the time the patient has achieved remission of his or her disease, only routine maintenance of oral and dental care is needed, along with stressing the fluoride decay prevention program. However, some oncologists defer any dental intervention until the child's disease has stabilized or until a less aggressive phase of chemotherapy is entered. Dental intervention during early treatment phases is done only when an acute problem arises.

The diminished intensity of maintenance chemotherapy is such that immunosuppression and myelosuppression occur less frequently. At this stage of cancer therapy, a more comprehensive and aggressive scope of dental treatment can be offered. If, for example, orthodontia had been interrupted to prevent complications, such dental care could be resumed. Extended dental care must always be done in consultation with the pediatric oncologist and with the understanding that extensive dental therapy (e.g., orthodontics) may have to be discontinued if more intensive chemotherapy is reinstituted, as in the case of relapse.

COMMENTS

As cure is achieved and pediatric oncology patients live longer, more physical and dental abnormalities are being created that must be recognized by the doctors administering cancer treatment. Dental malformations in the supporting root structure of the teeth induced by radiotherapy contraindicate orthodontic tooth movement. Malformation may also lead to early loss of affected teeth in adulthood.

Oral and dental preventive care measures should be part of the overall care for oncology patients. Diligence must be maintained in evaluating the oral cavity and related structures before, during, and even years after therapy. It is also important to monitor for and to inform the patient and family of the long-term effects of cancer therapy on the developing dentition, jaws, and associated facial structures. Oral hygiene and decay prevention protocols must be followed strictly and reinforced at each follow-up visit. Such oral care plans are critical to preserving dentition, particularly in patients who receive radiation to the head and neck.

REFERENCES

1. Abildgaard, C. F. Progress and Problems in the Hemophilia and von Willebrand's Disease. In L. A. Barness (ed.), *Advances in Pediatrics*. Chicago: Year Book, 1984.
2. Jaffe, N., et al. Dental and maxillofacial abnormalities in long-term survivors of childhood cancer: Effects of treatment with chemotherapy and radiation to the head and neck. *Pediatrics* 73:816, 1984.
3. Maguire, A., et al. The long-term effects of treatment on the dental condition of children surviving malignant disease. *Cancer* 60:2570, 1987.
4. Toth, B. B., and Hoar, R. E. Oral/dental care for the pediatric oncology patient. *Cancer Bull.* 34:66, 1982.
5. Fleming, T. J. Dental care for cancer patients receiving radiotherapy to the head and neck. *Cancer Bull.* 34:63, 1982.
6. Toth, B. B., and Frame, R. T. Dental oncology: The management of disease and treatment-related oral/dental complications associated with chemotherapy. *Curr. Probl. Cancer* 10:7, 1983.
7. Coombs, R., and Friedlander, G. (eds.). *Bone Tumor Management*. London: Butterworth, 1987.
8. Shulman, S. T., et al. Prevention of bacterial endocarditis. *Circulation* 70:1123, 1984.
9. Shulman, S. T., et al. Group C streptococcal endocarditis. *Pediatrics* 75:114, 1985.
10. Fleming, T. J. Use of topical fluoride by patients receiving cancer therapy. *Curr. Probl. Cancer* 7:37, 1983.
11. Marx, R. E. Osteoradionecrosis: A new concept of its pathophysiology. *J. Oral Maxillofac. Surg.* 41:283, 1983.
12. Marx, R. E., Johnson, R. P., and Kline, S. N. Prevention of osteoradionecrosis: A randomized prospective trial of hyperbaric oxygen versus penicillin. *J.A.M.A.* 111:49, 1985.

SELECTED READINGS

Aubertin, J., et al. *Opportunistic Infections in Cancer Patients.* New York: Masson, 1978.

Bodey, G. P. Infectious complications in the cancer patient. *Curr. Probl. Cancer* 1:1, 1977.

Rodriguez, V. Acute infections in cancer patients. *The University of Texas System Cancer Center, M. D. Anderson Hospital and Tumor Institute Newsletter* 23:4, 1978.

Hickey, A. J., Toth, B. B., and Lindquist, S. F. Effect of intravenous hyperalimentation and oral care on the development of oral stomatitis during cancer chemotherapy. *J. Prosthet. Dent.* 47:188, 1982.

26

Long-Term Consequences of Cancer Therapy

Margaret P. Sullivan

Late effects of cancer therapy have been thoroughly assessed in three groups of pediatric patients—those with acute leukemia receiving cranial radiation, those with Wilms' tumor, and those with Hodgkin's disease. The late effects of radiotherapy observed in patients with Wilms' tumor in the 1960s have profoundly influenced treatment policies for all pediatric tumors, particularly those reported by the National Wilms' Tumor Studies, with respect to radiation treatment field design and radiation dose [1,2], as well as concomitant chemotherapy. Information regarding the late effects of radiotherapy and combined modality therapy given to children with Hodgkin's disease is still incomplete with respect to sterility and the occurrence of second malignant tumors [3]. Available data, however, do provide a basis for predicting and evaluating late effects of therapy throughout the spectrum of pediatric tumors.

ALTERED BONE GROWTH

With decreasing age, late effects of radiotherapy are increased [3], being most severe in children treated when younger than 6 years. Treatment given during "growth spurts" also has a more profound effect, as seen in the early teenage group. Retardation in growth is a direct result of growth arrest in irradiated bone. When vertebrae are included in a treatment field, as in Wilms' tumor, the entire width of the bone is treated in an effort to prevent scoliosis. Because of the inclusion of many vertebrae in the treatment field among children receiving extended-field radiotherapy, growth retardation is primarily manifested as decreased sitting height. Figure 26-1 shows the relative shortening of the upper thorax following irradiation of a mantle field (40 Gy total dose) and the abdomen (20 Gy total dose) and chemotherapy. The lower torso appears elongated in comparison with the upper torso. The position of the elbows is lower than normal because of the shortening of the upper torso; this is reflected by a reduction in sitting height. With modern treatment techniques and reduced radiation doses used in combination with chemotherapy, height remains within two standard deviations of the norm [4].

Postradiation changes in the skull are dependent on the fields treated and dose delivered. Treatment of the entire cranium produces reduction in cranial volume, which relates to radiation dose and age. Treatment of limited fields subsequently produces distortions of the skull, which relate to dose and field sizes.

Bilateral necrosis of the head of the femur is a rare complication. Figure 26-2 demonstrates this complication in a teenaged girl who had previously received a regimen of sandwich chemotherapy plus radiotherapy. Prednisone therapy is believed to be the cause. Bilateral replacement of the femoral heads was subsequently performed.

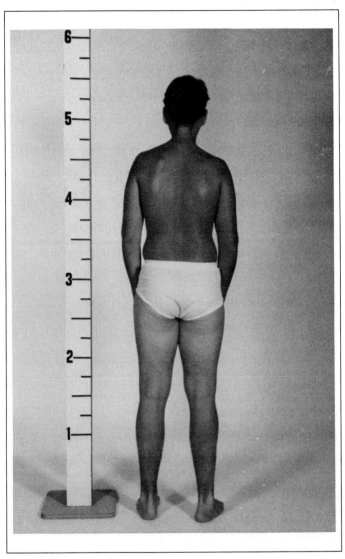

Fig. 26-1

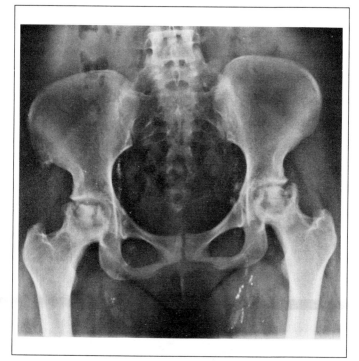

Fig. 26-2

SOFT-TISSUE CHANGES

Therapeutic doses of radiation delivered by supravoltage techniques spare the skin surface to a large extent. The underlying soft tissues are reduced in thickness and pliability. Underlying muscle becomes fibrotic. The margins of the treatment fields are often discernible. *Cobalt neck* is a term used to denote decreased diameter of the neck, inelasticity of the skin, and firmness of the soft tissues, including muscle, which suggests a likeness to a fence post (Fig. 26-3). Soft-tissue changes also occur in the supraclavicular tissues and the trapezius muscles when the neck and supraclavicular areas are irradiated [4].

BREAST CHANGES

Breast buds are very sensitive to radiation [3]. Figure 26-4A shows a radiation treatment portal for Hodgkin's disease involving the mediastinum and pleura. The effect of this radiotherapy on left breast development is pronounced, as evidenced by Figure 26-4B, taken 12 years after treatment.

SALIVARY GLAND EFFECTS

Irradiation of the neck in patients with Hodgkin's disease results in salivary gland changes that influence volume, consistency, and pH of the saliva. These changes, often augmented by chemotherapy,

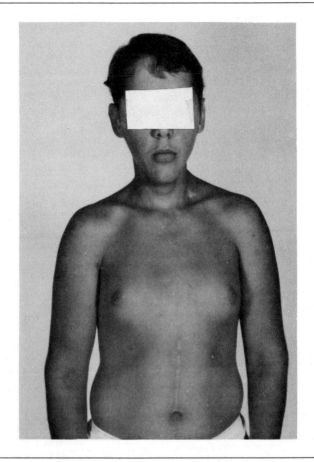

Fig. 26-3

promote cuspal or cervical caries [5] (Fig. 26-5). In neglected children, caries have resulted in loss of many or all of the teeth by early adulthood. Therefore, as outlined in Chap. 25, patients should be seen by the Pediatric Dental Service before treatment is initiated. The teeth are cleaned, caries are filled, and indicated extractions are performed so that conditions are optimum before treating cervical fields. After treatment, a fluoride carrier is used and dental surveillance continues.

LYMPHEDEMA

The inguinal node area is the usual biopsy site when Hodgkin's disease presents in the lower torso. Lymphangiogram on the side of the biopsy is usually unsuccessful or only partially successful because of disruption of lymphatic channels by the biopsy procedure, which results in a bizarre distribution of dye into the soft tissues

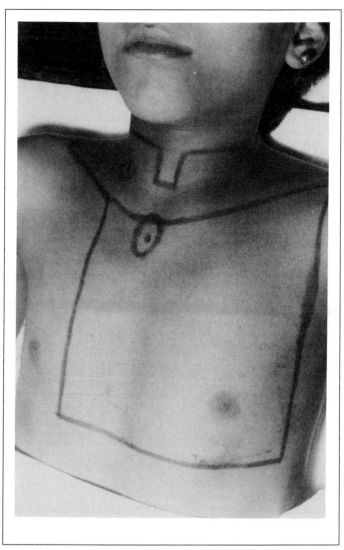

Fig. 26-4A

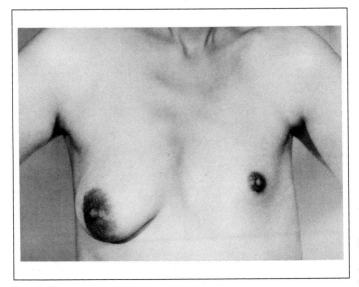

Fig. 26-4B

with little or no filling of the iliac lympatics above the biopsy site. After radiotherapy to the involved nodes, lymphedema is common (Fig. 26-6). Lymphedema can be controlled to a variable degree by using an elasticized garment that extends from the ankle to the waist on the involved side. Some patients will require pneumocompression from time to time, particularly following trauma or infection involving the edematous extremity. The use of the unilateral lower-extremity elasticized garment is very traumatic to patients, particularly school-aged boys who become the object of curiosity and are subjected to ridicule by classmates. There is often a financial burden of buying two pairs of shoes when the edema involves the foot.

ALTERED GONADAL FUNCTION

The ovaries are relatively resistant to both radiotherapy and chemotherapy. Girls with Hodgkin's disease usually have their ovaries moved outside the boundaries of a potential inverted Y field as a part of the staging procedure. Many births have been reported among women who have received three or six courses of mechlorethamine, vincristine (Oncovin), procarbazine, and prednisone (MOPP) chemotherapy [6]. Nonetheless, 26.4 percent of MOPP-treated women aged 36 years or younger have oligomenorrhea or amenorrhea; the age of the patient when chemotherapy is given appears to be the most important factor in the genesis of amenorrhea [6]. Among boys receiving irradiation and MOPP chemotherapy, the probability of return of spermatogenesis is low or absent [4].

CARDIOTOXICITY

Inclusion of the heart in a mediastinal radiation treatment field induces overt pericarditis in 15 percent or more of adults and sub-

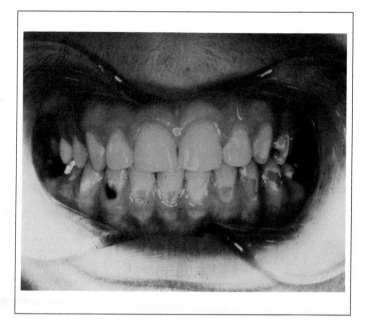

Fig. 26-5

clinical myocardial fibrosis in 50 percent. Chronic cardiomyopathy may occur after anthracycline therapy when the dose of doxorubicin exceeds 400 mg/sq m or less. Late cardiac toxicity occurring 10 years or more after treatment is now being observed [7,8]. It is hoped that cardiotoxicity may be averted by administering the anthracycline by slow intravenous drip or continuous infusion rather than by intravenous push or rapid injection (see Chap. 17).

PULMONARY TOXICITY

Bleomycin, a small molecular weight peptide isolated from a fungus, has little myelosuppressive toxicity, the primary toxicity being subacute and chronic pneumonitis that progresses to interstitial fibrosis. This toxicity is more common in the elderly, and its occurrence in children is unusual. Significant pulmonary toxicity occurs in 10 percent of patients receiving total doses of 450 mg or more [9]. Anecdotal cases suggest corticosteroid therapy can prevent the progression of pneumonitis to pulmonary fibrosis.

CHEMOTHERAPY-INDUCED HEMATURIA

Hemorrhagic cystitis and bladder fibrosis have occurred with MOPP therapy but are more commonly associated with cyclophosphamide or ifosfamide administration; an incidence of 7 to 12 percent has been observed. Concomitant administration of doxorubicin may aggravate cyclophosphamide bladder injury. The prophylactic use of 2-mercaptoethanesulfonate (MESNA) may be preventative; high fluid intake and bladder catheter drainage are useful in treatment [10].

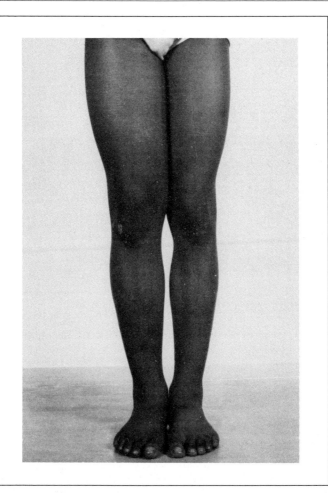

Fig. 26-6

SECOND MALIGNANT TUMORS

The incidence of second malignancies, primarily acute myeloid leukemia (AML), among young adults with Hodgkin's disease given MOPP chemotherapy is 3 to 4 percent within the first 10 years of follow-up. The risk is increased when radiation is included in the original treatment plan or given as salvage therapy. In a series of M. D. Anderson Cancer Center patients with Hodgkin's disease, approximately 7 percent have developed second malignant tumors; however, AML has been uncommon. Solid tumors are representative of those occurring in childhood.

Bones included in the radiation field have an increased incidence of malignant degeneration. Careful monitoring and prompt investigation of bony tumors is mandatory. A benign osteochondroma of the

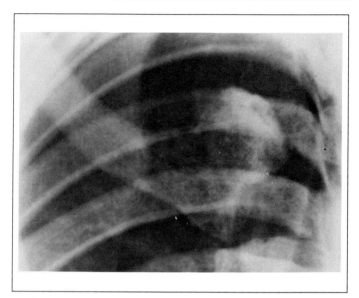

Fig. 26-7

medial end of the clavicle, which occurred in a radiotherapy field, is shown in Figure 26-7.

INFECTIOUS COMPLICATIONS

Herpes zoster has developed in 39 percent of splenectomized patients with Hodgkin's disease who received sandwich chemotherapy plus radiotherapy at the M. D. Anderson Cancer Center. Herpes zoster usually occurred during the first course of chemotherapy following radiotherapy. Prompt acyclovir therapy, given intravenously, has been effective. Oral acyclovir prophylaxis has not been studied.

The reported susceptibility of splenectomized patients to pneumococcal or *Haemophilus influenzae* septicemia has been publicized widely. However, the Intergroup Hodgkin's Disease Study showed an incidence of 4.5 percent for serious postsplenectomy infections. The infections occurred in patients who had received pneumococcal vaccine before splenectomy and prophylactic penicillin following splenectomy until they were 21 years old.

REFERENCES

1. Katzman, H., Haugh, T., and Berdon, W. Skeletal changes following irradiation of childhood tumors. *J. Bone Joint Surg [Am.]* 51:823, 1969.
2. D'Angio, G.J. Late adversities of treatment in long term survivors of childhood cancer. Proceedings of the National Conference on Human Values and Cancer of the American Cancer Society, Chicago, Sept. 7–9, 1977. Pp. 59–72.
3. Sullivan, M.P., Fuller, L.M., and Bulter, J.J. Hodgkin's Disease. In W.W. Sutow, D.F. Fernback, and T.J. Vietti (eds.), *Clinical Pediatric Oncology* (3rd ed.). St. Louis: Mosby, 1984. Pp. 437–442.

4. Donaldson, S.S., and Kaplan, H.S. Complications of treatment of Hodgkin's disease in children. *Cancer Treat. Rep.* 66:977, 1982.

5. Jaffe, N., et al. Dental and maxillofacial abnormalities in long-term survivors of childhood cancer: Effects of treatment with chemotherapy and radiation to the head and neck. *Pediatrics* 73:816, 1984.

6. Andrieu, J.M., and Ochoa-Molina, M.E. Menstrual cycle, pregnancies and offspring before and after MOPP therapy for Hodgkin's disease. *Cancer* 52:435, 1983.

7. Sullivan, M.P., et al. Comparative effectiveness of two combined modality regimens in the treatment of surgical stage III Hodgkin's disease in children; an eight-year follow-up. (Submitted to *Am. J. Pediatr. Hematol. Oncol.*)

8. Personal communication.

9. Blum, R.H., Carter, S.K., and Agre, K. A clinical review of bleomycin—a new anti-neoplastic agent. *Cancer* 31:903, 1973.

10. Javadpour, N., and Barakat, H.A. Bladder toxicity due to cyclophosphamide. *Urology* 2:634, 1973.

27

Psychosocial Issues

Maureen S. Sanger and Donna R. Copeland

THE DEVELOPING CHILD

Comprehensive care of children with cancer requires attention to their psychological as well as their physical needs. Children's beliefs and feelings about their malignancies not only influence their psychosocial adaptation to disease, but also can affect compliance with prescribed treatment regimens, the nature and severity of treatment-related side effects and, ultimately, the course of the cancer itself. We will provide an overview of the developmental and psychologic issues that the child with cancer must face and health care providers must confront.

The Infant

Cognitive Development

During the first 18 months of life, the infant is in a period of sensori-motor exploration. Through repeated interactions with the environment, the infant learns to attach meaning to sensory information. Although infants do not have the cognitive ability to understand concepts about their body or their illness, they do begin to associate objects and events. Thus, infants who have experienced painful injections from medical personnel may show signs of fear and distress at the sight of a white coat at their bedside.

Social and Emotional Development

The primary task of the infant is the development of trust in significant adults. When the quality and consistency of parental responsiveness to and care of the infant is high, the infant's trust in the world is fostered. As the attachment between parent and infant is strengthened, the child demonstrates a growing fear of strangers and anxiety regarding prolonged separation from caregivers. During this period, the infant may adopt a transitional object, such as a favorite blanket or toy, that serves to comfort the infant during periods of separation from the caregiver. Thumb sucking, genital play, and the use of a transitional object are all activities that the infant may initiate to decrease anxiety and produce greater self-calm in the absence of a parent [1].

Impact of Illness

The diagnosis and treatment of cancer in the infant results in a series of disruptions for both patient and family, some of which may threaten the infant's sense of trust in the environment and interfere with the normal processes of attachment and separation. Parents should be allowed to stay with the hospitalized child as much as possible and should participate in the physical care of their child. The medical team can facilitate parental involvement by establishing a trusting relationship with parents and teaching them strategies for meeting the special care needs of their infant [2].

The Toddler

Cognitive Development

Between the ages of 18 and 36 months, egocentric and magical thinking in children is evident. Toddlers ascribe great power to their thoughts and beliefs and often perceive the cause of events as resulting from their own actions, thoughts, or wishes. Thus, children this age often attribute illness to being bad or having bad thoughts and may view cancer or hospitalization as a punishment for transgressions.

Social and Emotional Development

The major developmental goal for toddlers is establishing autonomy and independence. Toddlers frequently test the limits of their emerging independence, and resistant behaviors, including temper tantrums, are common. Parents are challenged to foster their children's sense of autonomy by allowing them freedom to make choices while establishing firm limits to help guide and protect them [3].

Impact of Illness

The physical limitations and restrictions that accompany the treatment of cancer may interfere with the toddler's acquisition of independent behavior. The child may experience feelings of helplessness and loss of control over his or her environment, the reaction to which may be manifested by increased passivity and dependence, or by defiant, negativistic behavior. Parents often need assurance that treating their toddler as normally as possible, including setting appropriate limits, is the best way to facilitate adjustment to disease and attainment of a good developmental outcome.

The Preschool Child

Cognitive Development

Before age 6 or 7 years, children function at the preoperational stage of cognitive development. Preschoolers' notions about how their bodies work are very simple and concrete. Although they have a growing awareness of their specific body parts, they lack an understanding of how these parts function. Some preschoolers believe that all body parts, including hair, are vital to bodily integrity and survival. Hence, their anxiety may be heightened if a part of the body is altered, removed, or lost in surgery or the course of treatment [2]. Preschool children's understanding of illness is similarly incomplete and concrete. Although preschoolers are able to repeat information given to them by parents or medical staff, they often do not have an understanding of the facts they are verbalizing. It is important that health care providers elicit children's understanding of bodily functions and illness concepts and provide simple, concrete explanations to clarify misconceptions.

Social and Emotional Development

Acquiring a sense of initiative is the chief developmental task of the preschooler. Freedom to pursue activities and interests and master new skills fosters a sense of achievement in preschool children. Preschoolers work industriously to attain their desired goals and to receive social approval for their accomplishments. When children fail in their pursuit of self-selected goals, they may experience a sense of disappointment, frustration, and defeat that prevents them from identifying and pursuing future goals with confidence.

Impact of Illness

Limitations imposed by the diagnosis and treatment of cancer may reduce the preschooler's opportunity for consistent and sustained involvement in tasks in which the child is interested or skilled, thereby reducing the child's sense of initiative. As a consequence, the preschool child may feel guilty that he or she is not living up to expected standards of behavior. In times of stress, the child might revert to behaviors more appropriate to an earlier developmental level. Admonishments for regressive behavior may further weaken the preschooler's developing sense of competence and self-esteem.

The School-Age Child

Cognitive Development

During the elementary school period, children progress to the concrete operational stage of cognitive development and attain the ability to think in terms of cause and effect, make generalizations, understand relational terms, and reason about objects in systematic ways. School-age children can differentiate the structure and function of individual body parts, but they have only limited understanding of the connectedness of various organs or the interrelationships of different bodily systems. The cause of illness frequently is attributed to an external action, event, or object that effects a change inside the body, with little knowledge of the body's role in pathogenesis [4,5]. In discussing their illness with school-age children, medical personnel need to provide information in a descriptive and explanatory manner; such information may be conveyed most effectively with the use of models, drawings, or diagrams.

Social and Emotional Development

School-age children are faced with the task of developing a sense of industry. The acquisition of academic skills and skills in activities and sports is important to fostering their self-esteem and sense of competence. The school-age period is also a time of significant social growth. Peer acceptance is sought and sensitivity to peer response is heightened.

Impact of Illness

Irregular school attendance, as a consequence of clinic visits and absences due to treatment side effects, may limit the child's opportunities for academic achievement and success. The diagnosis of cancer often leads to alterations in peer relations as well. School-age children are aware of their differentness and worry about how their illness will be accepted by their classmates. Educating teachers and peers about a child's illness may facilitate the child's integration into academic and social activities.

The Adolescent

Cognitive Development

As the child moves into adolescence, the final cognitive developmental stage of formal operational thought is gradually attained. The adolescent can better understand and integrate the structure and function of individual body parts and is able to articulate more complex physiologic explanations of the relationships between organ systems. With their greater understanding of internal physiologic processes, adolescents can explain illness in terms of internal bodily dysfunction. Multiple causes of a disease can be considered, the interaction between host and agent can be recognized, and the causal processes resulting in illness onset or arrest can be delineated.

Social and Emotional Development

The central developmental task of adolescents is the establishment of a stable and autonomous identity. During this period, the adolescent strives to develop a secure self-concept and comfortable body image, to establish emotional and economic independence from parents, to foster peer relationships, to develop a sexual identity, and to prepare for a career. Teenagers are particularly preoccupied by their changing bodies and by the ways in which they are perceived by peers and may become absorbed with their appearance, sexuality, and ability to meet gender role expectations.

Impact of Illness

Challenges to the chronically ill adolescent's sense of autonomy come from many sources. The physical side effects of cancer and its treatment, which result in periods of weakness and debilitation, make it necessary for the adolescent to depend on others for care. Emotional dependence on parents also is intensified. Furthermore, medical treatment and hospitalization require a shift in control from the adolescent to the staff, as the patient must submit to procedures, regulations, and schedules. Adolescents may rebel against the lack of control and autonomy inherent in the cancer experience, which can make medical management more difficult. Allowing the adolescent to have some decision-making power, respecting his or her need for privacy, and encouraging the resumption of normal activities may help restore the adolescent's sense of autonomous functioning.

PSYCHOLOGICAL ISSUES IN MEDICAL MANAGEMENT

Side Effects of Chemotherapy

The side effects that children experience from the medical treatment of cancer can be divided into two types: pharmacologic and psychologically conditioned [6]. Pharmacologically induced side effects occur as a consequence of damage produced by toxic chemotherapeutic agents to noncancerous tissue. Conditioned side effects are symptomatically similar to drug-induced sequelae but are the result of conditioned learning. Conditioned side effects typically develop when an association is established between the postchemotherapy side effects and other stimuli in the environment in which the drugs are administered. Thus, previously neutral sights, smells, or thoughts that recur with the experience of pharmacologically based side effects may, in and of themselves, come to elicit those side effects.

Two of the most noxious and frequent side effects of cancer treatment are nausea and vomiting. Pharmacologically induced emesis results from the toxic action of chemotherapeutic agents on the gastrointestinal tract or the chemoreceptor triggering zone of the central nervous system and may be treated by antiemetic medications. Conditioned nausea and vomiting may occur before, during, or after chemotherapy. When these effects occur before the administration of treatment, they are referred to as anticipatory nausea and vomiting and are clearly identified as psychologic phenomena. When conditioned emesis follows treatment, it frequently occurs with, and is not easily differentiated from, pharmacologically induced vomiting.

Conditioned emesis is often a source of confusion, embarrassment, and distress to the child who develops it. Family and staff may not be supportive to the child who vomits outside of treatment and whose unpleasant side effects appear to be "all in his head." Therefore, children and their families need to be educated as to the etiology of conditioned nausea and vomiting and the ways in which these learned behaviors may be unlearned [7]. Psychologic interventions that have been found to be successful in helping children reduce conditioned emesis and its associated anxiety include hypnosis, relaxation training, and systematic desensitization.

Painful Procedures

Perhaps the most difficult and anxiety-producing components of the treatment regimen for the child with cancer and his or her parents are the painful procedures the child must undergo for the diagnostic evaluation and medical management of his or her disease. Bone marrow aspirations and lumbar punctures are perhaps the most traumatic procedures, although many children experience heightened anxiety over less invasive procedures as well. Managing children's distress associated with painful procedures is a constant challenge for pediatric oncology staff.

Children vary greatly in their experience and expression of pain. Physiologic factors that influence pain include the type, location, and extensiveness of the tumor; the integrity of the peripheral and central nervous system; and individual physiologic differences in pain thresholds [8]. Psychological factors also account for some variability in children's perceptions of pain. These factors include the perceived meaning of the pain, social response to the expression of pain, and anxiety.

There are two primary models of psychological intervention aimed at assisting children with painful procedures: (1) the education preparation model, and (2) the skills-building model.

The Education Preparation Model

The provision of preparatory information and activities is among the most frequently employed interventions for pediatric cancer patients undergoing medical and surgical procedures. The premise underlying this approach is that preparing children and their families for what to expect before, during, and after a procedure will decrease the fear and anxiety associated with the procedure and, consequently, reduce the pain and distress the child experiences.

Before a painful event, educating the child about the procedure is essential and must be done using words and concepts that the child is able to comprehend. Young children are particularly interested in knowing what will happen and how it will feel. They require brief, simple, and concrete explanations, since they cannot maintain focused attention in the face of threatening events. Older children also benefit from verbal descriptions of procedures. Their learning may be enhanced by visual aids including diagrams, dolls, observation of peer models, and films.

During the procedure, most (but not all) children benefit from having each step verbalized to them. Information about the mechanics of the procedure as well as the sensation to be experienced is helpful. Labeling and reinforcing specific positive behaviors that the child exhibits during the procedure will both enhance the child's sense of competence and help shape appropriate actions. It is best to ignore negative behaviors.

After the procedure, children need time to review the event and express their feelings about it. This helps the child integrate the experience and provides an opportunity to reflect on ways in which future adaptation to procedures may be facilitated.

The Skills-Building Model

An alternative or additional approach to assisting children with painful procedures is the skills-building model of intervention. Within the context of this model, children are taught specific coping skills for reducing pain and anxiety. These skills include the use of hypnosis, relaxation techniques, biofeedback, imagery, and distraction. The benefits of skills-building interventions lie not only in the alleviation of pain but in the sense of control and accomplishment they foster in the children who use them effectively. Armed with coping skills and techniques, children can become active participants in, rather than passive recipients of, the medical treatment of their disease.

Compliance with Treatment

Adherence is an important issue in the medical management of children with cancer. Patient noncompliance with prescribed therapeutic regimens undermines the effectiveness of treatment protocols and results in unnecessary morbidity, mortality, and cost [9]. Across the few studies that have investigated the rate of nonadherence to treatment among pediatric cancer patients, estimates of the incidence of children with significant compliance difficulties range from 14 to 55 percent [10]. Noncompliant behaviors include failure to take prescribed medications, failure to take medications properly, missing doses of medication, missing clinic appointments, and failure to heed medical restrictions.

Several factors that have been associated with noncompliance include the complexity, severity, and duration of the child's treatment [8]. The cost, inconvenience, and side effects of chemotherapeutic agents may impede adherence to treatment. Failure of parents to supervise drug administration may also increase the likelihood of noncompliance. The thoughts, feelings, and attitudes children and their families have about the disease may affect their rate of compliance as well. Denial of the illness or rationalization of unhealthy behaviors may interfere with adherence to medical regimens. Beliefs regarding the relative costs and benefits of treatment, the prognosis of the disease, the effectiveness of treatment, and one's ability to carry out medical recommendations also may influence compliance.

The physician's relationship with and behaviors toward the patient also influence compliance. Research indicates that patients who receive the information they seek and are treated in a caring manner by their physician are more satisfied with the help they receive, express more positive feelings about their physician, and are more compliant with recommended actions [11].

Three strategies that have been employed to increase patients' compliance with medical regimens are education, behavioral intervention, and relationship building between patient and physician.

Education

Educating children and their parents about the specific behaviors required by the children's treatment, and the reasons behind them, helps patients and families follow the requirements of the regimen. Children and parents must understand how and when to implement the treatment program and how to deal with problems when they develop. This information must be tailored to the patient's ability level and circumstances. Educating children and their parents about the benefits and consequences of compliance with medical recommendations also may increase treatment adherence.

Behavioral Intervention

Behavioral intervention strategies to enhance compliance can involve stimulus control or consequence control [12]. Stimulus control procedures may involve tailoring a child's medication schedule to normal behaviors in his or her routine, so that daily activities serve as cues for appropriate compliance behavior. Consequence control techniques function by manipulating the reinforcers that follow the child's compliant behaviors. Verbal praise, tangible rewards, token economies, and penalty systems may be effective consequence control procedures for promoting short-term increases in compliance. Self-monitoring, goal setting, and behavioral contracting also have been used to improve treatment adherence.

Relationship Building

Finally, enhancing the patient-physician relationship will facilitate compliance. By demonstrating understanding and empathy, and creating a conducive atmosphere wherein children and families can feel they are respected and cared for, the health care provider will foster a more effective working alliance with the patient [13]. Other behaviors in which physicians can engage to facilitate their relationship with children and parents include exploring families' concerns, goals, and expectations; listening to and answering all questions; avoiding the use of medical jargon; acknowledging and discussing the advantages and disadvantages of alternative evaluations and treatments; and eliciting patients' feelings, suggestions, and conflicts about treatment [11].

The Dying Child

When standard treatment protocols fail and prognosis becomes bleak, children with cancer must deal with the reality of their eventual and impending death. A child's reaction to and ability to cope with death depends on his or her intellectual and emotional maturity.

Children as young as 3 years of age begin to formulate a vague conceptualization of death. Death, to the toddler, is not understood as a permanent, irreversible condition but as a separation from those whom the child loves and on whom he or she depends for nurturance and safety. Thus, fear of separation, rather than fear of death, is the salient concern of the very young child, and he or she may exhibit sadness or anxiety in response to the depression or fear manifested by significant adults [1].

Like toddlers, preschool children are unable to understand the finality and irreversibility of death. Death is viewed as a departure or separation or as a kind of sleep. Children's observations of dead animals on the side of the road or fatal tragedies reported in the media may instill in some children a fear that death is painful and mutilating [1]. Such fears and perceptions should be explored in order to dispel misconceptions and decrease anxiety.

Children between the ages of 5 and 9 years often maintain a superstitious and personified view of death. Death is conceptualized as an objectified being such as a ghost, skeleton, or bogeyman. The cause of death is attributed to an entity external to the child rather than a process that occurs within oneself.

At approximately 9 years of age, children develop a recognition that death signals the end of life and is the consequence of bodily malfunction. They have an awareness that death is inevitable and irreversible, and consequently, they often exhibit strong affect in relation to death. With the emerging cognitive ability to think about alternative beliefs and future possibilities, the school-age child begins to wonder what happens after death and considers concepts such as heaven, hell, and an afterlife.

Adolescents have a cognitively sophisticated, adultlike concept of death but often do not have the emotional maturity to cope with death as would an adult. At the time in life when the child is striving to develop his or her identity and future, the adolescent has great difficulty accepting his or her own death. Consequently, dying adolescents may behave in daring or noncompliant ways, maintaining a belief in their own invincibility and denying the inevitability of death, or they may become depressed or angry with the prospect of having no future.

Honest and open communication between the health care provider and the dying child and his or her family is important in helping the child come to terms with his or her own death. Often, health care providers are reluctant to talk with children who are terminally ill, believing that it is better to protect them from the burden of information about their disease [14]. However, terminally ill children usually are aware of their fatal prognosis without being told. They observe and experience changes in their medical regimens, changes in the way family and staff respond to them, and changes within their own bodies. Thus, attempts to shield children from knowing they are fatally ill are rarely beneficial and, in some cases, may prevent children from expressing their feelings about death and from obtaining accurate information to allay unrealistic fears and concerns.

Encouraging the dying child to communicate his or her experiences gives the child a chance to vent his or her thoughts and feelings and concomitantly allows the listener to identify the child's fears and fantasies, correct misperceptions, and intervene in a manner that will alleviate the child's anxieties. By allowing dying children, when possible, to participate in decisions regarding treatment and to maintain their involvement in normal activities, terminally ill children may be helped to cope with the loss of control and self-esteem engendered by their condition.

THE PEDIATRIC ONCOLOGY PATIENT AND SCHOOL

The School Experience

Encouraging the child with cancer to maintain active involvement in the classroom is critical, because it is primarily within the context of school and peer interactions that children develop the cognitive and social skills necessary for a sense of competence, mastery, and independence. Although the development of these skills is important for all children, it is particularly relevant to children and adolescents with cancer whose illness has a tendency to foster passivity, dependence, and low self-esteem. Whatever type of differentness the child experiences as a result of the illness and treatment will be minimized by participation in school and school-related activities. Some of the difficulties children with cancer encounter at school are associated with changes in physical appearance and cognitive functioning, the stigma associated with cancer, school absenteeism, and educators' tendency to view school as a place for well children only.

Parents and teachers need to be encouraged by the physician to see that children stay in school. Teachers are uncertain about the child's physical status and need reassurance that it is appropriate for the child to be in the classroom. Parents must be reassured that their children are not likely to contract infections or be physically harmed at school. Physicians are in a key position to assess a child's readiness to return to school and to boost the confidence of parents and teachers in achieving this goal. It often requires specific medical guidelines provided by the physician.

Not all children with cancer will require special services. Most will require special education only in certain subjects or during certain periods in the course of treatment, and some may require only adjunct services such as counseling or periodic homebound instruction.

Neuropsychological and Academic Side Effects of Cancer and Its Treatment

Neuropyschological Effects

The neuropsychological effects of cancer and its treatment on children with tumors outside the central nervous system (CNS) have been studied extensively [15]. A review of these studies [15] shows that in general, these children perform within the average range during the treatment phase of the illness and even 5 or more years after treatment has been discontinued. Studies that have compared the performance of groups who received CNS treatment with those who did not have found significant between-group differences. The authors of the review article conclude that poorer performance tends to be associated with CNS prophylaxis that includes cranial radiotherapy (CRT). Leukemia patients whose CNS prophylaxis consists of chemotherapy alone perform generally at the same level as patients who receive no CNS treatment. Neuropsychologic deficits in CNS-irradiated children may be more apparent in attention capacities and other nonverbal cognitive processing skills, although results of some of the studies reviewed suggest a more generalized effect. Decrements in performance among CRT patients may be linked to white matter alterations, in that these changes have been detected on neural imaging scans following treatment of the CNS.

Before treatment, children with tumors outside the CNS usually perform at average levels relative to normative standards on tasks measuring intellect, language, memory, and other higher cortical functions. Longitudinal studies of these patients demonstrate that children retain these abilities across time, provided they are not treated with CRT. If they do receive CRT, their performance varies widely, although as a group, their scores still tend to be within one standard deviation of the mean [5].

Some systematically administered chemotherapies have neuropathic side effects that are detected on neuropsychological assessment. Vincristine has been associated with declines in fine-motor speed and coordination, and cisplatin with poorer performance on visual-motor integration and tactile-spatial (stereognosis) tasks [16]. The effects of vincristine appear to be transient and diminish once the drug is discontinued, whereas the effects of cisplatin tend to persist.

Because of the site of the tumor and the more intensive treatment required, children with brain tumors are at even greater risk for neurobehavioral impairments. Cumulative experience indicates that more than 50 percent of these children are significantly impaired in intellectual skills and academic achievement. Most will need some type of special educational assistance during their school years. Heterogeneity of diagnoses and characteristics of tumors, as well as varying sequelae as a result of treatment, make it difficult to generalize about this group of patients. Therefore, comprehensive neuropsychologic examinations at periodic intervals are useful in monitoring the children's progress and are essential for advising the school about special educational needs the patients may have.

Academic Effects

Academic deficits are not uncommon in children with cancer, although most perform within normal limits. Factors that may contribute to academic declines include treatment with cranial radiation, learning disabilities, cumulative effects of school absences, and psychosocial factors.

Specific skills required for academic achievement that are adversely affected by CRT include memory, visual-motor and fine-motor skills and arithmetic and attentional capacities [15]. Children who have received CRT perform less well in problem solving and planning ahead, learning new material, and following instructions with multiple components. They require a longer time to complete tasks, and they lack mental efficiency in information processing [17]. Deficiencies tend to be mild to moderate for leukemia patients and moderate to severe for children with brain tumors, although the extent of impairment varies widely. Pediatric CRT patients are more likely to need special educational assistance and to repeat grades in school.

Learning-based deficits are characterized by an ability-performance discrepancy. That is, children with a learning disability score within normal limits on IQ tests, but their academic achievement scores are below average because of impairments in learning skills (e.g., auditory processing, phonetic discrimination, and mental calculations). Learning disabilities may predate the diagnosis of cancer or may be acquired as a result of the illness and treatment, either directly or indirectly.

Children with cancer must miss school because of their illness and treatment. Therefore, school absences are likely to be a contributing factor in declines in academic achievement. During the year that cancer is diagnosed, children are expected to miss more than 40 days of school on the average. (Well children miss approximately 9 days per year.) Even 3 to 4 years after diagnosis, when it is likely that treatment has been completed and children are well, pediatric oncology patients still miss an average of 20 or more days per school year [18,19].

Clearly, the side effects of treatment for cancer and the disease itself, with its accompanying psychosocial sequelae, are likely to contribute to school absenteeism. However, there are other reasons for being absent, particularly for those who are no longer receiving treatment and who are doing well physically. The child may have become used to staying home from school during the period of active treatment and may have learned that physical symptoms are a legitimate excuse for not attending school. Thus, he or she may have developed a propensity for somatic complaints as well as an ability to use them for secondary gain. Additionally, parents who have cared for their children during the intensive period of treatment for cancer may become overly protective or may even become dependent on the child for their own sense of self-worth. These parents may unconsciously encourage their children to miss school and stay home with them.

In the child with cancer, psychosocial factors may contribute to lower performance and involvement at school. Alterations in physical appearance and limitations in stamina and physical capabilities may inhibit the child's desire and opportunity for successful performance at school and integration into the classroom. In addition, unrealistically high or low expectations on the part of parents and teachers may stifle the child's openness to learning.

According to parents who have completed the Personality Inventory for Children, children and adolescents with cancer do tend to focus more on physical symptomatology, as evidenced by high scores on the Somatic Concern scale [20,21]. Although it is not clear whether these concerns are more physically or more psychologically based, it is clear that children with cancer are more preoccupied with their bodies; and in one study, this type of concern correlated significantly with teacher-rated and parent-rated performance of the child at school [22].

The educational consequences of illness that are found among children with cancer occur among children with other types of chronic illness as well. That is, academic performance is likely to be lower than expected based on the child's IQ and below that of healthy children. Although these findings could be due in part to the children's compromised physical status or secondary to medical treatment, evidence [18,19] suggests that, in addition, lower performance at school may be the result of unnecessary school absences, a tendency toward somatization, and other psychosocial factors. This suggests that the medical treatment team, parents, and schools should monitor the academic progress of chronically ill children and arrange for tutorial assistance or special education when problems arise.

School absenteeism continues to be a problem for these children even after completion of medical treatment. The reasons for this should be examined more carefully. Each child's situation should be assessed with regard to disease status and ongoing treatment. If the child is well and treatment has been discontinued, then further investigation into psychosocial factors is warranted. Follow-up consultation with parents and schools is likely to be essential in helping overcome the barriers to school attendance and academic performance.

Timely assessments and preventive services are probably the most effective ways of addressing the problem. For instance, pediatricians might inquire about their young patients' attitude toward school and their academic progress. Given the tendency of these children's families to gloss over problems, however, this is probably not sufficient. Adequate assessments with well-standardized instruments administered by specialists are required to obtain a realistic picture of each child's progress. Even schoolteachers tend to overrate the performance of medically ill children. Thus, liaison work between hospital and school would be helpful in obtaining accurate information about a child's performance at school, as well as in educating the teachers about that child's medical situation.

For the more complicated and longer-term medical conditions, a comprehensive program is needed in which a range of services is provided and a coordinator is identified to maintain efficiency and quality control. Specifically with regard to their academic achievement, children may require neurocognitive assessments, speech and hearing assessment and follow-up, school consultation and intervention, tutorial and special education assistance, and individual or family counseling.

PSYCHOLOGICAL INTERVENTIONS

The acute and chronic stresses associated with the cancer experience place a child at risk for developing difficulties in psychosocial adaptation. Although many children and families are able to meet the challenges presented by the diagnosis and treatment of malignancies and utilize personal resources and social support to achieve a good developmental outcome, children and families often benefit from psychological intervention. Mental health interventions may be short-term or long-term, they may focus on specific treatment-related difficulties or more general issues of adjustment, and they may involve the child alone or the whole family system. Several modalities of psychological treatment have been used effectively to help children with cancer. These include individual, group, and family psychotherapy, hypnotherapy, and behavioral therapy.

Psychotherapy

Individual Therapy

The purpose of individual psychotherapy with pediatric cancer patients is to provide a safe, accepting environment within which children can freely express their feelings, fears, and fantasies and to help children cope effectively with the challenges of cancer and its treatment. For young children, therapeutic work is often done through the medium of play. In this context, play is not only an enjoyable activity but it is used as a means of building rapport with the child, a medium of observation and source of data, and a tool that promotes identification and interpretation of the child's conflicts so that the child becomes aware of them and can resolve them.

A special form of play therapy frequently used in hospital and clinic settings is medical play. This is a structured play activity in which children are provided with real medical equipment to manipulate and a doll on which to carry out treatment procedures. Medical play allows for active confrontation of feared stimuli and events and experimentation with alternative coping strategies.

With older children and adolescents, verbal therapies are typically employed in which patients are encouraged to explore their concerns and problems and come to a greater understanding of and, ultimately, a solution to their difficulties. Older children are often hesitant, initially, to see a mental health professional for assistance in coping with their illness. Recommendations for individual psychotherapy, when indicated, must be approached in a sensitive and tactful manner.

Group Therapy

Group therapy has also been found to be beneficial for pediatric cancer patients. Groups may be unstructured and oriented toward helping children deal with broad developmental and illness-related issues such as autonomy, identity, depression, and the search for meaning. Alternatively, groups may be structured, addressing specific issues such as answering questions from peers, accepting limitations, and setting realistic expectations, or teaching specific skills to cope with treatment. A group psychotherapeutic approach to treating children with cancer is beneficial in that it provides opportunities for fostering peer support, observing competent children, and promoting the development of mutual helping relationships [23].

Family Therapy

Given the profound impact childhood cancer has on the family and the power that parental coping has to influence children's health status, psychotherapeutic interventions that focus on the family's adaptation to illness often are beneficial in helping a child cope with cancer. This approach is particularly indicated when maladaptive family functioning interferes with successful treatment of the cancer or when the strain of the cancer experience exacerbates conflicts that existed in the family prior to diagnosis. Common goals in working with families in a pediatric oncology setting include: (1) modifying failures in family interactional patterns that prevent the development of mutually satisfying relationships and the fulfillment of needs; (2) helping families redefine roles and relationship demands that inevitably shift as a result of the illness; (3) facilitating the adaptive expression of grief; and (4) assisting in identifying areas of strength and competence on which they can draw to cope with the physical and emotional demands of the family member's disease [24].

Family therapy may be problem-focused and directive, with the purpose of changing the way family members relate to one another, or it may be oriented toward resolving problems by reorganizing the family structure (e.g., altering alignments, establishing boundaries, and shifting power within the family). In either case, the goal of family therapy is to help the family acquire the organization and skills needed to be flexible in meeting the demands of a chronic illness and the needs of its individual members.

Hypnotherapy

Hypnosis has been proved a useful and effective technique for children with cancer. Children tend to demonstrate high levels of susceptibility to and motivation for involvement with hypnosis and often enjoy the opportunities for fantasy and self-control provided by such therapeutic strategies. Hypnosis serves to support the child's sense of competence while teaching the child a variety of skills to help master pain and anxiety, thereby reducing the child's sense of helplessness.

Specific applications of hypnosis with pediatric oncology patients include the utilization of direct and indirect suggestion, relaxation, analgesia, dissociation, and fantasy and imagery. A variety of goals may be simultaneously addressed by hypnotherapeutic interventions. These include: (1) control of pain associated with the disease process and treatment procedures; (2) management of anxiety and related resistance; (3) modulation of nausea and vomiting associated with chemotherapy; (4) support of appetite and adequate food intake; (5) relaxation and maintenance of appropriate sleep patterns; (6) use of fantasy and imagery to escape the hospital environment; (7) support of coping strategies in coming to terms and dealing with the cancer experience; and (8) intervention to resolve or prevent psychiatric sequelae such as depression and transient regressive behavior [25]. Research suggests that between 60 and 90 percent of children with cancer can successfully manage some aspect of their discomfort and difficulty through the use of hypnosis [26,27].

Behavioral Therapy

Behavioral therapy techniques are among the most frequently employed intervention strategies in pediatric settings. Behavioral therapy has been used to help children with cancer deal with a variety of problematic illness-related issues including adhering to treatment, managing pain, reducing anxiety, decreasing fear, controlling weight, and enhancing social skills.

One of the most widely used behavioral techniques is the implementation of contingent reward or punishment programs. Contingent reinforcement has been effective in altering the frequency of behaviors such as food refusal, weight gain and loss, and tantrums. One type of contingent reward system is the token economy, in which children earn tokens for specified appropriate behaviors. Token economy programs are particulary well suited for dealing with difficult children on inpatient units.

Another effective behavioral intervention is modeling, or the learning of behavior through the observation of another's behavior and its consequences. Modeling techniques have been used to reduce fears in medical settings. Filmed modeling, in which common fears and ways in which children can adaptively cope with them are depicted, has been successfully used in preparing children for hospitalization, surgery, and painful procedures. Research indicates that the anxiety levels of children who view such films are markedly decreased compared with those children who view a control film [28].

Biofeedback and relaxation training programs are also commonly used in pediatric settings. These techniques are beneficial in promoting a reduction in pain and anxiety, as well as fostering a sense of active participation in and control over symptom managment.

THE PHYSICIAN'S ROLE

Communicating With Families

From the time the child's cancer is diagnosed and throughout the course of treatment, the physician plays an integral role in the adaptation of families of pediatric cancer patients. Open communication between the physician and family about the disease and its medical management is one of the most important elements in adjustment. This openness may be difficult for family members to accept initially, as they frequently desire to protect the child from knowledge of his or her condition and thereby avoid undue distress. However, the child who does not receive accurate information will fill in the gaps in his or her knowledge with unrealistic fears and misperceptions. As a result, this child is more likely to show signs of depression and anxiety.

In communicating with the family about the disease, particularly when the news is unexpected or unfavorable, the physician should present the information slowly and concisely, pausing to allow family members to react. It is usually necessary for the physician to repeat the same information a number of times and over several meetings, especially during the initial weeks. Anxious family members may deny the information until they can cope with it on an emotional level. Sometimes the emotional experience predominates and interferes with the family's intellectual processing of the information. Alternatively, the family may take an intellectualized approach and focus on technical aspects of treatment to avoid confronting the emotional concomitants. What is important is that the physician schedule a series of follow-up meetings with the family after the initial diagnostic conference to assess how the family is coping with the information, to answer questions, and to provide an opportunity to repeat what the family did not hear.

In addition to providing families with information, it is important for the physician to obtain feedback from the child and family regarding their understanding and beliefs about the illness so that any misconceptions they might have can be clarified. The physician should be attuned to parental feelings of guilt associated with the possible genetic etiology of the illness and self-recrimination for not recognizing symptoms or seeking medical attention more quickly. The physician can do much to alleviate the guilt if these feelings are recognized and attended to promptly. Allotting a "silent" period at the end of each informational meeting may be particularly helpful in allowing family members to process what they have heard and to seek clarification. Encouraging family members to ask questions about medical decisions and treatment options helps families gain a greater understanding of the disease and enhances the patient-physician relationship.

When imparting emotionally laden information, it is helpful to allow the child and family to express their grief, anger, and sadness. Although the physician may experience some discomfort in observing families' spontaneous demonstration of emotion, healing will begin more quickly if feelings are expressed rather than suppressed. Offering words of comfort and periods of silent support may facilitate this process.

Aspects of Effective Doctor-Patient Relationships

The relationship between doctor and patient is always special because it plays a large role in the patient's sense of security and well-being. This relationship has been examined in studies of psychotherapy to assess its influence on treatment outcome. These investigations have identified the quality of the doctor-patient relationship and personal characteristics of the therapist as key elements of successful treatment. In a medical context, the doctor-patient relationship is just as important. The physician's ability to form a positive working alliance with the child and the child's family will greatly influence their adherence to treatment protocols and medical recommendations. For instance, there is an important relationship between the patient's perceptions of the physician's friendliness and concern and the patient's satisfaction with service and compliance with the treatment plan [29]. Giving information to the patient and family and spending time with them heightens their satisfaction and fosters the development of a working alliance. As much as possible, it helps to phrase explanations in common language and to be frank, even if a family is anxious and upset. Families may need an opportunity to ask questions and express their emotions. The physician can demonstrate a willingness to understand by making open-ended statements (e.g., "Tell me about your main concerns") and by making sympathetic comments (e.g., "I know this is difficult for you").

An important and often overlooked way of winning the family's trust and confidence is to be consistent and dependable in contacts with them. Not knowing when to expect the physician's visit increases the uncertainty and anxiety a family may already be experiencing.

If an adversarial relationship develops, the family is likely to resist treatment by missing appointments and scheduled medications and by displaying discontent in their behavior. Should this occur, the physician can have a frank discussion with the family, allowing them to voice their concerns in order to try to resolve the problem. Sometimes, enlisting the aid of another staff member who can serve temporarily as a mediator may be most helpful.

The physician's personal qualities may enhance the therapeutic relationship or detract from it. Attributes such as being empathic and genuinely interested in people will be recognized and appreciated by the families. The physician who is psychologically mature, cares for patients without feeling possessive, and who is neutral toward patients' values and personal characteristics will be most effective. Although it is ethically and medically important for the physician to maintain a professional stance toward them, patients and families adjust more easily when they know the physician cares about them. When they sense detachment or exaggerated professionalism, they are likely to withdraw and, in turn, and not ask questions or provide useful information. They may infer from the detached attitude that their adherence to treatment is not especially important or that the doctor is not going to be conscientious about the care of the child.

In summary, the physician plays a key role in families' adjustment to illness, primarily through the therapeutic relationship. The alliance may be fostered by listening carefully and responding to the families' perceived needs; by providing support, guidance, and hope; by being honest and frank with information; and by encouraging family members to express their feelings in an atmosphere of neutrality and understanding.

Psychological Consultation

Most children and their families adjust remarkably well to the challenges presented by childhood cancer. However, a certain number will encounter difficulties that require extra attention from the physician and the medical treatment team. Prompt identification of problems and referral for psychological evaluation and intervention may make the difference between healthy adaptation and maladjustment. At the outset, during the diagnostic workup, the physician may assess the child and family's current level of functioning on the dimensions of communication, family structure, emotional expression, and doctor-patient relationship.

Communication

The physician should note how easily and effectively family members communicate with one another and with the physician. Are parents open and honest with the child or adolescent, or do they tend to be secretive and fearful of information? Do they comprehend what the physician tells them? If they have difficulty understanding, is it related to cognitive limitations or to anxiety? How reality-based are their responses to the doctor's information? Do they become illogical and tangential under stressful circumstances?

Family Structure

The preexisting organization of the family is predictive of how well family will respond and adapt to the stress of cancer. If family organization is chaotic or complex, family members will be more difficult to manage in a health care setting. For instance, if grandparents, stepparents, and other relatives are heavily involved with the primary family and their relationship is tinged with conflict, communications with them will be more difficult and more open to conflict. Chaotic families bring this aspect of themselves to the medical treatment setting and generally require increased structure, time, and attention on the part of staff members. Typically, boundaries in these families are diffuse with respect to roles, construction of reality (they are likely to distort what staff members tell them and have difficulty accepting the reality of the diagnosis), and emotional experience. Conflicts are likely to be obvious, and family members will have difficulty resolving them, in reference to both within-family disagreements and family-staff conflict. When the physician observes overprotectiveness on the part of parents as a function of enmeshment (merging of family members) or need for control, the family is likely to be rigid in their response to stress and conflict, and thus will have a more difficult time adjusting and adapting to an illness such as cancer.

Emotional Expression

The physician may assess how well family members express their feelings and whether parents encourage the children to do so. A family who does not express deep feelings during the diagnostic period is just as vulnerable to emotional problems as those who decompensate. Also important is whether family members are able to be supportive and comforting when a family member is distressed or whether they feel overwhelmed and helpless or angry and punitive. Notice the predominant emotions in a family's experience and whether these are primarily negative or positive in tone.

Doctor-Patient Relationship

Much information can be gained from observing how family members respond to the doctor. How well do they use empathic and sympathetic statements for their support? How well do they accept the physician's authority, and how much does that authority threaten their sense of control? How receptive are they to the diagnosis and treatment information, and how much confidence and trust do they place in the physician? Are they inclined to criticize previous health care providers and institutions, and do they precipitate conflict among the current staff members?

If the physician observes major problems in communication, family disorganization, protracted anxiety and depression, and problems with authority and compliance, a referral for psychologic consultation is justified and will generally be helpful in minimizing future problems and avoiding intensification of conflict. Presenting the recommendation for psychologic referral to the family must be done in a sensitive, tactful manner since many people still misinterpret the referral as evidence that they have done something wrong or that staff members believe they are "crazy." If the physician refers to the child's or family's needs for additional support or assistance in coping with the illness, the family is likely to be more receptive to counseling.

REFERENCES

1. Lewandowski, L. A. Psychosocial Aspects of Pediatric Critical Care. In M. F. Hazinski (ed.), *Nursing Care of the Critically Ill Child*. St. Louis: Mosby, 1984. Pp. 12–62.
2. O'Dougherty, M. M. *Counselling the Chronically Ill Child: Psychology Impact and Intervention*. Lexington, MA: Lewis Publishing, 1983.
3. Perrin, E. C., and Gerrity, P. S. Development of children with a chronic illness. *Pediat. Clin. North Am.* 31(1): 19–31, 1984.
4. Bibace, R., and Walsh, M. E. Development of children's concepts of illness. *Pediatrics* 66(6):912–917, 1980.
5. Perrin, E. C., and Gerrity, P. S. There's a demon in your belly: Children's understanding of illness. *Pediatrics* 67(6):841–849, 1981.
6. Burish, T. G., and Carey, M. P. Conditional aversive responses in cancer chemotherapy patients: Theoretical and developmental analysis. *Consult. Clin. Psychol.* 54(5):593–600, 1986.
7. Redd, W. H., and Hendler, C. S. Learned aversions to chemotherapy treatment. *Health Educ. Q.* 10:57–66, 1984.
8. McGrath, P. J., and Vair, C. Psychological aspects of pain management of the burned child. *Children's Health Care* 13(1):15–19, 1984.
9. Varni, J. W. *Clinical Behavioral Pediatrics: An Interdisciplinary Biobehavioral Approach*. New York: Pergamon Press, 1983.
10. Dolgin, M. J., et al. Caregiver's perceptions of medical compliance in adolescents with cancer. *Adolesc. Health Care* 7(1):22–27, 1986.
11. Meichenbaum, D., and Turk, D. C. *Facilitating Treatment Adherence*. New York: Plenum Press, 1987.
12. Hovanitz, C. A., Gerwell, E. L., and Russo, D. C. Behavioral Methods in Pediatric Chronic Illness. In B. B. Lahey and A. E. Kazdin (eds.), *Advances in Child Clinical Psychology*, Vol. 7. New York: Plenum Press, 1984. Pp. 253–293.
13. DiMatteo, M. R., and DiNicola, D. D. *Achieving Patient Compliance*. New York: Pergamon Press, 1982.
14. Spinetta, J. J. Disease-Related Communication: How to Tell. In J. Kellerman (ed.), *Psychological Aspects of Childhood Cancer*. Springfield, IL: Thomas, 1980. Pp. 257–269.
15. Fletcher, J. M., and Copeland, D. R. Neurobehavioral effects of central nervous system prophylactic treatment of cancer in children. *J. Clin. Exp. Neuropsychol.* 10:495–538, 1988.

16. Copeland, D. R., et al. Neuropsychological test performance of pediatric cancer patients at diagnosis and one year later. *J. Pediatr. Psychol.* 13(2):183–196, 1988.

17. Taylor, H. G., et al. Postirradiation treatment outcomes for children with acute lymphocytic leukemia: Clarification of risks. *J. Pediatr. Psychol.* 12(3):395–411, 1987.

18. Copeland, D. R., and Dowell, R. E., Jr. Cognitive and social problems of children who survive. In *Proceedings of the Fifth National Conference on Human Values and Cancer* of the American Cancer Society, San Francisco, 1987. Pp. 79–84.

19. Lansky, S. G., Cairns, N. U., and Zwartjes, W. School attendance among children with cancer: A report from two centers. *J. Psychosoc. Oncol.* 1:75–82, 1983.

20. Armstrong, G. D., et al. Multidimensional assessment of psychological problems in children with cancer. *Res. Nurs. Health* 5:205–211, 1982.

21. Sanger, M. S., Copeland, D. R., and Davidson, E. R. Unpublished data, 1989.

22. Sanger, M. S., Copeland, D. R., and Davidson, E. R. School-related social competencies in pediatric oncology patients. Presented at the Florida Conference on Child Health Psychology, Gainesville, FL, April 1988.

23. Mesibov, G. B., and Johnson, M. R. Intervention Techniques in Pediatric Psychology. In J. M. Tuma (ed.), *Handbook for the Practice of Pediatric Psychology*. New York: Wiley, 1982. Pp. 110–164.

24. Quinn, W. H., and Herndon, A. The family ecology of cancer. *Psychosoc. Oncol.* 4(1/2):45–59, 1986.

25. Copeland, D. R., and Baker, E. L. Hypnosis in Pediatric Oncology. In E. T. Healy and J. M. Healy (eds.), *Case Studies in Hypnotherapy*. New York: Guilford Press, 1985. Pp. 135–145.

26. Gardner, G. G., and Olness K. *Hypnosis and Hypnotherapy in Children*. New York: Grune & Stratton, 1981.

27. Zeltzer, L., and LeBaron, S. Hypnosis and non-hypnotic techniques for reduction of pain and anxiety during painful procedures in children and adolescents with cancer. *J. Pediatr.* 101:1032–1035, 1982.

28. Melamed, B. G., and Siegel, L. J. Reduction of anxiety in children facing hospitalization and surgery by use of filmed modeling. *J. Consult. Clin. Psychol.* 43:511–521, 1975.

29. Bartlett, E. E., et al. The effects of physician communications skills on patient satisfaction, recall, and adherence. *J. Chronic Dis.* 3(9/10):755–764, 1984.

28

Family Issues

Allison Stovall

THE FAMILY OF THE CHILD WITH CANCER

Parental Responses to the Child with Cancer

Initially, after parents learn that their child has cancer, they generally express shock and disbelief. Often, they have been through a period during which they have sought medical care for a seemingly routine childhood ailment or injury only to find, in the course of the investigation, that the child has cancer. The parents question how their child could have such a serious illness when they have carefully observed his or her health status. Parents feel responsible for their children's welfare and question their own competence as protectors when such a frightening illness is diagnosed. In angry moments following the diagnosis, parents may blame themselves or their child's physician for what they perceive to be delays in making the diagnosis. With time, and with the help of information about the etiology of the child's illness, most parents eventually understand that many cancers are difficult to detect.

The ability of each parent to cope with the emotional blow of the diagnosis depends on the parent's skills for managing prior family crises. Those who have experienced a great deal of guilt surrounding the diagnosis may develop an overprotective stance toward the ill child. Both during and after treatment, they may inhibit their child's normal strivings for mastery and control of his or her environment. Medical staff are rightfully concerned about the need for parents to understand infection control precautions and to comply with the treatment regimens. Parents who are especially anxious about adhering to the recommendations of the medical staff may become excessively restrictive of their child's exposure to peers. Overprotective parents are likely to have an especially difficult time with the sudden loss of usual parental control, because it has been replaced with the intervention of physicians and other health care providers.

Regardless of whether parents' involvement with their ill child is excessive, they must dedicate more time than is normally necessary to their child's welfare. In some families, each parent may choose to accompany the child to the treatment center on alternate days, whereas others may choose to accompany their child together. In many instances, because of her role as primary nurturer, it is the mother who brings the child to the treatment center. In the case of a single-parent family, the single parent may have to depend on a grandparent to assist in attending to the child's needs at the treatment center. When it is one parent who consistently brings the child to the treatment center, the usual roles of the other parent are altered as well. For example, the father who is accustomed to being the primary breadwinner in the family may not be used to taking responsibility for household management tasks. Parents may also experience changes in the roles they assume with their children. The parent at the treatment center becomes the family spokesperson with the medical staff, sometimes leaving the parent at home with insufficient information about the progress of the child's treatment. At times, the parent remaining at home may feel emotionally isolated from both the parent at the treatment center and the ill child. Parents often relinquish their roles in community activities while their children are undergoing treatment and thus lose access to important extrafamilial relationships with adults. If they do not replace these losses with relationships with other parents at the treatment center, they are at risk for becoming excessively involved with the ill child.

Sibling Responses to the Child with Cancer

Brothers and sisters of a child with cancer have their own unique responses to the news of the child's diagnosis. Certainly, their reactions depend on their developmental levels and commensurate levels of conceptualization of illness. It is common for brothers and sisters to experience confusion at the conflicting feelings they have about their sibling's illness. They may be very fearful about the other child's welfare and display this fear through anxious behaviors. At the same time that they are fearful of the well-being of the ill child, siblings often fear that they, too, will become ill. They may have difficulty understanding explanations given by their parents and medical staff regarding the unknown etiology of the disease and may be tempted to blame the child's illness on their parents, themselves, or some forces external to the family. Siblings often have angry feelings toward the ill child for consuming so much parental attention and for getting the opportunity to travel away from home to the treatment center. When conscious of these feelings of jealousy, siblings may experience guilt if they are aware of the gravity of the other child's illness.

Changes in parental expectations of all the children in the family can generate additional sibling responses. During times when the ill child is away from home for treatment, the children at home may have to assume responsibility for some of his or her usual chores as well as some duties usually carried out by the absent parent. Older siblings, especially, may carry a heavy load of child care and household management tasks. Even when the ill child is at home during treatment or between treatments, the parents may expect a disproportionate amount of effort from siblings. Although it is common for siblings to understand the need to take on extra responsibilities at times, they may develop resentment toward the child with cancer when parents lower expectations of that child too much.

Responses of the Extended Family to the Child with Cancer

Members of the ill child's extended family and the friendship network that surrounds the child and his or her immediate family are also affected by the child's diagnosis and treatment. Grandparents may become more actively involved in the family by providing child care for either the ill child or the siblings. The opinions of grandparents regarding the parents' approach to caring for an ill child may produce conflict between parents and grandparents. Again, this can lead to parents feeling their parental control is threatened if the grandparents try to intervene rather than support them. Relatives or friends with young children may withdraw from the family fearing that their children are somehow vulnerable. On the other hand, they may want to be involved with the child and family and have some difficulty understanding when it is medically necessary for the child to have limited contacts with others. The best support comes from family members and friends who trust the child's parents to give them the proper cues regarding their readiness and that of the child for social interaction.

Interaction Between Families and Medical Staff

It is important for physicians to be aware of each family's needs for information and support as they address the needs of the ill child. Physicians can rely on child-life specialists and social workers for routine interventions designed to facilitate patient and family adaptation. These mental health professionals can alert parents to common issues that arise in families of children with cancer. At times, it may be necessary to refer family members to psychotherapy with staff members (e. g., psychologists or psychiatrists) (see Chap. 27).

Staff members need to make the ill children and parents the focal point for communication of medical information and to include the siblings whenever possible. Families need clear, complete accounts of the diagnostic findings, the treatment plan, and the potential side effects of treatment. The medical staff should use descriptive language that is meaningful to the parties involved and give a simplified account to young children. Physicians and other caregivers need to assist families in their adaptation to the hospital system by explaining the roles of the various staff members and trainees involved in the care of their child. House officers and students need to prepare children and families for the changes in rotations. Families rely on the daily contacts that they have with these caregivers and need to prepare for the loss of their attention and support.

SOCIOCULTURAL FACTORS

Family Background

The life experiences of the families who bring their children to a cancer treatment center vary considerably. Physicians need to individualize their approaches to families according to each family's educational and vocational background and the personalities involved. When families come from a rural area to a treatment center located in an urban environment, they are dealing at the outset with culture shock as well as the shock of the diagnosis. Throughout the treatment course and especially in terminal care, it is important to remember that the hospital is an alien environment no matter how familiar it has become. Every effort should be made to assist families with caring for their children at home as much of the time as possible.

Ethnic Minorities

When the patient is a member of an ethnic minority, there are several issues that physicians must consider as they develop a working relationship with the patient and family. In the United States, communication may be hampered if the primary language of the patient or any of the immediate family members is not English. Children of first-generation immigrants may be accustomed to serving as translators for their parents, but they should not be put in this position when it is time for discussion of their own health care or that of a sibling. If at all possible, use a professional translator, preferably one employed by the hospital, for all communication of medical information and treatment planning. If it is necessary to use a translator from the community, either one of the family's choosing or one recruited by a hospital employee, discuss the matter to be translated first with the translator. When you do this, you can respond to the translator's reaction to the nature of the message and you can assist the translator with medical terminology as needed. When family members have capability in English but are not fluent, it is advisable to use a translator periodically when discussing the diagnosis, treatment alternatives, and complications of treatment.

Communication with a child about the diagnosis of cancer may also be inhibited by the culturally acquired view of cancer held by the family. In many cultures, a diagnosis of cancer is still viewed as a death sentence because many people do not have access to adequate medical care. If the adults in the family are frightened by the fact that the child has cancer, they may choose to withhold that information from the child. It is important that the physician clearly sanction the sharing of information about the diagnosis and treatment with the child. Families usually respond well to the explanation that the child will undoubtedly discover the truth and would fare better on hearing it from the parents, perhaps in conjunction with the physician. When working with a family from another culture, it can be helpful to try to understand how people from that culture value children. This can give the health care provider a better understanding of the family's perspective on caring for the child during treatment and afterward.

INTERVENTIONS WITH FAMILIES

The Child and Family at Diagnosis

All families need information about the diagnosis, the recommended treatment, and the usual side effects and probable outcome of treatment. This information should be imparted in a way that provides the family with a basic understanding of what they are facing as they attempt to support the child through treatment. The staff members need to assure the family of their availability for handling the numerous questions that may arise. The medical, nursing, and mental health professionals involved from the outset need to reinforce the coping skills that the family members exhibit. Parents often believe that they will be inadequate caregivers when they face supporting their child through painful procedures and the noxious side effects of treatment. During the first phase of treatment, staff members need to intervene in ways that bolster the parents' confidence in their ability to return the lives of family members to as normal a state as possible.

These guidelines for intervention with families apply in all cases but they are, in some cases, difficult to implement. Children in whom cancer has been diagnosed come from all types of family situations, and many times they do not have the kind of secure parental support needed for the most effective adaptation to the diagnosis and treatment. The pediatric oncology social worker's family history and preliminary psychosocial assessment can serve as a guide to the medical team working with the family. In cases in which the family has been dysfunctional prior to the child's diagnosis and the child's health status exacerbates existing family problems, it is advisable to refer the family to psychotherapy. The social worker can serve as a liaison between medical staff and mental health resources in the treatment center or the home community.

Reentry Into the Home Community

After the initial phase of treatment and the family's recovery from the shock of the diagnosis, there is a period of reentry into life in the family home and community. Families must begin to make the necessary changes in the routines they have known at home, in school, at church, and in the neighborhood. They must often become acquainted with another set of health care providers in the hometown. These health care providers have been designated to collaborate with the staff at the cancer treatment center on behalf of the ill child. Prior to being discharged from the first stay at the cancer treatment center, the ill child and his or her family need social workers and child-life staff to help them prepare for the reactions of friends and neighbors as well as for the possible changes in the balance of family functioning. Physicians and nurses must take the lead in preparing parents to handle the medical needs of their child. At the time of the child's first return appointment to the cancer treatment center, the primary treatment team should review with the child and family the period of reentry into the home community. This review can expose any adaptation problems that need attention.

TREATMENT COMPLICATIONS

Throughout the child's course of therapy at a cancer treatment center, staff need to be alert for signs of problematic emotional or social functioning of children and family members. There are treatment complications that challenge the coping skills of even the most functional families. As described earlier, children may have problems coping with painful procedures and the parents may find it difficult to support the child through such procedures. Some children experience treatment complications that create pronounced discomfort or require tiresome, lengthy stays in the hospital. They and their parents are likely to become angry or depressed over these unplanned developments in the course of treatment and will need extra attention from social workers and child-life staff to work through these feelings.

The most devastating complication of treatment is a relapse of the cancer. When the news of a relapse is conveyed to the child and family, their reactions may be similar to those that they experienced at the time of diagnosis: profound shock, disbelief, and distress. The social worker and child-life worker can assist the physicians and nurses in providing support for the family by assuring the family of their presence and offering them new perspectives on the possibilities of hope for the child's future.

PREPARATION FOR THE END OF THERAPY

Several months before the scheduled end of therapy, staff need to provide children and families with opportunities to explore their feelings and questions about the termination of therapy. Whereas children may express only relief at the prospect of discontinuing treatment, parents often express some ambivalence about this event. Parents are grateful that their children will be free of the side effects of treatment, but they fear that the termination of therapy will leave the children more vulnerable to relapse. It is important that mental health and medical professionals at the cancer treatment center validate the parents' ambivalence as an expected reaction. A family may need some extra time with medical staff to address their questions about likely changes in their child's physical, emotional, or social status after the completion of therapy.

THE FAMILY OF THE DYING CHILD

When the child has had multiple relapses and has disease that is resistant to therapy, it is time for the physician, aided by the social worker and nurse, to address treatment planning in a new way. At the time of diagnosis, families generally accept the physician's recommendation for treatment by protocol. With multiply relapsed patients, it is important to emphasize that the patient and parents need to let the physician know when it is time to terminate treatment.

The physician can assist the family in this decision-making process by acknowledging that withdrawal from treatment or the use of palliative measures only are acceptable alternatives to experimental treatment. As the child becomes increasingly symptomatic, the social worker and other support personnel can assist with anticipatory grief work. At this time, the patient and family may be amenable to a hospice referral or preliminary funeral planning.

Following the death of a child, hospital staff who have known the child during treatment can help the family by maintaining telephone contact. Bereavement counseling for individuals or groups is an important service to offer if the families live close enough to take advantage of it. Hospital social workers may make referrals to bereavement groups in the hometown area as well.

SUPPORT SERVICES

Self-Help Groups

In addition to the support available to families from professional staff, relatives, and friends, there is a very special kind of support that families derive from knowing other families of children with cancer. Some families appreciate the opportunity to participate in a support group with regularly planned meetings. There are many such groups both across the United States and in several foreign countries that are part of the Candlelighters' Childhood Cancer Foundation based in Washington, D.C. The missions of the various groups vary from fund raising to education to social activities to advocacy. Inherent in all the groups in this network is the common bond of having a child with cancer and the mutual support generated by that bond. More recently, a new organization has formed to focus on issues pertinent to survivors of cancer: The National Coalition for Cancer Survivorship is an advocacy network composed of individuals and groups and has its headquarters in Albuquerque, N.M. Bereaved parents often choose to affiliate with the Compassionate Friends, an association of support groups for parents who have lost children to deaths from various causes.

Professionally Led Groups

In hospitals, private counseling services, and voluntary health agencies, there are support groups facilitated by mental health professionals for cancer patients and their families. The American Cancer Society sponsors support groups in many localities as part of its Dialogue program. In addition, this society also sponsors support groups for bereaved families. The Leukemia Society of America has established a Family Support Group program on the national level and has a staff member dedicated to promoting the establishment of such groups at chapters across the United States. There are also group programs devoted to the emotional and spiritual support of families stricken with catastrophic illness in the Centers for Attitudinal Healing in various cities across the country.

Educational Services

Families are better able to provide support for one another when they are well informed about the nature of childhood cancers and their treatments. Patient education departments at university teaching hospitals provide extensive educational resources for families of children with cancer. Some of the literature and audiovisual resources they provide come from a federal agency, the National Cancer Institute, as well as private sources. The best known of these are the voluntary health agencies, the American Cancer Society, and the Leukemia Society of America.

Financial Support Services

In addition to needing specialized social support systems, families of children with cancer often need financial support services. Parents have to adjust to a loss of income when employers refuse to give them leave with pay when they take time to be with their children during treatment. Those who are granted leave often use their allotted amount long before the child's treatment ends. Often, one parent chooses to withdraw from the work force in order to accompany the child to treatment. At the same time that the family income is reduced, the family must manage new expenses incurred by the circumstances surrounding treatment for the child. Out-of-pocket expenses for travel, lodging and food, and extra clothing can amount to 25 percent of the family income. In the year that a child dies, the family is likely to have out-of-pocket expenses of 35 percent of the family income, including funeral expenses. Some parents find that they are unable to make desirable career moves since it is very difficult to make changes in insurance coverage for their children.

There are both public and private sources of financial assistance for families of children with cancer. For those who meet the income limits, the U.S. federal government offers the Social Supplementary Income–Disabled Children's Program (SSI-DCP) through the Social Security Administration. Children eligible for this program receive a monthly stipend and coverage by their state's Medicaid program. Many states provide assistance to lower-income and middle-income families through a program based in the state health department and designed to meet the needs of children with serious chronic illnesses. The titles of these state-funded programs vary from state to state, and not every state makes provisions in its program for coverage of children with cancer. One of the best-known private sources of aid is the Patient Aid Program sponsored by the Leukemia Society of America, which assists with the cost of outpatient chemotherapy, outpatient blood transfusions, and travel reimbursement. The American Cancer Society assists patients with housing programs and loans them durable medical equipment if needed at home. Ronald McDonald Houses across the United States provide a "home away from home" for nominal fees for children with cancer and their families. Service groups in the community support the Ronald McDonald Houses both by providing volunteers and by raising funds to underwrite the operating expenses. There are numerous local groups that can assist families of children with cancer with material assistance. The pediatric oncology social worker can make the referrals that are appropriate to each family's needs. Some of the primary support services for families of children with cancer are listed in the appendix.

SELECTED READINGS

Adams, D. W., and Deveau, E. J. *Coping with Childhood Cancer: Where Do We Go from Here?* Hamilton, Ontario: Reston Publishing, 1984

Bloom, B. S., Knorr, R. S., and Evans, A. E. The epidemiology of disease expenses. *J.A.M.A.* 253(16):2393, 1985.

Chester, M. A., and Barbarin, O. A. *Childhood Cancer and the Family.* New York: Brunner/Mazel, 1987.

Kellerman, J. (ed.). *Psychological Aspects of Childhood Cancer.* Springfield, IL: Thomas, 1980.

Spinetta, J. J., and Deasy-Spinetta, P. (eds.). *Living with Childhood Cancer.* St. Louis: Mosby, 1981.

V

Genetics and Pediatric Oncology

29

Genetic Etiology of Pediatric Cancer

Louise C. Strong

PERSPECTIVE

Numerous studies of experimental and natural cancer etiology have demonstrated that cancer may be considered a genetic disease, at least at the cellular level. Initial genetic changes may be inherited or acquired, and predispose to cancer. However, data from epidemiologic studies and experimental carcinogenesis indicate that the development of cancer requires more than a single discrete cellular change, suggesting that further acquired genetic events are necessary for tumor development. Hereditary or environmental factors may influence the probability of such genetic changes. For pediatric cancers, there are unique opportunities to investigate the environmental as well as the hereditary predisposing factors, given the relatively short latent period or time for tumor to develop and the readily available and cooperative parents who can report both environmental exposures and familial histories. Nevertheless, only a small fraction of pediatric cancers are attributable to known genetic or environmental factors.

If only rare cancers in children can be attributed to known genetic factors, then what is important to know about genetics and pediatric cancer? It is important to know the contribution from the study of rare hereditary tumors to the understanding of cancer in general, which will be outlined in this chapter with particular emphasis on the observations from retinoblastoma. Studies of rare tumors have not only led to the identification of specific genes that are involved in cancer in general, but they have clearly created opportunities for genetic counseling, for medical surveillance, and for early cancer detection. Hence, some degree of screening pediatric cancer patients for evidence of a rare genetic predisposition is valuable for that rare patient and family with a genetic predisposition as well as for the more common patient with no evidence of genetic predisposition.

In the latter and more common situation, there is the opportunity to offer reassuring information to parents of pediatric cancer patients who have probably scrutinized the pregnancy and years preceding the cancer to try to identify an etiologic factor. Screening information can lead to further genetic evaluation of rare cases in which there may be a genetic predisposition but, for the most part, it can offer reassurance to otherwise concerned and perhaps guilt-ridden parents.

Finally, there is the recognition that pediatric cancer today represents a potentially curable disease. Given that the success in cancer treatment has been largely achieved by multimodal therapy, which involves cytotoxic and genotoxic effects, it is ironic that those individuals who have been helped the most by such therapy are the same individuals who have the greatest potential to suffer long-term consequences of genetic damage. There are questions regarding the long-term effects of such therapy on reproduction and long-term survival. Because at this time data are somewhat limited, the available experience of survivors of pediatric and adolescent cancers, with respect to the genetic consequences of pediatric cancer, should be reviewed.

RETINOBLASTOMA AS A MODEL

In general, cancer is considered a genetic disease at the cellular level. For most human cancers, there may be both hereditary and nonhereditary forms of the tumor. Although the fraction of cases that may occur in the hereditary form may be small, it is these cancers that have yielded the most information about cancer development. The most informative of such cancers has been retinoblastoma in childhood. This tumor occurs in approximately 1 in 20,000 live births. It has been a unique model for genetic studies for many reasons: The diagnosis of childhood retinoblastoma is fairly straightforward, and the tumor occurs at an early age and in a paired organ. Multiple primary tumors can be readily detected, and new tumors rarely arise after the age of 5 years. Retinoblastoma has been successfully treated without ill effects on the patients' reproductive ability; consequently, the patients have had the opportunity to reproduce, providing information on the familial nature of the cancer in some cases [1, 2].

Heritable and Nonheritable Form

Surveys of the reproductive outcome in retinoblastoma patients, according to the patients' unilateral (single) or bilateral tumors, have revealed that the frequency of retinoblastoma in the offspring of patients with bilateral retinoblastoma is very near 50 percent. Among the affected offspring, nearly 90 percent will also develop bilateral tumors. These findings are compatible with an autosomal dominant gene with very high penetrance and clearly indicate the need for monitoring all offspring of a bilateral retinoblastoma patient. The risk of tumor in the offspring of patients with unilateral sporadic (nonfamilial) retinoblastoma is very much lower, however, at 3 to 7 percent. These findings suggest that all bilateral retinoblastomas should be considered heritable, due to a germ cell mutation that can be transmitted in an autosomal dominant manner to the next generation, regardless of the previous family history. Although the findings also indicate that unilateral retinoblastoma may be heterogeneous, with a small percentage of cases heritable and the same high probability of transmitting the predisposition to offspring, the large majority of cases are due to nonheritable factors. It has long been suggested that the genetic event at the cellular level might be the same in both the heritable and nonheritable tumors; however, in heritable retinoblastoma, the initial genetic mutation occurs in a germ cell and is present in all cells of the individual, which gives rise to a high frequency of early-onset and multiple primary tumors.

Localizing the Gene

Further insight into the nature and localization of these genetic events was achieved by cytogenetic analysis of rare patients with retinoblastoma who also showed marked developmental delay. Whereas most patients with retinoblastoma are of normal intelligence and exhibit normal development, some 1 percent of patients will have pronounced developmental delay. Chromosomal analysis of the normal cells from such patients showed a deletion of chromosome 13 involving the 13q14 region. Identification of this chromosome region in those rare patients with retinoblastoma and developmental delay provided a genetic locus for further study.

Most patients with familial or bilateral retinoblastoma have normal-appearing constitutional chromosomes and normal growth and development; however, by using genetic markers with multiple alleles (variants) from the 13q14 region, which can be tracked in families along with the inheritance of retinoblastoma, linkage between genetic markers in the 13q14 region and the retinoblastoma gene was demonstrated. These findings indicated that the more common autosomal dominant gene for retinoblastoma was also located in the 13q14 region. Hence, the same genetic region may predispose to retinoblastoma when grossly absent (as in the cases of visible chromosome deletion and associated developmental delay) or when associated with a normal-appearing chromosome 13 and normal development. Application of genetic markers may be useful in studies of families for genetic counseling or prenatal diagnosis when multiple affected family members are available for study.

Additional Somatic Genetic Events in Tumor Development

These studies of children with both rare retinoblastoma and developmental delay and the families with multiple cases of retinoblastoma localized the gene for the hereditary type of retinoblastoma. However, if one inherits this retinoblastoma gene, one is predisposed to tumor even though tumor occurrence is still a relatively rare event at the cellular level. Gene carriers are not necessarily born with tumors in both eyes, and certainly not every predisposed retinal cell will develop into a tumor. Clearly, additional genetic events must occur. To determine whether these tumor-specific changes occur on chromosome 13, cytogenetic, biochemical, and molecular studies of tumor cell and normal cells from the same patient have been conducted. These studies have revealed that most retinoblastoma tumors show further alterations on chromosome 13. The findings suggest that all retinoblastomas, hereditary or nonhereditary, occur because of a sequence of two genetic events, one on each chromosome 13 [3]. In hereditary cases, a mutation or gross chromosomal deletion has occurred in an earlier generation or in a germ cell and is present in all cells of the individual, and it can be transmitted to the next generation with a 50 : 50 probability. However, the cells still retain one normal chromosome 13. In nonhereditary cases, the chromosome 13 mutation may occur in an embryonal retinal cell, in which case it is not passed on to the next generation. For tumor development, it appears that the remaining normal chromosome 13, or at least that region of the retinoblastoma gene, must be altered in the retinal cells by chromosome loss, deletion, recombination, or mutation to eliminate normal retinoblastoma gene function. The loss of function of both genes then permits tumor development [3,4].

These findings indicate that complete absence of the retinoblastoma gene and its product is related to tumor development. In normal tissue the retinoblastoma gene is present and, presumably, makes a product that has some critical function. With this background, researchers looked for evidence of genes from chromosome 13q14 expressed in normal tissue and not expressed in retinoblastoma tumors, and eventually cloned the gene [5] and identified the protein product [6,7]. Further study has confirmed that the normal protein product is absent or altered in virtually all retinoblastoma tumors [8].

Risk of New Tumor

Follow-up of patients with heritable retinoblastoma has also been informative because it has revealed an exceptionally high risk of a new tumor. Initially, the new tumors were observed primarily in patients treated with high doses of radiotherapy. However, over time, it has become very clear that these patients have a high risk of a second tumor in areas not exposed to radiotherapy. Follow-up has revealed that patients with hereditary bilateral retinoblastoma who were treated with radiation have at least a 6 to 12 percent probability of a second malignant tumor arising in the irradiated area within 18 years of follow-up. The majority of these tumors are osteosarcomas, but soft-tissue sarcomas, brain tumors, and other tumors have also been observed. In the absence of radiotherapy, the risk of a second tumor appears to be in the range of 3 percent over 18 years. Again, most second tumors are osteosarcomas, but soft-tissue sarcomas, melanomas, and other cancers have been observed. All long-term follow-up studies of retinoblastoma patients have confirmed an exceptionally high risk of a second malignant neoplasm among the hereditary subgroups [9,10].

Recent studies suggest that radiation increases the risk of a second tumor in bilateral retinoblastoma patients with about the same relative effect as in other pediatric cancer patients; however, given that the background risk for a patient with bilateral retinoblastoma is already elevated, increasing that rate by some three- to fivefold yields a much higher cumulative rate of a second tumor for bilateral retinoblastoma patients than for other pediatric cancer patients [9]. Available data suggest that a survivor of heritable retinoblastoma should be considered at risk for a new malignant neoplasm not only during adolescence but throughout his or her life. Such patients should undergo close medical surveillance and have biopsied any suspicious lesions. Nevertheless, second malignant neoplasms in retinoblastoma patients may be treated very effectively if they are detected in a timely manner.

Retinoblastoma, Osteosarcoma, and Other Tumors

Given the close association of retinoblastoma and osteosarcoma occurring in the same patient with a known genetic predisposition, it was natural to ask whether the development of osteosarcoma followed the same molecular genetic events as in retinoblastoma. Available evidence from the study of osteosarcoma following retinoblastoma and osteosarcoma occurring independent of retinoblastoma suggests that the same gene on chromosome 13q14 is indeed involved in the development of osteosarcoma. Although it has not been demonstrated that a mutation in that gene can be inherited and predispose to osteosarcoma in the absence of retinoblastoma, tumor-specific alterations of the retinoblastoma gene are observed in most osteosarcoma tumors [11]. Presumably, in most cases these are somatic and acquired and do not necessarily imply any germline mutation that would affect the cancer risk to the offspring of an osteosarcoma patient.

More recently, studies of soft-tissue sarcomas following retinoblastoma and soft-tissue sarcomas in the absence of retinoblastoma have also shown tumor-specific alterations of the retinoblastoma gene [12]. Perhaps more surprisingly, a considerable fraction of common adult cancers, including lung cancer (small-cell lung cancer and non-small-cell lung cancer) [13], ductal cell carcinoma of the breast (primarily premenopausal breast cancer) [14], and bladder tumor [15], have also been shown to have an alteration in the retinoblastoma gene. It seems, therefore, that from the study of a rare cancer in childhood—retinoblastoma, which occurs occasionally in patients with a detectable chromosomal deletion and more frequently in multiple family members—we have identified a gene that may play a role not only in pediatric cancer but in the onset of many common adult tumors as well.

Salient Features of the Retinoblastoma Model for Genetic Study of Childhood Cancer

The important findings from retinoblastoma that may carry over to investigation into the genetic etiology of other pediatric cancers include the following:

1. There appears to be both a hereditary and a nonhereditary subgroup for retinoblastoma and, perhaps, for must human cancers. The hereditary subgroup varies with respect to the fraction of total cases but is generally a rather small percentage of cases of a given tumor type.
2. The hereditary subgroup is characterized by an early age at diagnosis with a high frequency of multifocal (in paired organs, bilateral) tumors and a familial pattern of cancer consistent with an autosomal dominant mode of transmission.
3. Rare cases of pediatric cancer associated with congenital anomalies may be attributed to a gross chromosome deletion, which may also pinpoint the site of the gene in general.
4. Genetic linkage studies confirmed the site of the retinoblastoma gene at 13q14, the same region deleted in patients with developmental delay and retinoblastoma, using variable or polymorphic genetic markers in family studies. Similar approaches may be informative in studying other familial cancers.
5. Study of tumor-specific genetic alterations in retinoblastoma revealed subsequent alterations at the normal or wild type retinoblastoma gene on 13q14 to produce a tumor cell without a normal retinoblastoma gene or gene product.
6. Characteristics of the retinoblastoma gene, therefore, include expression in most normal tissues but absent or aberrant expression in nearly all retinoblastomas, osteosarcomas, and lung cancers, and in some breast cancers (primarily duct-cell premenopausal), soft-tissue sarcomas, and perhaps other tumors as well.

OTHER CANCERS IN CHILDHOOD

For no other tumor in childhood is the genetic etiology so well defined as for retinoblastoma. Nonetheless, for many cancers in childhood, there are limited data suggesting genetic predisposition that is at least somewhat analogous to retinoblastoma. Selected examples are discussed here.

Wilms' Tumor of the Kidney

Like retinoblastoma, Wilms' tumor is an embryonal tumor that occurs in young children, arises in paired organs, and can be unilateral or multifocal (including bilateral). Most tumors occur in patients with normal karyotypes, no family history of Wilms' tumor, and no congenital anomalies or developmental delay. Approximately 1 percent of patients report a family history of Wilms' tumor, most often in siblings, cousins, or other family members. The familial pattern of tumors is far less predictable than in families with retinoblastoma, although as in retinoblastoma, the bilateral and familial cases occur at an earlier-than-average age and the bilateral cases are far more frequent in familial Wilms' tumor. These findings suggest that there might be an autosomal dominant gene analogous to that of retinoblastoma that predisposes to Wilms' tumor but has a markedly lower penetrance than the retinoblastoma-predisposing gene (for a review see [16]).

Further evidence to support a genetic predisposition in at least a small fraction of Wilms' tumor patients comes from observing Wilms' tumor patients with congenital anomalies, specifically aniridia. Roughly 1 in 100 Wilms' tumor patients also have aniridia (absence or maldevelopment of the iris of the eye), and an estimated one-third of patients with severe sporadic aniridia (that requires hospitalization) will develop Wilms' tumor. The Wilms' tumors in these patients are frequently bilateral (approximately 15–20% of cases) and occur at a strikingly early age. These patients have been found to have a constitutional chromosome deletion involving chromosome 11 in the p13 region. Rare patients in whom the chromosomes appear normal can be shown to have a deletion of genetic material at the molecular level. All patients with aniridia should have a chromosomal analysis and, as it becomes feasible, molecular analysis of this region to identify those patients with 11p13 deletions and a predisposition to Wilms' tumor.

The identification of a specific chromosome region in which a deletion seems to predispose to Wilms' tumor again provided a specific region on which to focus to study tumor-specific genetic alterations. An estimated 50 percent of Wilms' tumors show alterations in the 11p13 region. Somewhat surprisingly, however, when rare familial clusters of Wilms' tumor were studied with markers for the 11p13 region, it was demonstrated that 11p13 was not the region of a Wilms' tumor–predisposing lesion [17]. There may be other critical alterations involved in the development of at least some Wilms' tumors. Further study is clearly indicated.

For the sake of research, probably all Wilms' tumor patients should be examined using molecular genetic techniques. Clearly, patients with Wilms' tumor and aniridia, or Wilms' tumor and other abnormalities such as genitourinary anomalies (most frequently cryptorchidism or hypospadias) or hemihypertrophy should certainly be studied with these techniques.

Soft-Tissue Sarcoma

In 1969, following a review of some 400 medical records of pediatric embryonal rhabdomyosarcoma patients, a familial cancer syndrome now termed the *Li Fraumeni syndrome* was identified. From that survey, four families in which there were siblings or cousins with pediatric soft-tissue sarcoma were identified. Further study of those families revealed a high frequency of breast cancer in the mothers, with the features of early onset (premenopausal) and a high frequency of bilaterality. A high frequency of other tumor types was also observed in the families, including brain tumors, other sarcomas, and a diverse array of other neoplasms. At the University of Texas M.D. Anderson Cancer Center, I have recently surveyed 3-

year survivors of pediatric soft-tissue sarcoma [18]. The study determined that some 6 to 7 percent of patients appear to be from families in which there is evidence of an autosomal dominant gene predisposing to multiple tumor types at young ages, with an estimated 30 percent probability of cancer by the age of 15 years and a 50 percent probability of cancer by the age of 30 years. Those surviving their first cancer have an extremely high incidence of second malignant neoplasms [19]. Conversely, the study of risk factors for second malignant neoplasms in these patients indicated that this autosomal dominant genetic predisposing factor was an overwhelming risk factor. Radiotherapy was an additional risk factor. The risk of a second tumor in soft-tissue sarcoma survivors may be somewhat analogous to that in retinoblastoma survivors, in that those patients with a genetic predisposition of the Li Fraumeni syndrome type have a high risk for developing a second tumor and radiotherapy may further increase that already high risk.

The most common second tumors that have been observed are osteosarcoma, soft-tissue sarcoma, and breast cancer, the same tumor types observed in other family members [18]. It may be that the majority of the second tumors arise in those patients with the genetic predisposition. To date, the gene has not been localized to a given chromosome, and there are no specific sarcoma/congenital malformation syndromes that have yielded information on a specific chromosome region. Patients with multiple primary tumors or with a family history of early onset sarcomas, brain tumors, or premenopausal breast cancer should be candidates for further study. In addition, study of tumor-specific genetic changes may be informative (for review see [18–20]).

Neuroblastoma

Neuroblastoma, also an embryonal tumor, occurs most often in very young children. Limited evidence also suggests that there may be a rare hereditary subgroup and a far more common nonhereditary subgroup. In the rare familial cases, a younger-than-average age at onset and a pattern of multiple primary tumors are often observed. There are limited data suggesting that genes in the 11q23 region may be involved in neuroblastoma, based on one family with multiple cases of neuroblastoma and a balanced translocation involving that region, and other sporadic cases that also have a chromosome rearrangement in that region in their normal cells. However, tumor-specific alterations most frequently involve deletions of chromosome 1p. Other cytogenetic alterations are discussed in the section on Genetics in the Diagnosis and Prognosis of Pediatric Cancer with respect to the prognosis of neuroblastoma patients.

Neuroblastoma is occasionally associated with other disorders of neural crest origin, including neurofibromatosis or Hirschsprung's disease (aganglionosis of the colon). Certainly, patients with neural crest abnormalities and neuroblastoma, familial neuroblastoma, or neuroblastoma with any congenital anomaly should be considered candidates for genetic study.

For a review, see reference 2.

Other Solid Tumors in Childhood

For many other cancers in childhood, there are at least some features—including association with congenital anomalies, rare familial cancer aggregations, or occurrence in known familial cancer syndromes—that may provide clues to the tumor etiology. In some cases, the cancer may be the first manifestation of a familial syndrome, such as a child with hepatoblastoma who may later be found to have familial polyposis coli or Gardner's syndrome. The finding of a pediatric cancer patient with any associated congenital anomalies or unusual familial cancers (including an unusually early age at onset) should be an indication for genetic referral. A summary of the epidemiologic and genetic features of some tumors of childhood and of the possible chromosomal localization of genes involved in some pediatric cancers is presented in Tables 29-1 and 29-2. Table 29-3 indicates the specific genetic syndromes that are frequently associated with pediatric cancer and Table 29-4 the specific chromosomal anomalies that are sometimes associated with pediatric cancers. Although the conditions listed in Tables 29-3 and 29-4 represent hereditary conditions with an increased risk of specific pediatric cancers, the degree of risk varies tremendously. In most cases, the cancer is still a rare event even among those with the given syndrome listed. Nevertheless, these associations may provide important clues to the tumor etiology. In addition, they provide significant "flags" for individuals at high risk who should be carefully monitored for pediatric cancer development.

For a review and references, see reference 2.

Hematopoietic Tumors in Childhood

Little is known about the genetic etiology of the most common neoplasms occurring in white children in the United States. A very high risk of leukemia in identical twins when leukemia is diagnosed before the age of 4 years has long been observed. Recent use of cytogenetic markers has shown that the high concordance of leukemia in infant twins is due to the sharing of a common leukemogenic event with the establishment of the same malignant clone in both twins. Therefore, the high probability of leukemia in each of the identical twins is related not to a genetic predisposition but to the probability of the comingling of cells and the spread of the single leukemic clone from one twin to the other in utero.

An increased risk of leukemia in siblings and relatives of leukemic patients has been observed. However, no consistent heritable pattern outside of the rare hereditary syndromes, which are described in Tables 29-3 and 29-4, has emerged. Further cytogenetic, molecular genetic, and immunogenetic studies may be informative.

For a review and references, see reference 2.

Hodgkin's Disease

Overall, an increased risk of Hodgkin's disease has been observed in relatives of Hodgkin's disease patients. In some reported families, the affected siblings or cousins have had identical or haploidentical HLA types, suggesting that the disease susceptibility is associated with the major histocompatibility system. Other studies have suggested the possibility of an autosomal recessive genetic locus associated with the susceptibility to Hodgkin's disease and/or generalized immunodeficiency [21]. Still other studies suggest that the fairly common age at onset of Hodgkin's disease in multiply affected family members of the same kindred is more indicative of the effect of some common environmental exposure. At present, it seems likely that there may be an underlying genetic predisposition in some

Table 29-1. Summary of epidemiologic and genetic features of some childhood tumors

Tumor type	Demographic characteristics	Associated conditions
Teratomas and germ cell tumors overall	Increasing incidence in England, 1954–1978	Neural tube defects in patients and siblings; may be familial, site-specific; XXY
Intracranial teratomas	Excess in Japan	
Sacrococcygeal teratomas	Female excess; peak incidence before 3 years of age	Central nervous system, genitourinary, anorectal, lower vertebral congenital anomalies
Testicular cancer	Relative deficit in U.S. and African blacks, less pronounced in children; increasing incidence in Japan, U.S.; small age peak in early childhood, larger peak begins near puberty	Cryptorchidism, genitourinary anomalies, congenital adrenal hyperplasia, Down's syndrome, dysgenetic gonads; may be familial
Ovarian cancer	Increasing incidence after age 6 years; no deficit in blacks	Genitourinary anomalies; granulosa-theca cell tumor with Peutz-Jeghers syndrome; gonadal dysgenesis
Ewing's sarcoma	Extremely rare in U.S. and African blacks; peak during adolescent growth spurt in susceptible population; more common in Australia	High risk of osteosarcoma following radiotherapy and chemotherapy
Liver cancer		
Hepatoblastoma	Peak in infancy; male predominance	Hemihypertrophy, hemangioma, Beckwith-Wiedemann syndrome, Gardner's syndrome (familial polyposis coli)
Hepatocellular carcinoma	Increasing incidence after age 6 years; male predominance	Cirrhosis—familial, metabolic, or acquired, especially biliary; hepatitis B surface antigenemia
Adrenocortical adenocarcinoma	Female excess	Familial and multiple primary association with brain tumors, sarcomas, breast cancers; hemihypertrophy; Beckwith-Wiedemann syndrome; adrenocortical hyperplasia; Gardner's syndrome (familial polyposis coli)
Thyroid cancer	Female excess; Jewish excess	Radiation exposure; multiple endocrine adenomatosis II (medullary thyroid cancer)

Table 29-1. (continued)

Tumor type	Demographic characteristics	Associated conditions
Colonic cancer	Rare before 15 years of age; slight excess in males and black children	Familial association with brain tumors, lymphomas, leukemia; familial cancer syndrome; multiple polyposis coli
Melanoma		Dysplastic nevi; hereditary retinoblastoma; congenital nevi; xeroderma pigmentosum

Source: Modified from L.C. Strong. Genetics, Etiology, and Epidemiology of Childhood Cancer. In W.W. Sutow, D.J. Fernbach, and T.J. Vietti (eds.), *Clinical Pediatric Oncology* (3rd ed.). St. Louis, 1984, The C.V. Mosby Co.

families, further triggered by an environmental (possibly infectious) exposure.

For a review and other references, see reference 2.

PROGNOSIS OF PEDIATRIC CANCERS OCCURRING AS PART OF GENETIC SYNDROMES

In most instances, it appears that the pediatric cancer that occurs in a patient with a genetic syndrome behaves in the same biological manner as the sporadic form of that same pediatric cancer. Differences may involve the patient's age at diagnosis or the probability of multiple primary tumors of the same or different organ systems; however, in general the treatment and overall prognosis are similar. An exception to this general notion is that of leukemia occurring in infants with Down's syndrome. Infants with Down's syndrome have an increased incidence of acute leukemia; in addition, they also are at a significantly increased risk of a transient myeloproliferative disorder, difficult to distinguish from acute nonlymphocytic leukemia, which can undergo spontaneous resolution. The biological basis for this resolution is unknown [22].

Patients with unique metabolic disease or chromosomal instability syndromes (see Table 29-3) and pediatric cancer should be carefully monitored for unusual responses to radiotherapy (ataxia telangiectasia) (for a review see [2]) or chemotherapy as a result of their underlying genetic disease.

INDICATIONS FOR GENETIC STUDY OF PEDIATRIC CANCER PATIENTS

The following is a list of suggested indications for genetic study of pediatric cancer patients. With increasing use of molecular genetic techniques in the diagnosis and study of childhood tumors, this list may expand rapidly.

1. Pediatric cancer in a patient with a congenital anomaly or developmental delay
2. Childhood cancers in siblings, cousins, or parent and child
3. Family history of early onset of cancer or multiple primary can-

Table 29-2. Chromosomal localization of non-random genetic changes in tumor development based on consistent tumor-specific loss of heterozygosity (LOH), localization of cancer predisposition by genetic linkage, or constitutional chromosome alteration

Chromosomal site (gene)	Solid tumor	Type of study — Tumor-specific LOH or rearrangement	Type of study — Family study (linkage)	Constitutional deletion or rearrangement	References*
1p	Multiple endocrine adenomatosis IIa	+	−	−	Ponder, 1988
1pter-p36	Melanoma, cutaneous	−	+	−	Bale, et al., 1989
1p36	Neuroblastoma	+	−	−	Fong, et al., 1989
2	Melanoma, uveal	+	−	−	Mukai and Dryja, 1986
3p14.2-p25	Renal cell carcinoma	+	+	+	Ponder, 1988
3p25	von Hippel-Lindau disease (renal cell carcinoma)	+	+	−	Ponder, 1988
3p14-23	Small-cell lung carcinoma, other lung cancer	+	−	−	Ponder, 1988
5q21-23	Colonic carcinoma (polyposis coli)	+	+	+	Ponder, 1988
8q24.1	Multiple exostosis (Langer-Giedion syndrome)	−	−	+	Fryns, et al., 1983
10	Glioblastoma multiforme	+	−	−	James, et al., 1988
10q21.1	Multiple endocrine adenomatosis IIa	−	+	−	Ponder, 1988
11p15.5-11pter	Rhabdomyosarcoma, embryonal	+	−	−	Scrable, et al., 1987
11p15	Adrenocortical carcinoma	+	−	−	Henry, et al., 1989
11p15 (?Hras)	Breast carcinoma	+	−	−	Ponder, 1988; Liu, 1988
11p15	Wilms' tumor	+	−	−	Henry, et al., 1989
11p15	Hepatoblastoma	+	−	−	Ponder, 1988
11p	Bladder carcinoma	+	−	−	Ponder, 1988
11p	Lung cancer	+	−	−	Ponder, 1988
11p13	Wilms' tumor	+	−	+	Shiraishi, et al., 1987; Ponder, 1988; Huff, et al., 1989
11q13	Multiple endocrine adenomatosis I	+	+	−	Ponder, 1988

Table 29-2. (continued)

Chromosomal site (gene)	Solid tumor	Type of study			References*
		Tumor-specific LOH or rearrangement	Family study (linkage)	Constitutional deletion or rearrangement	
11q24	Ewing's sarcoma (cytogenetics)	+	—	—	McKeon, et al., 1988
12q13-14	Liposarcoma, lipoma (cytogenetics)	+	—	—	Mandahl, et al., 1987; Mertens, et al., 1987
13q14.1(Rb)	Lung cancer	+	—	—	Harbour, et al., 1988
13q14.1(Rb)	Breast carcinoma	+	—	—	T'Ang, et al., 1988
13q14.1(Rb)	Bladder carcinoma	+	—	—	Horowitz, et al., 1989
13q14.1(Rb)	Osteosarcoma	+	—	—	Ponder, 1988
13q14.1(Rb)	Retinoblastoma	+	+	+	Ponder, 1988
13q14.1(Rb)	Soft-tissue sarcoma	+	—	—	Friend, et al., 1987
13q14	Rhabdomyosarcoma, alveolar (cytogenetics)	+	—	—	Wang-Wuu, et al., 1988
13q	Brain tumor	+	—	—	James, et al., 1988
13q	Gastric carcinoma	+	—	—	Motomura, et al., 1988
14q	Neuroblastoma	+	—	—	Suzuki, et al., 1989

Locus	Tumor type			Reference
17p13(p53)	Colonic carcinoma	+	—	Baker, et al., 1989
17p	Breast carcinoma	+	—	Mackay, et al., 1988
17p	Adrenocortical carcinoma	+	—	Henry, et al., 1989
17p13(p53)	Osteosarcoma	+	—	Masuda, et al., 1987
17p	Lung cancer	+	—	Ponder, 1988
17p	Brain tumor (astrocytoma grade II–IV)	+	—	James, et al., 1989
17q12-22	von Recklinghausen's neurofibromatosis	—	+	Ponder, 1988; Fountain, et al., 1989
18q	Colonic cancer	+	—	Ponder, 1988
22q11	Acoustic neuroma } Bilateral acoustic neurofibromatosis	+	+	Ponder, 1988
22q11	Meningioma } Bilateral acoustic neurofibromatosis	+	+	Ponder, 1988
22q	Colonic cancer	+	—	Ponder, 1988
22q	Brain tumor	+	—	James, et al., 1988
22q	Medullary thyroid carcinoma, pheochromocytoma	+	—	Takai, et al., 1987
22q22	Ewing's sarcoma (cytogenetics)	+	—	McKeon, et al., 1988

Key: Rb = retinoblastoma gene; p53 = p53 tumor protein on chromosome 17p13.

*Where possible, reference is made to a review article, rather than the original article, to limit the extensive referencing otherwise required. Complete references are available in review articles. Complete information on the references in this column is given in the list of Table References at the end of the chapter unless otherwise noted.

Table 29-3. Hereditary conditions associated with childhood cancer

Hereditary condition	Mode of inheritance	Chromosomal localization	Childhood tumor	References*
von Recklinghausen's neurofibromatosis	AD	17q12	Optic neuroma, brain tumor, neurogenic and nonneurogenic sarcoma, neuroblastoma, Wilms' tumor, nonlymphoid leukemia, melanoma, hepatoma	Barker, et al., 1987
Bilateral acoustic neurofibromatosis	AD	22q11	Meningioma, schwannoma, neurofibroma, glioma, acoustic neurofibroma	Rouleau, et al., 1987
Tuberous sclerosis	AD	9q	Brain tumor, renal cell carcinoma	Fryer, et al., 1987
Nevoid basal cell carcinoma syndrome	AD	1p	Basal cell carcinoma, medulloblastoma, ovarian fibroma	Weinblatt, et al., 1987
Familial polyposis coli (Gardner's syndrome)	AD	5q21-q23	Colonic adenocarcinoma, brain tumor, sarcoma, adrenocortical adenocarcinoma, thyroid, pituitary or other endocrine tumor, hepatoblastoma	Bodmer, et al., 1987
Beckwith-Wiedemann syndrome	AD	11p15.5	Wilms' tumor, adrenocortical adenocarcinoma, hepatoblastoma, brain tumor, sarcoma	Koufos, et al., 1987
Multiple endocrine adenomatosis I	AD	11q13	Parathyroid, pituitary, pancreatic islet cell, carcinoid, adrenal tumors, schwannoma	Nakamura, et al., 1989
Multiple endocrine adenomatosis II (a & b)	AD	10	Medullary thyroid carcinoma, pheochromocytoma	Mathew, et al., 1987
von Hippel-Lindau disease	AD	3p25	Renal cell carcinoma, central nervous system tumor, hemangioblastoma, pheochromocytoma	Seizenger, et al., 1988
21-Hydroxylase deficiency congenital adrenal hyperplasia	AR	6p21.3	Adrenocortical carcinoma, testicular tumor, mesodermal or neurogenic tumor	White, et al., 1988

Familial cholestatic cirrhosis of childhood	AR	?	Postcirrhotic hepatocellular carcinoma	
Glycogen storage disease 1a	AR	?	Hepatoblastoma, postcirrhotic hepatocellular carcinoma	Ito, et al., 1987
Hereditary tyrosinemia	AR	?	Postcirrhotic hepatocellular carcinoma	
Genetic hemochromatosis	AR	6p21.3	Postcirrhotic hepatocellular carcinoma	Bradbear, et al., 1985
Galactosemia	AR	?	Postcirrhotic hepatocellular carcinoma	
Hypermethioninemia	AR	?	Postcirrhotic hepatocellular carcinoma	
Alpha-1-antitrypsin deficiency	AR	14q32	Postcirrhotic hepatocellular carcinoma	Cox, et al., 1987
Shwachman syndrome	AR	?	Leukemia	
Immunodeficiency disorders				
X-linked lymphoproliferative disease	SR	Xq24–q27	Lymphoma	
Bruton's agammaglobulinemia	SR	Xq21	Lymphoma, leukemia, brain tumor	
Severe combined immunodeficiency	SR	X	Lymphoma, leukemia	
Wiskott-Aldrich syndrome	SR	Xp11-q12	Lymphoma, leukemia (including myeloid), brain tumor	
IgA deficiency	?AD	?	Lymphoma, leukemia, gastrointestinal or brain tumor	
Common variable immunodeficiency	?	?	Lymphoma, gastrointestinal or brain tumor	

Table 29-3. (continued)

Hereditary condition	Mode of inheritance	Chromosomal localization	Childhood tumor	References
DiGeorge's syndrome	AD	del 22q	Brain tumor, oral squamous cell carcinoma	Gatti, et al., 1988
Ataxia telangiectasia	AR	11q23	Lymphoma, leukemia, Hodgkin's disease, brain, gastric, ovarian, or other epithelial tumors	
Genetic instability and DNA repair disorders				
Xeroderma pigmentosum	AR	?	Basal and squamous cell carcinoma of skin, melanoma, squamous cell carcinoma of tongue	
Bloom's syndrome	AR	?	Leukemia, lymphoma, gastrointestinal tumor, other epithelial tumors	
Fanconi's anemia	AR	?	Leukemia, hepatoma, squamous cell carcinoma	Gatti, et al., 1988
Ataxia telangiectasia	AR	11q23	Lymphoma, leukemia, Hodgkin's disease, brain, gastric, ovarian, or other epithelial tumors	

Key: AD = autosomal dominant; AR = autosomal recessive; SR = sex-linked recessive; del = chromosome deletion.
*See review for clinical references. Updated references on chromosomal assignment are referenced in far right column in the table. Complete information on these references is given in the list of Table References at the end of the chapter.
Source: Modified from L.C. Strong. Genetics, Etiology, and Epidemiology of Childhood Cancer. In W.W. Sutow, D.J. Fernbach, and T.J. Vietti (eds.), *Clinical Pediatric Oncology.* St. Louis, 1984, The C.V. Mosby Co.

Table 29-4. Constitutional chromosomal disorders associated with childhood cancer

Chromosomal abnormality	Childhood tumor
Down's syndrome	Leukemia, testicular tumor, retinoblastoma[a]
Turner's syndrome	Neurogenic tumors, postestrogen endometrial tumor, leukemia, gonadal tumor
Klinefelter's syndrome	Nonlymphoid leukemia, germ-cell tumor (gonadal and mediastinal)
Other sex aneuploidy (XXYY, XXXY, XXX including XXY)	Retinoblastoma[a]
XY gonadal dygenesis	Gonadoblastoma, dysgerminoma
Trisomy 13	Teratoma, leukemia, neurogenic tumors
Trisomy 18	Neurogenic tumor, Wilms' tumor
XYY, XYY mosaic	Osteosarcoma (1),[b] medulloblastoma (1), chronic myeloid leukemia (2), acute leukemia (1)

[a]Occurs often in trisomy 21 associated with sex chromosome aneuploidy.
[b]Numbers given in parentheses represent cases reported.
Source: Modified from L.C. Strong. Genetics, Etiology, and Epidemiology of Childhood Cancer. In W.W. Sutow, D.J. Fernbach, and T.J. Vietti (eds.), *Clinical Pediatric Oncology* (3rd ed.). St. Louis, 1984, The C.V. Mosby Co. (See review for complete references.)

cers (e.g., cancer before 35 years of age in grandparents, parents, aunts, uncles, siblings, and cousins)
4. Second or multiple malignant neoplasms or benign neoplasms in pediatric cancer patient
5. Cancer-predisposing conditions in patient or family (see *Table 29-3*)
6. Family request for genetic counseling regarding risk of cancer in siblings or offspring of patient
7. Patient with childhood cancer for which specific genes have been suspected, localized, or cloned, including retinoblastoma, osteosarcoma, Wilms' tumor, and soft-tissue sarcoma
8. Same-sex twins, one or both of whom have childhood cancers

REFERENCES

1. Tapley, N.duV. Strong, L.C., and Sutow, W.W. Retinoblastoma. In W.W. Sutow, D.J. Fernbach, and T.J. Vietti (eds.), *Clinical Pediatric Oncology* (3rd ed.). St. Louis: Mosby, 1984. Pp. 539–558.
2. Strong, L.C. Genetics, Etiology, and Epidemiology of Childhood Cancer. In W.W. Sutow, D.J. Fernbach, and T.J. Vietti (eds.), *Clinical Pediatric Oncology* (3rd ed.). St. Louis: Mosby, 1984.
3. Cavenee, W.K., et al. Expression of recessive alleles by chromosomal mechanisms in retinoblastoma. *Nature* 305:779, 1983.
4. Cavenee, W.K., et al. Genetic origin of mutations predisposing to retinoblastoma. *Science* 228:501, 1985.
5. Friend, S.H., et al. A human DNA segment with properties of the gene that predisposes to retinoblastoma and osteosarcoma. *Nature* 323:643, 1986.

6. Lee, W.H., et al. Human retinoblastoma susceptibility gene: Cloning, identification, and sequence. *Science* 235:1394, 1987.
7. Lee, W.H., et al. The retinoblastoma susceptibility gene encodes a nuclear phosphoprotein associated with DNA binding activity, *Nature* 329:642, 1987.
8. Dunn, J.M., et al. Identification of germline and somatic mutations affecting the retinoblastoma gene. *Science* 241:1797, 1988.
9. Tucker, M.A., et al. Bone sarcomas linked to radiotherapy and chemotherapy in children. *N. Engl. J. Med.* 317:588, 1987.
10. Draper, G.J., Sanders, B.M., and Kingston, J.E.. Second primary neoplasms in patients with retinoblastoma. *Br. J. Cancer* 53:661, 1986.
11. Hansen, M.F., et al. Osteosarcoma and retinoblastoma: A shared chromosomal mechanism revealing recessive predisposition. *Proc. Natl. Acad. Sci. USA* 82:6216, 1985.
12. Friend, S.H., et al. Deletions of a DNA sequence in retinoblastomas and mesenchymal tumors: Organization of the sequence and its encoded protein. *Proc. Natl. Acad. Sci. USA* 84:9059, 1987.
13. Harbour, J.W., et al. Abnormalities in structure and expression of the human retinoblastoma gene in SCLC. *Science* 241:353, 1988.
14. Lee, E.Y.-H.P., et al. Inactivation of the retinoblastoma susceptibility gene in human breast cancers. *Science* 241:218, 1988.
15. Horowitz, J.M., et al. Point mutational inactivation of the retinoblastoma antioncogene. *Science* 243:937, 1989.
16. Huff, V., et al. Molecular Genetics of Wilms' Tumor. In L.E. Cenedo, et al. (eds.), *Cell Function and Disease.* New York: Plenum, 1989 (in press).
17. Huff, V., et al. Lack of linkage of familial Wilms' tumour to chromosomal band 11p13. *Nature* 336:377, 1988.
18. Strong, L.C., Stine, M., and Norsted, T.L. Cancer in survivors of childhood soft tissue sarcoma and their relatives *J. Natl. Cancer Inst.* 79:1213, 1987.
19. Williams, W.R., and Strong, L.C. Genetic Epidemiology of Soft Tissue Sarcomas in Children. In H. Muller and W. Weber (eds.), *Familial Cancer: First International Research Conference.* Basel: Karger, 1985. Pp. 151–153.
20. Lustbader, E.D., Williams, W.R., and Strong, L.C. Analysis of cohort data with uncertainty in stratification. *Biometrics* (in press, 1989).
21. Cimino, G., et al. Immune-deficiency in Hodgkin's disease (HD): A study of patients and healthy relatives in families with multiple cases. *Eur. J. Cancer Clin. Oncol.* 24:1595, 1988.
22. Hayashi, Y., et al. Cytogenetic findings and clinical features in acute leukemia and transient myeloproliferative disorder in Down's syndrome. *Blood* 72:15, 1988.

TABLE REFERENCES

Baker, S.J., et al. Chromosome 17 deletions and p53 gene mutations in colorectal carcinomas. *Science* 244:217, 1989.
Bale, S.J., et al. Mapping the gene for hereditary cutaneous malignant melanoma-dysplastic nevus to chromosome lp. *N. Engl. J. Med.* 320:1367, 1989.
Barker, D., et al. Gene for von Recklinghausen neurofibromatosis is in the pericentromeric region of chromosome 17. *Science* 236:1100, 1987.
Bodmer, W.F., et al. Localization of the gene for familiar adenomatous polyposis on chromosome 5. *Nature* 328:614, 1987.
Bradbear, R.A., et al. Cohort study of internal malignancy in genetic

hemochromatosis and other chronic nonalcoholic liver diseases. *J. Natl. Cancer Inst.* 75:81–84, 1985.

Cox, D.W., Billingsley, G.D., and Mansfield, T. DNA restriction-site polymorphisms associated with the alpha$_1$-antitrypsin gene. *Am. J. Hum. Genet.* 41:891, 1987.

Fong, C.T., et al. Loss of heterozygosity for the short arm of chromosome 1 in human neuroblastomas: Correlation with N-myc amplification. *Proc. Natl. Acad. Sci. USA* 86:3753, 1989.

Fountain, J.W., et al. Physical mapping of a translocation breakpoint in neurofibromatosis. *Science* 244: 1085, 1989.

Friend, S.H., et al. Deletions of a DNA sequence in retinoblastomas and mesenchymal tumors; Organization of the sequence and its encoded protein. *Proc. Natl. Acad. Sci. USA* 84:9059, 1987.

Fryer, A.E., et al. Evidence that the gene for tuberous sclerosis is on chromosome 9. *Lancet* 1:659, 1987.

Fryns, J.P., et al. Langer-Giedion syndrome and deletion of the long arm of chromosome 8. Confirmation of the critical segment to 8q23. *Hum. Genet.* 64:194, 1983.

Gatti, R.A., et al. Localization of an ataxia-telangiectasia gene to chromosome 11q22–23. *Nature* 336:577, 1988.

Harbour, J.W., et al. Abnormalities in structure and expression of the human retinoblastoma gene in SCLC. *Science* 241:353, 1988.

Henry, I., et al. Tumor-specific loss of 11p15.5 alleles in del11p13 Wilms' tumor and in familial adrenocortical carcinoma. *Proc. Natl. Acad. Sci. USA* 86:3247, 1989.

Horowitz, J.M., et al. Point mutational inactivation of the retinoblastoma antioncogene. *Science* 243:937, 1989.

Huff, V., et al. Molecular Genetics of Wilms' Tumor. In L.E. Cenedo, et al. (eds.), *Cell Function and Disease.* New York: Plenum, 1989 (in press).

Ito, E. Type 1a glycogen storage disease with hepatoblastoma in siblings. *Cancer* 59:1776–1780, 1987.

James, C.D., et al. Clonal genomic alterations in glioma malignancy stages. *Cancer Res.* 48:5546, 1988.

James, C.D., et al. Mitotic recombination of chromosome 17 in astrocytomas. *Proc. Natl. Acad. Sci. USA* 86:2858, 1989.

Koufos, A. Familial Wiedemann-Beckwith syndrome and a second Wilms' tumor locus both map to 11p15.5. *Am. J. Hum. Genet.* 44:711, 1989.

Liu, E., et al. Molecular lesions involved in the progression of a human breast cancer. *Oncogene* 3:323, 1988.

Mackay, J., et al. Allele loss on short arm of chromosome 17 in breast cancers. *Lancet* 2:1384, 1988.

Mandahl, N., et al. Lipomas have characteristic structural chromosomal rearrangements of 12q13–q14. *Int. J. Cancer* 39:685, 1987.

Masuda, H., et al. Rearrangement of the p53 gene in human osteogenic sarcomas. *Proc. Natl. Acad. Sci. USA* 7716, 1987.

Mathew, C.G.P., et al. A linked genetic marker for multiple endocrine neoplasia type 2A on chromosome 10. *Nature* 328:527, 1987.

McKeon, C., et al. Indistinguishable patterns of protooncogene expression in two distinct but closely related tumors: Ewing's sarcoma and neuroepithelioma. *Cancer Res.* 48:4307, 1988.

Mertens, F., et al. Clonal chromosome abnormalities in two liposarcomas. *Cancer Genet. Cytogenet.* 28:137, 1987.

Motomura, K., et al. Loss of alleles at loci on chromosome 13 in human primary gastric cancers. *Genomics* 2:180, 1988.

Mukai, S., and Dryja, T.P. Loss of alleles at polymorphic loci on chromosome 2 in uveal melanoma. *Cancer Genet. Cytogenet.* 22:45, 1986.

Nakamura, Y., et al. Localization of the genetic defect in multiple endocrine neoplasia type 1 within a small region of chromosome 11. *Am. J. Hum. Genet.* 44:751, 1989.

Ponder, B. Gene losses in human tumours. *Nature* 335:400, 1988.

Rouleau, G.A., et al. Genetic linkage of bilateral acoustic neurofibromatosis to a DNA marker on chromosome 22. *Nature* 329:246, 1987.

Scrable, H.J., et al. Chromosomal localization of the human rhabdomyosarcoma locus by mitotic recombination mapping. *Nature* 329:645, 1987.

Seizinger, B.R., et al. Von Hippel-Lindau disease maps to the region of chromosome 3 associated with renal cell carcinoma. *Nature* 332:268, 1988.

Shiraishi, M., et al. Loss of genes on the short arm of chromosome 11 in human lung carcinomas. *Jpn. J. Cancer Res.* 78:1302, 1987.

Suzuki, T., et al. Frequent loss of heterozygosity on chromosome 14q in neuroblastoma. *Cancer Res.* 49:1095, 1989.

Takai, S., et al. Loss of genes on chromosome 22 in medullary thyroid carcinoma and pheochromocytoma. *Jpn. J. Cancer Res.* 78:894, 1987.

T'Ang, A., et al. Structural rearrangement of the retinoblastoma gene in human breast carcinoma. *Science* 242:263, 1988.

Wang-Wuu, S., et al. Chromosomal analysis of sixteen human rhabdomyosarcomas. *Cancer Res.* 48:983, 1988.

Weinblatt, M.E., Kahn, E., and Kochen, J. Renal cell carcinoma in patients with tuberous sclerosis. *Pediatrics* 80:898, 1987.

White, P.C., et al. Characterization of frequent deletions causing steroid 21-hydroxylase deficiency. *Proc. Natl. Acad. Sci. USA* 85:4436, 1988.

SELECTED READINGS

Green, A.R. Recessive mechanisms of malignancy. *Br. J. Cancer* 58:115, 1988.

Huff, V., et al. Molecular Genetics of Wilms' Tumor. In L.E. Cenedo, et al. (eds.), *Cell Function and Disease.* New York: Plenum, 1988.

Ponder, B. Gene losses in human tumours. *Nature* 335:400, 1988.

Strong, L. C. Genetics, Etiology, and Epidemiology of Childhood Cancer. In W. W. Sutow, D. J. Fernbach, and T. J. Vietti (eds.), *Clinical Pediatric Oncology* (3rd ed.). St. Louis: Mosby, 1984. Pp. 14–41.

Strong, L. C. Mutational Models for Cancer Etiology. In R. S. K. Chaganti and J. German (eds.), *Genetics in Clinical Oncology.* New York: Oxford University, 1985. Pp. 39–59.

This review was written to be used as an in-house pediatric oncology training manual, and therefore, where possible, references have been made to review articles rather than to original reports. Readers will find more thorough references in the review articles cited. This training chapter is not intended to include a comprehensive or encyclopedic reference list. Readers with interest in more detailed references should first check the review articles cited; if further questions arise, contact Dr. Louise C. Strong.

30

Genetics in the Diagnosis and Prognosis of Pediatric Cancer

Louise C. Strong

DIAGNOSTIC SIGNIFICANCE OF GENETIC FACTORS

Cytogenetic and molecular genetic tools have markedly contributed to the diagnosis of hematologic malignancies and have more recently provided new insights into the diagnosis and prognosis of solid pediatric tumors. Cytogenetic and molecular alterations may assist in the diagnosis of histopathologically indistinguishable tumors with different responses to treatment, as in the case of neuroblastoma and peripheral neuroectodermal tumors (PNET). Certain tumors occurring in older children, outside the adrenal gland, resembled neuroblastoma histologically but showed no response to neuroblastoma therapy. A distinct cytogenetic alteration, a chromosomal translocation (11;22) (q24q12), was identified in these tumors that was identical to the chromosomal alteration observed in Ewing's sarcoma. The lack of response of these PNET to neuroblastoma therapy and the suggestive evidence for an etiologic relationship to Ewing's sarcoma led to a clinical trial of a Ewing's sarcoma protocol in PNET patients. The outcome was a much improved response rate. Thus, the cytogenetic finding permitted development of a new classification of the tumors and a rational approach to an improved therapeutic response [1, 2].

PROGNOSTIC SIGNIFICANCE OF GENETIC FACTORS

Genetic analysis may also provide important prognostic information, as in neuroblastoma, for which the tumor-specific findings of amplification of the N-*myc* oncogene carries a poor prognosis independent of other staging information [3]. Furthermore, for the astrocytoma family of brain tumors, genetic analysis has revealed specific molecular alteration associated with the stage of disease, including alteration in chromosome 17 in astrocytomas and loss of chromosome 10 associated with tumor progression [4,5]. Altered or overly abundant gene products, such as those associated with multiple drug resistance or activated oncogenes, may identify patients with different therapeutic needs and, eventually, those gene products may be specific targets for therapy. It is likely that genetic analysis will play an important role in diagnosis and disease "staging" in the future (Table 30-1).

GENETIC CONSEQUENCES OF PEDIATRIC CANCER AND ITS TREATMENT

Survivors of pediatric cancer who have undergone treatment before the completion of active growth and before reproduction have the greatest opportunity to experience the ill effects of the potentially mutagenic and carcinogenic agents used in their treatment. These genetic ill effects include both the risk of a second tumor in the patient and the risk of genetic damage that may give rise to genetic abnormalities in subsequent generations. In addition, for those pa-

Table 30-1. Genetic alterations in childhood cancers with diagnostic and/or prognostic implications

Tumor type	Genetic alterations	Implications
Neuroblastoma	Amplification or over-expression of N-*myc* oncogene; may be evidenced cytogenetically by double minute chromosomes or homogeneous staining regions	Poor prognosis regardless of stage
Peripheral neuro-ectodermal tumor (PNET), formerly neuroblastoma, adult neuroblastoma, medulloepithelioma, neuroepithelioma, etc.	Chromosome 11:22 translocation (11;22) (q24;12)	1. New diagnostic classification of PNET separate from neuroblastoma 2. Cytogenetic identity with Ewing's sarcoma led to clinical trial with Ewing's sarcoma protocol and good response

tients with a genetic predisposition to cancer, there is the risk of transmitting that genetic predisposition to the next generation and, consequently, the risk of pediatric cancer in the patients' offspring. Some of these risks are summarized in Tables 30-2 and 30-3.

Risk of Second Tumors in the Patient
Risk factors for second tumors in the patient include both the genetic background, the patient's age, and the type and duration of treatment (see Table 30-2). Overall, the cumulative risk of a second tumor observed in large follow-up studies of childhood cancer patients has been approximately 12 percent by 25 years of follow-up [6,7].

Risk to Subsequent Generations
The risk to subsequent generations includes consideration of the risk of a heritable cancer and the risk of treatment-induced genetic damage. The heritable cancer risk has been discussed in some detail with reference to retinoblastoma, and other potential genetic syndromes were indicated in Chapter 29. However, for most pediatric cancer patients, the hereditary fraction appears to be small, and hence the overall risk of cancer in the offspring of pediatric cancer patients is very small [8].

Given the increasing numbers of pediatric cancer survivors and concerns about the late effects of treatment, we at the University of Texas M.D. Anderson Cancer Center participated in a large study to examine the characteristics of pediatric cancer survivors as compared with their siblings. The findings are summarized in Table 30-3 [9]. The study included five institutions, more than 2500 pediatric cancer survivors, and a comparison group of more than 3500 brothers and sisters of the pediatric cancer patients. The patients were all treated before 1975 for an invasive cancer or for any type of brain tumor diagnosed before the age of 20 years. Patients had to survive at least 5 years from diagnosis and had to reach the age of 21 years by 1979. In general, this study revealed a very high quality of life among the pediatric cancer survivors.

Table 30-2. Risk of second malignant neoplasms in childhood cancer patients

Risk factor	Major tissue at risk
Genetic predisposition	
Bilateral retinoblastoma	Osteosarcoma
	Soft tissue sarcoma
	Melanoma
	Other
Li Fraumeni syndrome	Osteosarcoma
(embryonal	Breast cancer
rhabdomyosarcoma, etc.)	Soft tissue sarcoma
Other	?
Radiation (dose dependent)	Osteosarcoma
	Thyroid carcinoma
	Breast, brain, soft tissue, etc.
Chemotherapy, alkylating agents	Nonlymphocytic leukemia
	Osteosarcoma

Table 30-3. Genetic and other considerations for childhood cancer survivors: Available data (1988) based on multi-institutional study of 2500 childhood cancer survivors and 3500 brothers and sisters

1. Criteria for childhood/adolescent cancer long-term survivor study: Invasive cancer or any brain tumor diagnosed before age 20 years
   Survival from diagnosis ≥ 5 years by 1979
   Achievement of age ≥ 21 years by 1979
2. Study outcome: Characteristics of childhood cancer survivors as compared with their siblings
   Quality of life: Very good (exception: childhood brain tumor patients)
   Educational achievement: At least as good as siblings (exception: childhood brain tumor patients)
   Marriage rate: Slightly less than siblings, primarily due to lower marriage rates for childhood brain tumor patients and for males with Hodgkin's disease
   Psychiatric disease rate: No different from siblings for depression, running away, psychiatric hospitalization, and suicide
   Insurance: Much greater difficulty obtaining health and life insurance
   Military: Less likely to be accepted
   Reproductive history posttreatment:
      Male fertility: Significantly reduced in males treated with alkylating agents or trunk radiation below diaphragm, especially Hodgkin's disease and genital tumor patients (consider cryopreservation of sperm)
      Female fertility: Increased frequency of surgical menopause. Increased frequency of non-surgical menopause in patients treated with alkylating agents or radiation below diaphragm. For patients with normal spontaneous menses posttreatment, normal fertility observed although preliminary data suggest possible earlier onset of menopause in alkylating agent-treated patients
   Reproductive outcome (3000 pregnancies): No significant increase in spontaneous abortion or stillbirth
   Offspring health history: No significant increase in childhood cancer, birth defects in general, or specific genetic conditions such as chromosomal anomalies or specific genetic diseases

Sources: Adapted from J. J. Mulvihill, et al. Cancer in offspring of long-term survivors of childhood and adolescent cancer. *Lancet* 2:813, 1987; and J. Byrne, et al. Effects of treatment on fertility in long-term survivors of childhood or adolescent cancer. *N. Engl. J. Med.* 317:1315, 1987.

The major goal of the study was to determine the effect of cancer therapy on fertility and reproduction. Alkylating agents and irradiation below the diaphragm significantly reduced fertility, particularly in male patients. However, for those patients who were able to conceive (representing 3000 pregnancies), no increase in the incidence of spontaneous abortion, stillbirth, or untoward pregnancy outcome was observed. Overall, no increase in the incidence of congenital anomalies or genetic disease was observed in the offspring. Furthermore, no appreciable increase in pediatric cancer has been observed in the offspring. However, follow-up of the offspring has only been maintained for relatively few years and, for the most part, the offspring have not achieved the age at which their parents suffered their cancer during childhood. Hence, while the available data do not indicate a major reproductive risk, further follow-up is indicated.

For further review of late effects of childhood cancer therapy, see reference 10.

COMMENTS

In recent years, advances in cytogenetics and molecular genetic techniques have permitted much more effective study of genes transmitted in families and of tumor-specific genetic alterations. An international effort to map the human genome, or at least to develop markers spaced in such a way that disease-related genes can be mapped between available markers, is ongoing. New techniques detect unique variations in DNA that can be used to follow the transmission of genetic disease in families or in tumor-specific alterations. In rare cases in which the specific gene is known, the structure of the gene itself or its protein product can be examined. If the gene itself is not known but has been localized to a specific chromosome, then the inheritance of that chromosomal region may be followed in families using neighboring genetic variant markers.

The use of molecular genetic techniques to diagnose genetic disease and to uncover the genetic events in pediatric cancer will continue to develop rapidly. Molecular analysis of the tumor and normal tissue will assume an increasingly important role in the diagnosis, treatment, and counseling of the pediatric cancer patient.

REFERENCES

1. McKeon, C., et al. Indistinguishable patterns of protooncogene expression in two distinct but closely related tumors: Ewing's sarcoma and neuroepithelioma. *Cancer Res.* 48:4307, 1988.
2. Miser, J.S., et al. Treatment of peripheral neuroepithelioma in children and young adults. *J. Clin. Oncol* 5:1752, 1987.
3. Seeger, R.C., et al. Association of multiple copies of the N-*myc* oncogene with rapid progression of neuroblastomas. *N. Engl. J. Med.* 313:1111, 1985.
4. James, C.D., et al. Clonal genomic alterations in glioma malignancy stages. *Cancer Res.* 48:5546, 1988.
5. James, C.D., et al. Mitotic recombination of chromosome 17 in astrocytomas. *Proc. Natl. Acad. Sci. USA* 86:2858, 1989.
6. Tucker, M.A., et al. Cancer Risk Following Treatment of Childhood Cancer. In J.D. Boice, Jr., and J.F. Fraumeni, Jr., (eds.), *Radiation Carcinogenesis: Epidemiology and Biological Significance. Progress in Cancer Research and Therapy.* New York: Raven, 1984. Pp. 211–224.

7. deVathaire, F., et al. Long-term risk of second malignant neoplasm after a cancer in childhood. *Br. J. Cancer* 59:448, 1989.
8. Mulvihill, J.J., et al. Cancer in offspring of long-term survivors of childhood and adolescent cancer. *Lancet* 2:813, 1987.
9. Byrne, J., et al. Effects of treatment on fertility in long-term survivors of childhood or adolescent cancer. *N. Engl. J. Med.* 317:1315, 1987.
10. Green, D.M. *Long-Term Complications of Therapy for Cancer in Childhood and Adolescence.* Baltimore: Johns Hopkins University Press, 1989. Pp. 1–171.

SELECTED READING

Strong, L. C. Genetic Considerations. In *Proceedings of the American Cancer Society: Second National Conference on Human Values and Cancer.* Chicago: American Cancer Society, 1978. Pp. 210–219.

This review was written to be used as an in-house pediatric oncology training manual, and therefore, where possible, references have been made to review articles rather than to original reports. Readers will find more thorough references in the review articles cited. This training chapter is not intended to include a comprehensive or encyclopedic reference list. Readers with interest in more detailed references should first check the review articles cited; if further questions arise, contact Dr. Louise C. Strong.

The work in Chaps. 29 and 30 was supported in part by Public Health Service grant number CA34936, awarded by the National Cancer Institute.

VI

Appendixes

Appendix 1

Commonly Used Emergency Medications

Medication	Dosage	Route of administration	Comments
Albumin 25%, 5%	0.5–1.0 gm/kg	IV	1.0 gm=4.0 ml of 25%
Atropine	0.01 mg/kg	ET, IV	Minimum dose 0.1 mg
Bicarbonate	1–2 mEq/kg	IV	q5minutes (½ dose)
Bretylium	5 mg/kg	IV	6 doses maximum
Calcium gluconate 10%	50–100 mg/kg	IV	q10minutes, slow
Chloral hydrate	25–50 mg/kg	PO, PR	For sedation
Dexamethasone	0.25–1.50 mg/kg	IV	For increased intracranial pressure
Dextrose 50%	0.5 gm/kg	IV	0.5 gm=1.0 ml
Diazepam	0.1–0.3 mg/kg	IV slow	Maximum 2 mg/minute
Diazoxide	3–5 mg/kg	IV push	Rapid push
Diphenhydramine hydrochloride	1–2 mg/kg	IV, IM	For anaphylaxis
Epinephrine	0.1 ml/kg of 1:10,000	ET, IV, SC	q5–10minutes
Racemic	0.25–0.50 ml 2.25% sol.	Inhaled	
Furosemide	1–3 mg/kg	IV, IM, PO	
Glucagon	0.025–0.100 mg/kg	IV, IM, SC	For hypoglycemia
Hydralazine	0.2 mg/kg	IV, IM	Initial dose
KayExalate	1 gm/kg	PO, PR	PO with sorbitol
Lidocaine	0.5–1.0 mg/kg	ET, IV	Bolus dose
Mannitol	0.25–1.00 gm/kg	IV	For CNS herniation
Methylprednisolone	30 mg/kg	IV	Septic shock
Morphine	0.1 mg/kg	IV, IM, SC	q1–3hours
Naloxone	0.01 mg/kg	IV, IM	Up to 0.1 mg/kg
Paraldehyde	300 mg (0.3 ml)/kg	PR	Mix 1:1 with oil
Pancuronium bromide	0.1 mg/kg	IV	Short-acting paralytic
Phenobarbital	5–10 mg/kg	IV	q20minutes
Phenytoin	10–15 mg/kg	IV slow	3 divided doses

Medication	Dosage	Route of administration	Comments
Propranolol	0.1 mg/kg	IV	Repeat after 10 minutes, maximum 10 mg
Succinylcholine	1 mg/kg	IV, IM	2 times dose IM
Thiopental	2–6 mg/kg	IV	For increased intracranial pressure
Verapamil	0.1–0.2 mg/kg	IV	Maximum 2.5 mg

Continuous infusions

Aminophylline	Load 3–6 mg/kg 1.0 mg/kg/hour
Dobutamine	0.5–20 μg/kg/minute
Dopamine	Low 1–5 μg/kg/minute Moderate 5–15 μg/kg/minute High > 15 μg/kg/minute
Epinephrine	0.05–1.00 μg/kg/minute
Heparin	Load 50–100 U/kg 10–50 U/kg/hour
Isoproterenol	0.05–2.00 μg/kg/minute
Lidocaine	20–40 μg/kg/minute
Nitroprusside	0.5–8.0 μg/kg/minute
Norepinephrine	0.05–1.00 μg/kg/minute
Tolazoline	Test 1.0 mg/kg 1–2 mg/kg/hour

Transfusions

PRBC	10–20 ml/kg
Platelets	0.2 U/kg for rise 60,000–90,000/μl
Plasma (FFP)	10 ml/kg
Factor VIII	1 U/kg for 2% rise in serum activity
Cryoprecipitate	1 bag/5.0 kg for 50% rise in serum activity

Source: James A. Griffith, M.D., Assistant Professor, Division of Pediatric Intensive Care, University of Texas Medical School at Houston

Appendix 2

Resources for Educational, Financial, and Psychosocial Support Services

Allison Stovall

1. American Cancer Society, National Office, 1599 Clifton Road N.E., Atlanta, GA 30329. *Provides patient and family educational services, loans of durable medical equipment, and support group services.*
2. Association for the Care of Children's Health, 3615 Wisconsin Avenue, N.W., Washington, D.C. 20016. *A multidisciplinary professional organization that encourages parent participation. The topical bibliographies that the group publishes are helpful to professionals and parents alike.*
3. Candelighters' Childhood Cancer Foundation, 1901 Pennsylvania Avenue, N.W., Washington, D.C. 20006. *A self-help group founded by parents of children with cancer. It has affiliated groups throughout the nation that provide support to families. The group's three very informative newsletters are useful to patients, families, and professionals.*
4. Leukemia Society of America, Inc., 733 Third Avenue, New York, N.Y. 10017. *The Patient Aid Program of this agency provides assistance with the costs of outpatient treatment and transportation to outpatient appointments, educational materials, and support groups for patients with leukemia, lymphoma, or Hodgkin's disease.*
5. Ronald McDonald Houses. For information contact: Henry Lienau, Ronald McDonald House Coordinator, Golin/Harris, 500 N. Michigan Avenue, Chicago, IL 60611. *The McDonald's Children's Charities assist local community groups in creating "homes away from home" for children with serious illnesses and their families.*
6. Social Supplementary Income–Disabled Children's Program (SSI-DCP), Social Security Administration. *Provides stipends to income-eligible families in whose children the diagnoses are expected to create disabling conditions for 1 year or more. Children eligible for this program are also eligible for Medicaid, which is administered through each state's public welfare agency.*
7. State Health Department. *At the state level, the health department in many states includes a program that addresses the needs of children with major chronic illnesses. Children may be eligible for financial assistance and social services depending on the diagnoses and family income.*
8. U.S. Department of Health and Human Services, Public Health Service, National Institutes of Health, Office of Cancer Communications, National Cancer Institute, Bethesda, MD. *The federal office provides an extensive range of patient and professional educational materials.*

Index

Index